BIOREVERSIBLE CARRIERS IN DRUG DESIGN

Pergamon Titles of Related Interest

Dunn et al. PARTITION COEFFICIENT
Auriche et al. DRUG SAFETY: PROGRESS AND CONTROVERSIES
Patel PHARMACEUTICALS AND HEALTH IN THE THIRD WORLD

Related Journals
(Free sample copies available upon request)

JOURNAL OF PHARMACEUTICAL & BIOMEDICAL ANALYSIS
CURRENT ADVANCES IN PHARMACOLOGY & TOXICOLOGY
BIOMEDICAL PHARMACOLOGY
PHARMACOLOGY & THERAPEUTICS
GENERAL PHARMACOLOGY

BIOREVERSIBLE CARRIERS IN DRUG DESIGN
Theory and Application

Edited by Edward B. Roche
University of Nebraska Medical Center
College of Pharmacy

PERGAMON PRESS
New York Oxford Beijing Frankfurt São Paulo Sydney Tokyo Toronto

Pergamon Press Offices:

U.S.A.	Pergamon Press, Maxwell House, Fairview Park, Elmsford, New York 10523, U.S.A.
U.K.	Pergamon Press, Headington Hill Hall, Oxford OX3 0BW, England
PEOPLE'S REPUBLIC OF CHINA	Pergamon Press, Qianmen Hotel, Beijing, People's Republic of China
FEDERAL REPUBLIC OF GERMANY	Pergamon Press, Hammerweg 6, D-6242 Kronberg, Federal Republic of Germany
BRAZIL	Pergamon Editora, Rua Eça de Queiros, 346, CEP 04011, São Paulo, Brazil
AUSTRALIA	Pergamon Press (Aust.) Pty., P.O. Box 544, Potts Point, NSW 2011, Australia
JAPAN	Pergamon Press, 8th Floor, Matsuoka Central Building, 1-7-1 Nishishinjuku, Shinjuku-ku, Tokyo 160, Japan
CANADA	Pergamon Press Canada, Suite 104, 150 Consumers Road, Willowdale, Ontario M2J 1P9, Canada

Copyright © 1987 American Pharmaceutical Association

All rights reserved. No part of this publication may be reproduced, stored in a retrieval system or transmitted in any form or by any means: electronic, electrostatic, magnetic tape, mechanical, photocopying, recording or otherwise, without permission in writing from the publishers.

First printing 1987

Library of Congress Cataloging in Publication Data

Bioreversible carriers in drug design.

    Includes index.
    1. Prodrugs. 2. Drugs--Vehicles.
I. Roche, Edward B.
RM301.57.B56   1986   615.5'8   86-30354
ISBN 0-08-034681-2

In order to make this volume available as economically and as rapidly as possible, the authors' typescripts have been reproduced in their original forms. This method unfortunately has its typographical limitations but it is hoped that they in no way distract the reader.

Printed in Great Britain by A. Wheaton & Co. Ltd., Exeter

CONTENTS

Preface vii

Chapter

1. Prodrug and Drug Delivery, An Overview 1
   Takeru Higuchi

2. Design of Bioreversible Drug Derivatives and the Utility of the Double Prodrug Concept 13
   Hans Bundgaard

3. Chemical Drug Delivery Systems 95
   Nicholas Bodor

4. Application of Physical Organic Concepts to In Vitro and In Vivo Lability Design of Water Soluble Prodrugs 121
   Bradley D. Anderson
   Robert A. Conradi

5. Physical Model Based Optimization of Local and Systemic Delivery of Prodrugs 164
   Jeffery L. Fox

6. Biological Evaluation of Soluble Macromolecules as Bioreversible Drug Carriers 196
   Ruth Duncan
   J. Kopecek
   J. B. Lloyd

7. Preferential Membrane Permeation and Recognition in Drug Targeting 214
   T. Y. Shen

8. Carrier Mediated and Receptor Transport 226
across the Endothelial Cells of the
Vasculature
    Kenneth L. Audus
    Ronald T. Borchardt

9. Intestinal Aminopeptidase Distribution 243
and Specificity: Basis for a Prodrug
Strategy
    Gordon L. Amidon
    Kevin C. Johnson

10. Drug Delivery Systems Research from an 262
Industrial Perspective
    Anthony A. Sinkula

Index   281

Biographical Sketches of the Authors   287

PREFACE

The focus of this volume is on underlying concepts in physical organic chemistry, physical chemistry, biochemistry, cell biology, and immunology as they relate to bioreversible carrier design. The authors have created chapters which should well serve those who are working and studying in the various areas of drug design. It is our hope that this volume will serve as an instructional work for the serious student, and a stimulus for the scientist beginning to work in this area of research. The phrase "theory and application" in the title brings forth this intent.

In the first chapter, Professor Takeru Higuchi, whose pioneering research in this area is well known, gives us an overview of prodrugs and drug delivery systems. His discussion introduces aspects of specificity leading into the later chapters, and provides thoughts on the regulatory aspects of prodrug development including efficacy testing and patents.

The design of bioreversible derivatives and "chemical drug delivery systems" are discussed in detail in the next two chapters by Professors Bundgaard and Bodor, respectively. These discussions relate the state of the art in the design of chemical entities that are selective or specific for particular target tissues or systems.

The application of physical and chemical properties to the design of bioreversible compounds is discussed in the two chapters by Professor Anderson and Drs. Conradi and Fox, respectively. The importance of physicochemical considerations and the detailed analysis of physically based models is brought clearly into focus by these authors.

Professor Duncan and her colleagues discuss the use of synthetic soluble polymers, e.g., HPMA co-polymers, as specific intracellular macromolecular carriers. This is followed by Dr. Shen's chapter on targeting cell surface receptors and achieving selective permeation of cell membranes. This topic is discussed in another sense in the chapter by Audus and Borchardt on transport across the blood-brain barrier. The unique nature of vascular endothelial cells is discussed with regard to the design of carrier systems for drugs intended to be transported across the cerebral vasculature.

Targeting the enzymes of the gastro-intestinal tract as sites of bioconversion of carrier systems is the subject of the chapter by Amidon and Johnson. The location and specificity of these systems is discussed in detail. The closing chapter by Dr. Sinkula brings the industrial perspective into focus. The organization of multidisciplinary research groups to bring input from all of the cognizant sciences to bear on problems surrounding the selective targeting of drug entities and bioreversible carriers is discussed in detail.

It has been a pleasure for me to be involved with all of these authors, and with the editorial phase of the production of this book. I thank them for their efforts and cooperation. I would also like to thank Mrs. Andrea Steele for her invaluable assistance in the preparation of this volume.

Edward B. Roche
University of Nebraska Medical Center
College of Pharmacy
Omaha, Nebraska
November, 1985

Chapter 1
Prodrug and Drug Delivery—An Overview

Takeru Higuchi

Department of Pharmaceutical Chemistry
University of Kansas
Lawrence, KS 66045

It has now been more than a decade since we helped organize a symposium on prodrugs as a part of an ACS meeting at Atlantic City. Although the interest in the approach even at that time led to a standing-room-only crowd, the concept probably has gained a far greater number of advocates today. The recent mainstream recognition of the importance of effective delivery in the development of new therapeutic agents has given major impetus to the growth of prodrug technology. This is because the approach permits, for a number of drug areas, a useful separation of the structural needs associated with optimal biological activity at the target site from the structural requirements associated with the best delivery of these agents to that site.

Delivery technology, in general, will play an increasing role in the near and indefinite future of new drug development. More complex and higher molecular weight chemical species are now being considered as new drug candidates; these bioactive agents are generally poorly absorbed -- being difficultly transported across various biological barriers. Development of many of the products of biotechnology into therapeutically useful dosages, for example, will particularly require new drug delivery technology. The prodrug concept will, without question, play an increasing major role in this respect.

It has already been well demonstrated that chemical modification of an active agent can significantly influence its availability to its targetted biospace. Thus, the dipivalyl ester of epinephrine developed for improved ocular delivery illustrates a recent success along this line. Another program which took place in our own laboratories demonstrated that 2-PAM, an antidote for nerve gas poisoning, in its dihydro form was able to regenerate esterase activity in the brain following exposure of the whole animal to the choline esterase inhibitor. The parent drug, 2-PAM, in its quarternary form, is unable to penetrate the BBB and affect the enzyme system.

Since no serious student of drug activity would today suggest action at a distance, the effect induced at the target site by a given dose of drug will be the product of the drug's intrinsic activity and the efficiency with which it is delivered to the site. The two factors are thus of equal importance in the development of any new drug. And because of the structural orthogonality of those molecular attributes which would tend to optimize each of the factors, the prodrug approach which would often permit independent treatment of the two by separating them temporally offers real advantages.

Thus, for example, in the development of dipivalyl epinephrine as an agent for treatment of glaucoma, the intent was not to alter or improve the activity of epinephrine at its target site within the eye, but rather to confer on the drug those physical properties by chemical modifications which would permit its ready delivery into the intraocular space. During or after transit across the corneal barrier, the ester is cleaved to regenerate the active species. It is evident that the approach, when the basic technology is better developed, will certainly lead to significantly more useful drug substances.

There are two research directions related to future prodrug application which, I feel, need substantially greater effort. The first is concerned with the chemistry of chemical modifications which convert readily to the desired active species. The second relates to increasing our understanding of endogenous enzymic systems which can be used to trigger the generation of these active agents and the specificity of these enzymes. I will use the remainder of my time to elaborate on these points.

Prodrug Chemistry

Much of the earlier efforts on prodrugs has been based on simple esterification of the active substance. Thus, the ester aspirin was developed from salicylic acid nearly a century ago with the intent to deliver the acid without its corrosive effect. More recent examples are chloramphenicol palmitate, triacetyloleandomycin, etc. These esters were developed essentially by trial and error and underwent hydrolysis to varying degrees on their journey to the circulating blood.

More recently, newer chemistry has been developed which permits use of endogenous esterases to convert derivatized drugs to their active forms. Thus, a number of amines, amides and imides have been converted to esterase-sensitive prodrugs. Some of these are shown in Figure 1 and Figure 2.

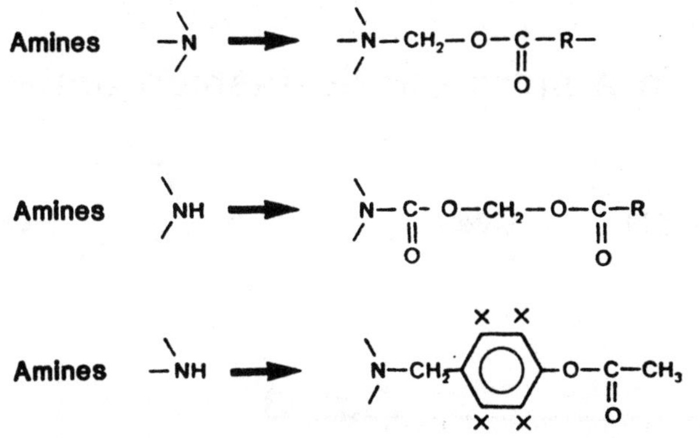

Fig. 1

Some Chemistry Leading to Esterase Sensitive Prodrug Forms of Amines.

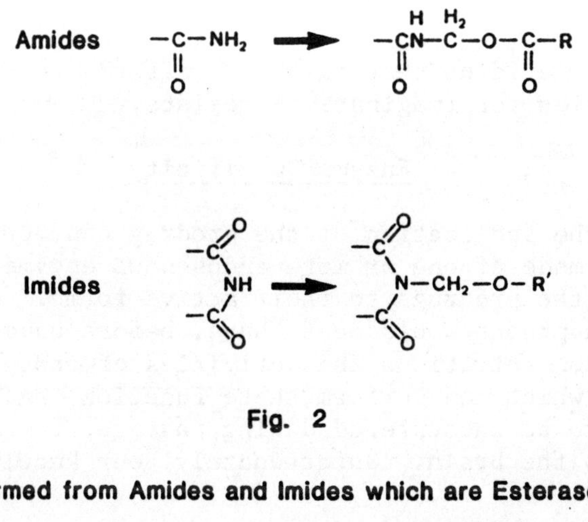

Fig. 2

Prodrugs Formed from Amides and Imides which are Esterase Sensitive.

Other similar contrived chemistry can be imagined. For example, thiols can be simply acylated or soft alkylated.

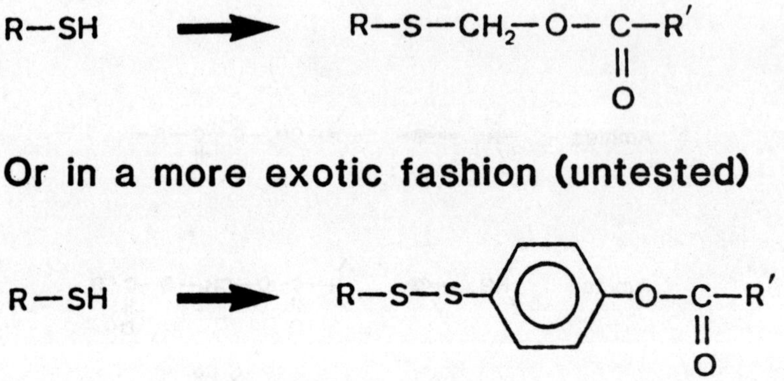

$$R-SH \longrightarrow R-S-CH_2-O-\underset{\underset{O}{\|}}{C}-R'$$

Or in a more exotic fashion (untested)

$$R-SH \longrightarrow R-S-S-\underset{}{\bigcirc}-O-\underset{\underset{O}{\|}}{C}-R'$$

Fig. 3

Derivitization of Sulfahydryl Drugs.

It is evident that this area affords a multitude of opportunities for imaginative chemists.

<u>Enzyme Specificity</u>

In the application of the prodrug concept, use is generally made of one or more endogenous enzymes to transform the prodrugs to their active forms. A truly rational approach would be to have, before hand, the relative concentrations and activities of those biological catalysts which can perform these functions and can be expected to be encountered during passage, for example, from the gut to the brain. Unfortunately, our knowledge in this area is still very limited. Specificity, for example, of various esterases toward variations in substrate structures is as yet poorly known. Recently, for this reason, we have been looking at the relative sensitivities of a limited number of structurally different esters toward several esterases which may be encountered during and after gut absorption. I would, at this point, like to share with you some of the results of this study.

We looked at the hydrolytic behavior of some acetaminophen esters in the presence of various crude esterases. The system had been studied in some detail by Lew Dittert, Cliff Wong and Joe Swintosky here in Philadelphia nearly twenty years ago. Our recent effort had been directed primarily toward evaluation of the relative catalytic activities of esterases obtained from the gut wall, the liver, and the blood with variation in substrate structure. The program was designed to test the possibility of designing esters (prodrugs) which would cleave more or less specifically at a selected point along the absorption pathway.

```
    Gut     }    Gut    }    Liver    }    Blood
    Lumen   }    Wall   }             }
```

In these studies, enzymic activities toward different esters were in all instances compared directly to that toward APAP propionate. Since the activities of crude tissue homogenates, for example, cannot be easily reproduced, each preparation was run with APAP proprianate as well as with the ester under study and the results expressed as the ratio of the two rates obtained at substrate concentrations usually well below saturation.

The esters studied are shown in Table I, along with their observed hydrolytic half lives at pH 7.0 and 25° under nonenzymatic conditions. In Figs. 4, 5, 6, 7, and 8, their relative susceptibilities toward rat intestinal homogenate, rat liver homogenate, commercial partly purified porcine liver esterase, rat plasma and partly purified horse serum butyrl cholinesterase are shown. It is evident that the susceptibility profiles are relatively reproducible and distinctly different. It is of interest to note the very close similarity between that obtained for rat liver homogenate and that for the porcine liver esterse. Essentially the same response was observed for similar structural changes in related reverse esters (P-acetamido benzoic acid ester series).

TABLE I. Structure and Chemical Hydrolytic Half – Lives of APAP Esters Studied

Compound	Structure	Half-Life (hrs.) pH=7.0 T=25°
E-1	$-\text{O}-\underset{\underset{\text{O}}{\parallel}}{\text{C}}\text{CH}_2\text{CH}_3$	>250
E-2	$-\text{O}-\underset{\underset{\text{O}}{\parallel}}{\text{C}}(\text{CH}_2)_2\text{CH}_3$	>460
E-3	$-\text{O}-\underset{\underset{\text{O}}{\parallel}}{\text{C}}\text{C}(\text{CH}_3)_3$	>1400
E-4	$-\text{O}-\text{CH}_2-\underset{\underset{\text{O}}{\parallel}}{\text{O}}\text{C}(\text{CH}_3)_3$	>3500
E-5	$-\text{O}-\underset{\underset{\text{O}}{\parallel}}{\text{C}}\text{CH}_2\text{CH}_2-\text{N}(\text{CH}_2\text{CH}_2\text{CH}_3)_2 \cdot \text{HCl}$	0.65
E-6	$-\text{O}-\underset{\underset{\text{O}}{\parallel}}{\text{C}}\text{CH}_2\text{CH}_2-\text{N}(\text{Et})_2 \cdot \text{HCl}$	0.69

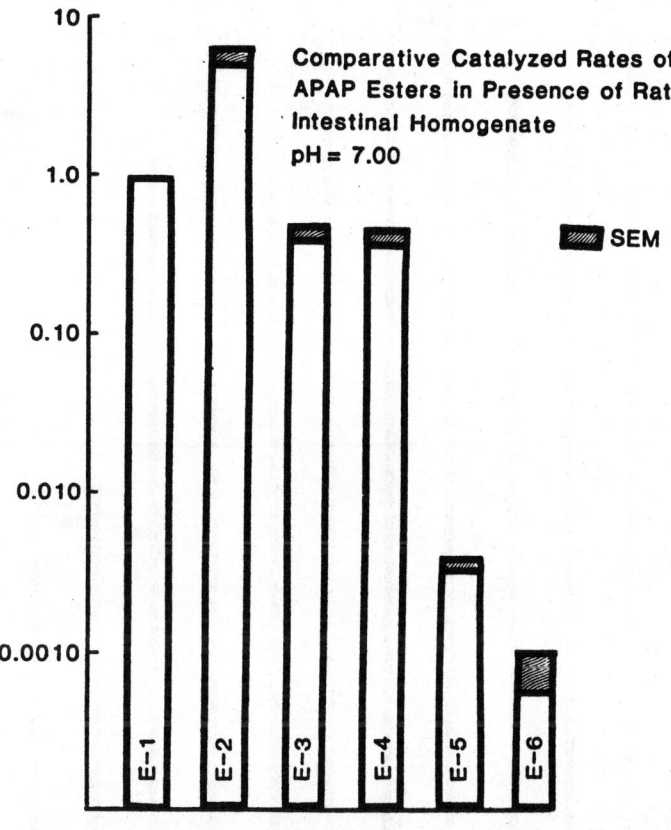

Fig. 4

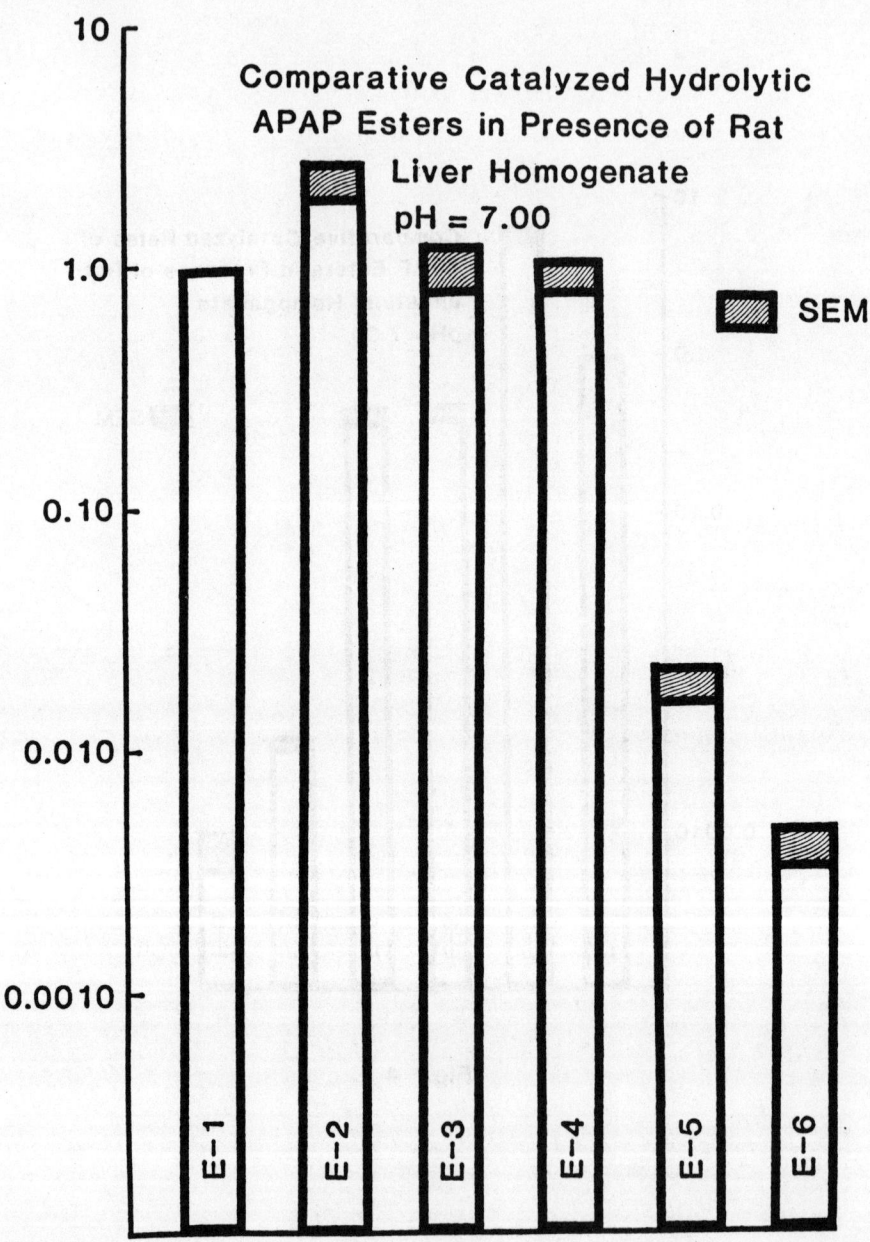

Fig. 5

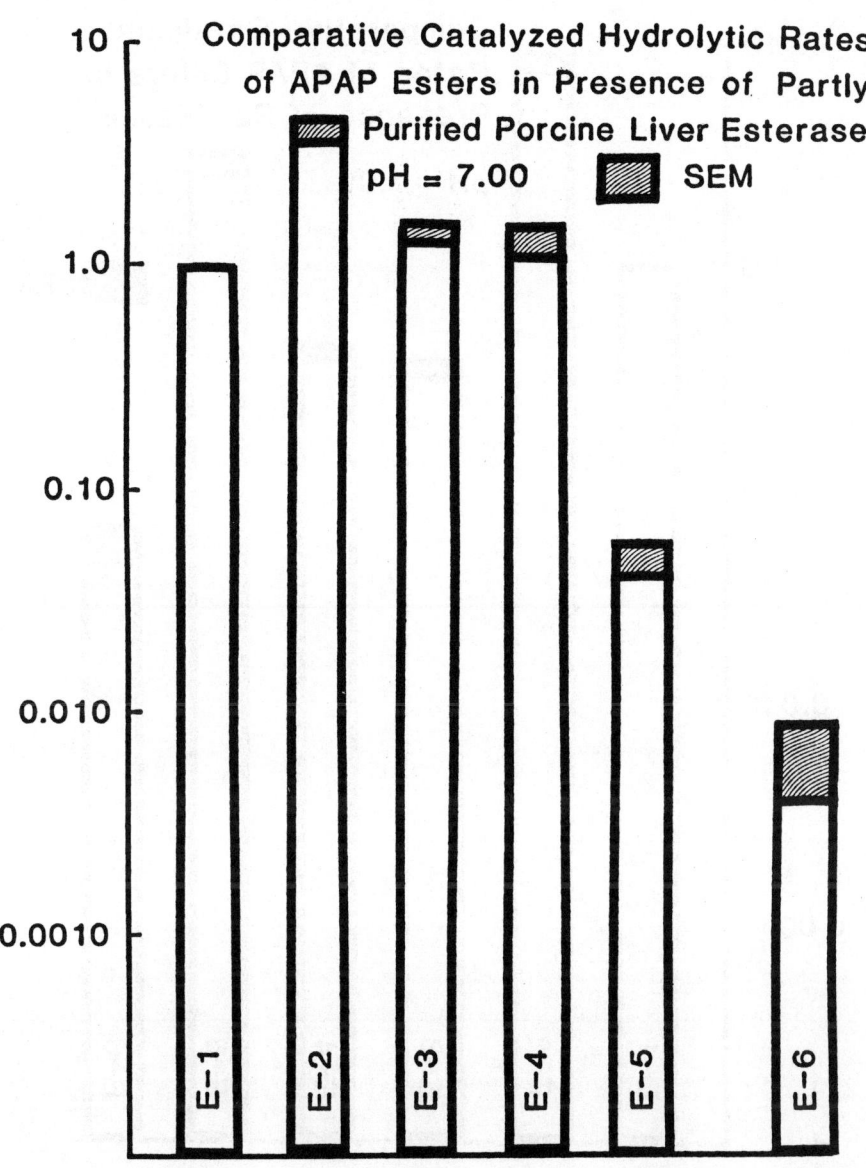

Fig. 6

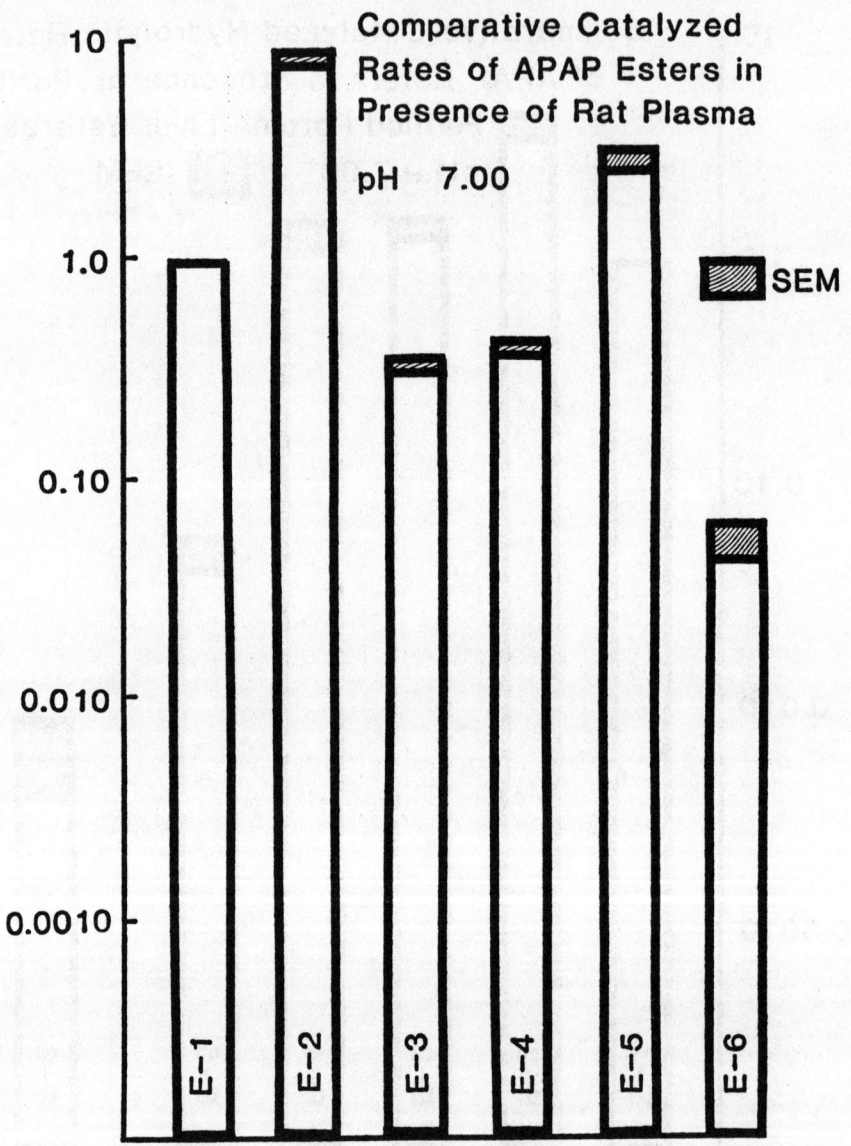

Fig. 7

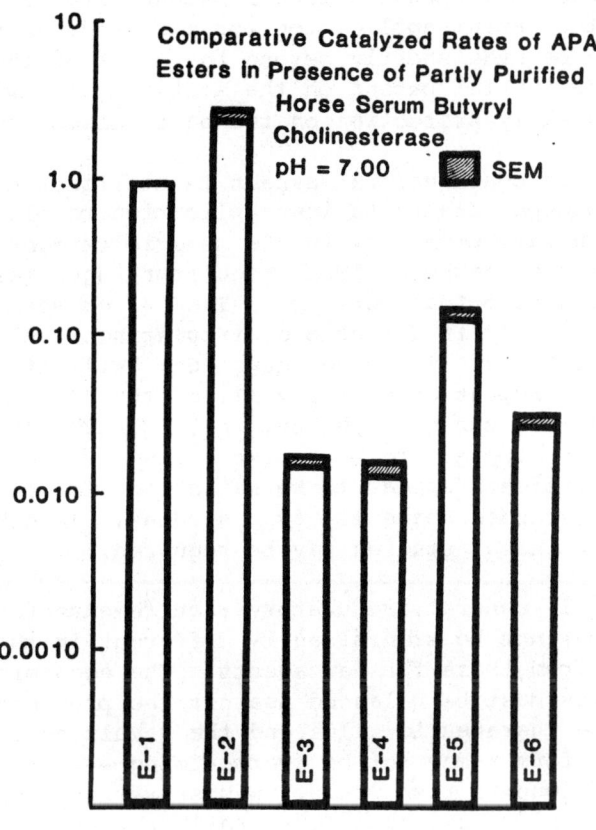

Fig. 8

It is evident that much more needs to be done to understand the relative specificity of such esterases if we are to use these agents in activating our prodrugs.

Prodrug Approach and Regulatory Aspects

The merit of the basic thesis underlying the prodrug approach is so self evident that most of the new drugs which will be introduced henceforth no doubt will either be prodrugs or, at the least, closely examined as to possible application of the concept. Regulatory consideration of prodrug modifications of new agents will probably be the same as that for any new drug substance and will require the usual level of safety and efficacy testing. For economic reasons, these may be brought into clinical testing some years after patenting of the original parent compound since this approach will provide longer patent life to the NDA end product, the patent application for the prodrugs being assumed to be made shortly before the start of the clinical phase. The initial patent on the active moiety will provide the needed early protection on the basic discovery.

The more controversial aspect in utilization of the prodrug concept relates to its application to old drugs, drugs which fall primarily in the generic category. The usual question has been, "Will regulatory agencies require the full toxicological work up?" The answer seems to be yes, particularly if detectable circulating levels of the prodrug are found. The other question, "Will it be necessary to repeat essentially all of the clinical efficacy studies carried out with the original agent?" The answer to this question appears to be somewhat less defined; in some cases requirements appear to be satisfied with carefully conceived extended Phase II_B type studies. In others, more extensive clinical studies may be required.

Thus, in general, regulatory requirements for these prodrugs may not be significantly different in these instances from those for new agents. The economic cost of such studies must be balanced against the presumed improvement in the therapeutic value and the resulting commercial gain. The former may not be overwhelming -- on the other hand, the economic risk would, in most rational situations, be substantially less than for totally new agents since the likelihood of totally unanticipated side effects is limited.

In summary, the prodrug concept will be widely practiced in the development of new chemical agents as drugs. For older drugs, we need to pick and choose our opportunities.

Chapter 2
Design of Bioreversible Drug Derivatives and the Utility of the Double Prodrug Concept

Hans Bundgaard

Royal Danish School of Pharmacy
Department of Pharmaceutical Chemistry AD
2 Universitetsparken
DK-2100 Copenhagen, Denmark

Introduction

A basal requisite for the prodrug approach to be useful in solving drug delivery problems is the ready availability of chemical derivative types satisfying the prodrug requirements, the most prominent of these being reconversion of the prodrug to the parent drug in vivo. This prodrug-drug conversion may take place before absorption (e.g. in the gastro - intestinal tract), during absorption, after absorption or at the specific site of drug action in the body, all dependent upon the specific goal for which the prodrug is designed. Ideally, the prodrug should be converted to the drug as soon as the goal is achieved. The prodrug per se is an inactive species and therefore, once its job is completed, intact prodrug represents unavailable drug. For example, prodrugs designed to overcome solubility problems in formulating intravenous injection solutions should preferably be converted immediately to drug following injection so that the concentration of circulating prodrug would rapidly become insignificant in relation to that of the active drug. Conversely, if the objective of the prodrug is to produce a sustained drug action through rate-limiting prodrug conversion the rate of the conversion should not be too high.

The necessary conversion or activation of prodrugs to the parent drug molecules in the body can take place by a variety of reactions. The most common prodrugs are those requiring a hydrolytic cleavage mediated by enzymic catalysis. Active drug species containing hydroxyl or carboxyl groups can often be converted to prodrug esters from which the active forms are regenerated by esterases within the body, e.g. in the blood. In other cases, active drug substances are regenerated from their prodrugs by biochemical reductive or oxidative processes. Besides usage of the various enzyme systems of the body to carry out the necessary activation of prodrugs, the buffered and relatively constant value of the physiological pH (7.4) may be useful in triggering the release of a drug from a prodrug. In these cases, the prodrugs are characterized by a high degree of chemical lability at pH 7.4 while preferably exhibiting a higher stability at for example pH 3-4.

Several types of bioreversible derivatives have been exploited for utilization in designing prodrugs. The purpose of the present chapter is to discuss some chemical approaches to obtain prodrug forms with due attention to the potential therapeutic and pharmaceutical benefits achievable by the prodrug approach and with emphasis on recently developed types of bioreversible derivatives including double prodrugs. Additional information on the subject can be gathered from other reviews (1-8). A more extensive coverage of various types of bioreversible derivatives is published elsewhere (9).

Esters as prodrugs for compounds containing carboxyl and hydroxyl groups

The popularity of using esters as a prodrug type for drugs containing carboxyl or hydroxyl functions (or thiol groups) stems primarily from the fact that the organism is rich in enzymes capable of hydrolyzing esters. The distribution of esterases is ubiquitous and several types can be found in the blood, liver and other organs or tissues. In addition, by appropriate esterification of molecules containing a hydroxyl or carboxyl group it is feasible to obtain derivatives with almost any desirable hydrophilicity or lipophilicity as well as in vivo lability, the latter being dictated by electronic and steric factors. Accordingly, a great number of alcoholic or carboxylic acid drugs have been modified for a multitude of reasons using the ester prodrug approach. Several examples can be found in various reviews (1-5, 9).

Sometimes, simple aliphatic or aromatic esters may not be sufficiently labile in vivo to ensure a sufficiently high rate and extent of prodrug conversion. This is thus the case for penicillin esters. Although various simple alkyl and aryl esters of the thiazolidine carboxyl groups are rapidly hydrolyzed to the free penicillin acid in animals, such as rodents, they proved to be far too stable in man to have any therapeutic potential (10). This illustrates also - as do many other examples - the occurrence of marked species differences in the in vivo hydrolysis of ester prodrugs. A solution to the problem was found in 1965 by Jansen and Russell (11) who showed that a special double ester type (acyloxymethyl ester) of benzylpenicillin was hydrolyzed rapidly in the blood and tissues of several species including man. The first step in the hydrolysis of such an ester is enzymatic cleavage of the terminal ester bond with formation of a highly unstable hydroxymethyl ester which rapidly dissociates to the parent penicillin and formaldehyde (Scheme 1). A reason for the different enzymatic stabilities of the acyloxymethyl ester and simple alkyl esters of penicillins is certainly that the penicillin carboxyl group is highly sterically hindered. The terminal ester in the acyloxymethyl derivative is less hindered and thus should be more accessible to enzymatic attack.

$$Drug\text{-}COO\text{-}CH_2\text{-}OCOR \xrightarrow{enzymatic} Drug\text{-}COO\text{-}CH_2OH + R\text{-}COOH$$

$$\downarrow fast$$

$$Drug\text{-}COOH + CH_2O$$

Scheme 1

The principle has been used successfully to improve the oral bioavailability of ampicillin (1), and no fewer than three ampicillin prodrug forms are now on the market, namely the pivaloyloxymethyl ester (2) (pivampicillin) (12), the phthalidyl ester (3) (talampicillin) (13, 14) and the ethoxycarbonyloxyethyl ester (4) (bacampicillin) (15), the latter containing a terminal carbonate ester moiety. The properties of these prodrugs as well as of other similar acyloxyalkyl esters of β-lactam antibiotics such as mecillinam and cephalosporins have been extensively reviewed (10).

In more recent years the applicability of this double ester concept in prodrug design has been further expanded. Thus, similar esters have been prepared from cromoglycicacid (16), isoguvacine (17), methyldopa (18-20) and tyrosine (21). Whereas methyldopa (5) is variably and incompletely absorbed its pivaloyloxyethyl ester (6) is almost completely and more uniformly absorbed in man following oral administration and is rapidly hydrolyzed on the first pass to the parent drug (19, 20). A different ester type of methyldopa, a (5-methyl-2-oxo-1,3-dioxol-4-yl)methyl derivative (7) was recently reported to be another potentially useful prodrug for improving the oral bioavailability (22). A similar ester type of ampicillin has recently been described and shown to be an orally well absorbed prodrug (23).

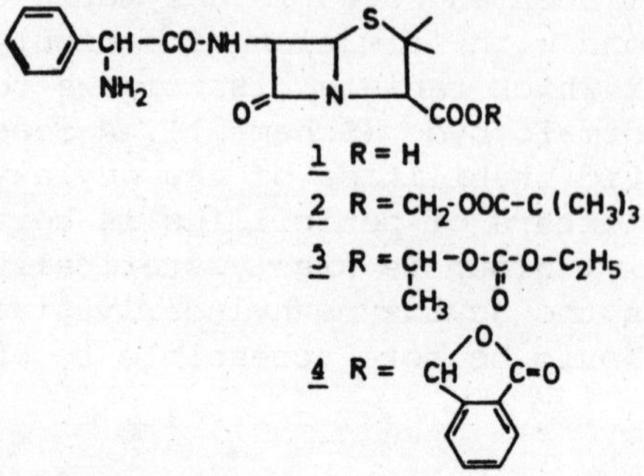

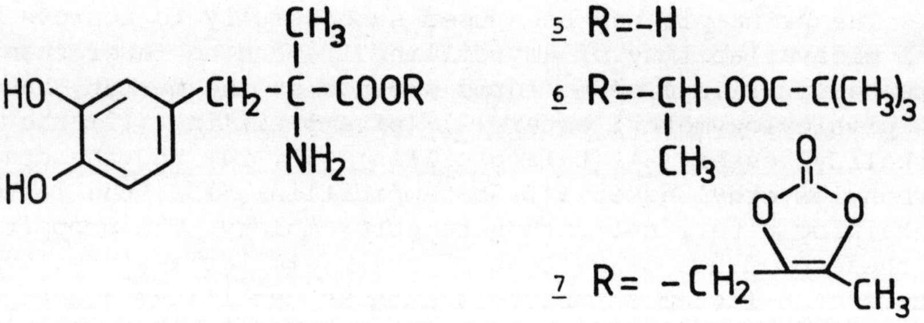

[Structures of compounds 1–4: ampicillin derivatives]

1 R = H
2 R = CH$_2$-OOC-C(CH$_3$)$_3$
3 R = CH-O-C-O-C$_2$H$_5$
         | ‖
         CH$_3$ O
4 R = CH—O
         | \
         (phthalide) C=O

[Structure of α-methyldopa derivatives 5–7]

5 R = -H
6 R = -CH-OOC-C(CH$_3$)$_3$
         |
         CH$_3$
7 R = -CH$_2$—(4-methyl-1,3-dioxol-2-one-5-yl)

The applicability of acyloxyalkyl esters as biologically reversible transport forms has been extended to include phenolic drugs, the derivatives being acyloxyalkyl ethers (8). Bodor and co-workers (24, 25) have recently prepared such acyloxyalkyl ethers of various phenols (e.g. β-estradiol and phenylephrine), thiophenol and catechols (e.g. dopamine and epinephrine). The derivatives are hydrolyzed by a sequential reaction involving the formation of an unstable hemiacetal intermediate (Scheme 2) and they are as susceptible as normal phenol esters to undergo enzymatic hydrolysis by e.g. human plasma enzymes. However, the acyloxyalkyl ethers appear to be more stable against chemical (hydroxide ion-catalyzed) hydrolysis than phenolate esters and this may make them more favorable in prodrug design (24).

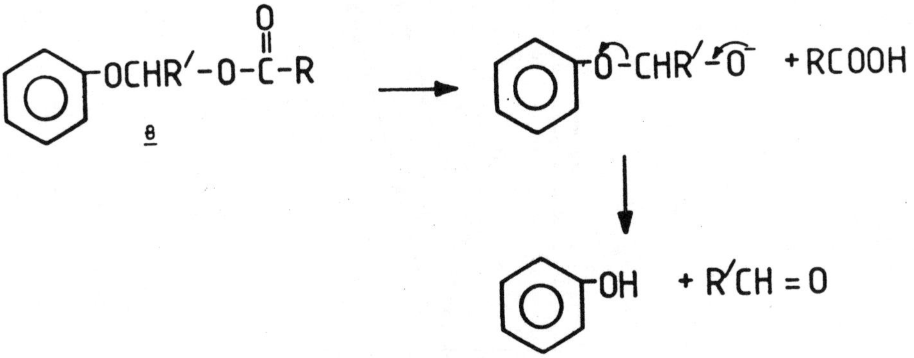

Scheme 2

Carbamate esters may be promising prodrug candidates for phenolic drugs. The enzymatic hydrolytic behaviour of carbamate esters have been examined by Digenis and Swintosky (1). N-Unsubstituted or N-monosubstituted carbamates derived from phenols showed high lability and strong enzymatic catalysis whereas most N-disubstituted carbamates proved highly stable as did carbamates of aliphatic hydroxy compounds. The kinetics and mechanism of the non-enzymatic hydrolysis of carbamates have been thoroughly studied (26-31).

Whereas carbamates of alcohols in general appear to be of no value in prodrug design due to their high stability certain activated carbamates may be useful. Imidazole-1-carboxylic acid esters belong to this category and such derivatives of hydrocortisone (9) and testosterone (10) have recent-

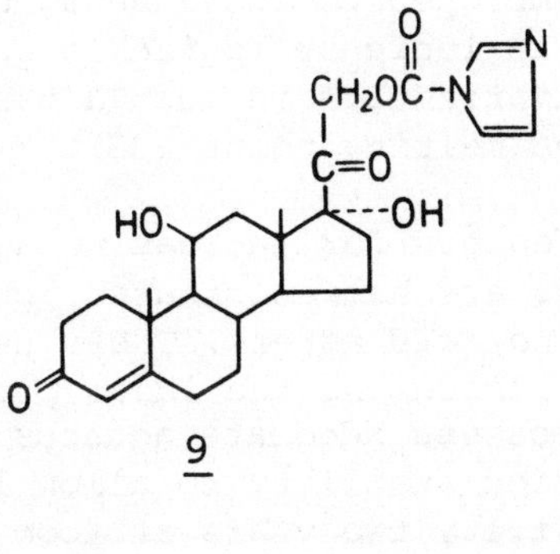

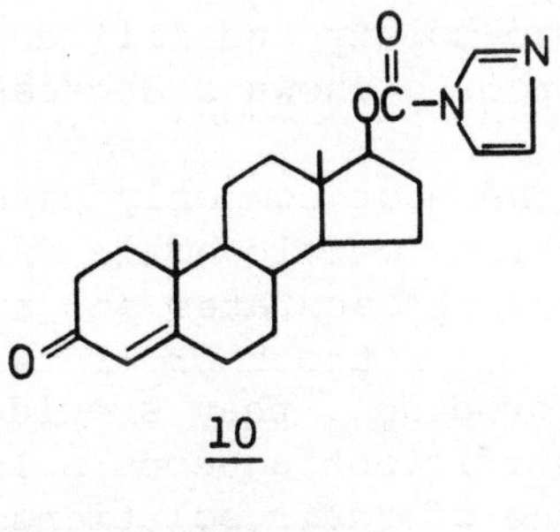

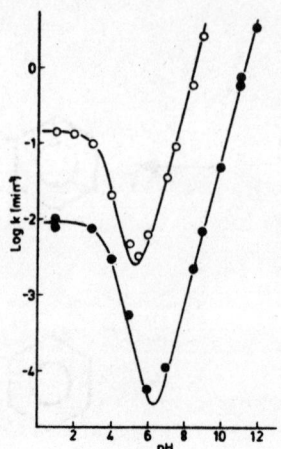

Fig. 1. The pH-rate profiles for the hydrolysis of compound 9 (o) and 10 (●) at 37°C (32).

ly been shown to undergo a relatively facile hydrolysis in aqueous buffer solutions (32). At pH 7.4 and 37°C the half-life of hydrolysis of the hydrocortisone derivative was found to be 8 min and that for the testosterone derivative 65 h, the different reactivity being ascribed to the different steric hindrance in the alcohol portions of the steroids. The pH-rate profiles for the hydrolysis of the derivatives are shown in Fig. 1. No enzymatic catalysis by human plasma was observed. Due to protonation of the imidazole group (pK_a ~3.5) the derivatives showed increased solubility in acidic solution relative to the parent steroids (32).

Ester formation has long been recognized as an effective means of increasing the aqueous solubility of drugs containing a hydroxyl group with the aim of developing prodrug preparations suitable for parenteral administration. Two physicochemical strategies can be employed to increase aqueous solubility: (i) introduction of an ionic or ionizable group by the pro-moiety and (ii) derivatization in such a manner that the prodrug shows a decreased melting point (33).

The most commonly used esters for increasing aqueous solubility of alcoholic drugs are hemisuccinates, phosphates, dialkylaminoacetates and amino acid esters. Their use is, however, not without problems considering the ideal properties of such prodrugs: they should possess adequate aqueous solubility, sufficient aqueous solution stability to allow long term storage of their solutions (i.e., two years at room temperature) and yet they should be converted rapidly in vivo to the active parent drug. For example, succinate esters are not good substrates for hydrolytic enzymes (34) and often show relatively slow and incomplete cleavage in vivo as has been described for such esters of various corticosteroids (35) and chloramphenicol (36-39). Besides, their solution stability is limited due to intramolecular reactions (e.g. catalysis of ester hydrolysis or O-acyl migration in corticosteroids) of the terminal succinate carboxyl group (40, 41). Phosphate esters as sodium salts are freely water soluble and are so stable in vitro that solutions with practical shelf-lives often can be formulated (42-45). Thus, a shelf-life of more than 10 years for an aqueous solution of vidarabine-5'-phosphate at pH 6.8 and 25°C has been predicted (43). They are also rapidly hydrolyzed enzymatically in vivo (e.g. 46-48) although exceptions exist. Thus, the phosphate ester (12) of metronidazole (11) shows a rather slow rate of conversion in human serum, the hydrolysis exhibiting apparent zero-order kinetics (49). The hemisuccinate ester of metronidazole has been shown to be highly stable in 80% human plasma, the half-life at 37°C being 440 h (50). For the third type of water-soluble ester derivatives, i.e. esters with an ionizable amino function in the acid portion, only sparse information is available on their enzymatic hydrolysis. Bundgaard et al. (51, 52) have prepared eight amino acid esters of metronidazole and evaluated their potentiality as water-soluble parenteral delivery forms of the parent drug whose solubility in water is limited (~ 1% w/v). Hydrochloride salts of all the esters exhibited a water solubility greater than 20% w/v but their susceptibility to undergo enzymatic hydrolysis varied widely as seen from the data in Table 1. For the sake of comparison rate data for the hydrolysis of other metronidazole esters are included in Table 1. Due to its facile cleavage in plasma, excellent solubility properties (> 50 w/v in water), and ease of synthesis and purification, the hydrochloride salt of metronidazole N,N-dimethylglycinate (13) appeared to be the most promising prodrug candidate (51). Following intravenous administration to dogs the ester was rapidly ($t_{\frac{1}{2}}$~5 min) and completely converted to metronidazole (52). It is of interest to compare the in vivo half-life in dogs (5 min) to that observed in vitro in dog plasma (25 min). A disadvantage of this prodrug is that it is not sufficiently stable for formulation as a ready-to-use solution (52) and must be used as a formulation to be reconstituted as a solution prior to use. Recently, some kinds of water-soluble amino acid 21-esters of corticosteroids possessing both a high in vitro stability and a high susceptibility of undergoing enzymatic hydrolysis have been developed by Anderson et al. (53).

Table 1. Half-lives for the hydrolysis of various amino acid esters as well as other esters of metronidazole in 80% human plasma (pH 7.4) and 0.05 M phosphate buffer pH 7.40 at 37°C

Ester	$t_{\frac{1}{2}}$ in human plasma (min)	$t_{\frac{1}{2}}$ in buffer (min)
N,N-Dimethylglycinate[a]	12	250
Glycinate[a]	41	115
N-Propylglycinate[a]	8	90
3-Aminopropionate[a]	207	315
3-Dimethylaminopropionate[a]	46	52
3-Dimethylaminobutyrate[a]	334	580
4-Morpholinoacetate[a]	30	1880
4-Methyl-1-piperazinoacetate[a]	523	1720
Benzoate[b]	4	1000 h
Butyrate[c]	1.5	890 h
Valerate[c]	1.5	800 h
Hemisuccinate[c]	630 h	440 h

[a]From Bundgaard et al. (51). [b]H. Bundgaard (unpublished).
[c]From Johansen and Larsen (50).

Sulphate esters of alcohols and phenols have long been considered as prodrug forms useful for obtaining injectable preparations (3). However, recent studies indicate that such esters may be very resistant to undergo hydrolysis in vivo and accordingly, would not be suitable prodrugs. Thus, Miyabo et al. (48) found that dexamethasone-21-sulphate produced virtually no free dexamethasone in plasma and urine following intravenous injection in man but was largely excreted unchanged in urine. Similarly, Williams et al. (54) have found that the sulphate esters of paracetamol and 3-hydroxymethyl-phenytoin do not generate the parent drugs when administered parenterally to mice or rats.

A high crystal lattice energy of solid compounds, as manifested in a high melting point, results in poor solubility (in all solvents). Therefore, an approach to reduce this energy may result in improved aqueous solubility. An example of the usefulness of this approach in prodrug design concerns vidarabine (14). It has a low water solubility (0.5 mg ml^{-1}) primarily due to the occurrence of intramolecular hydrogen bonding in the crystalline state as reflected in its melting point of 260°C. By esterification of the 5'-hydroxyl group this bonding is reduced and by further choosing an only

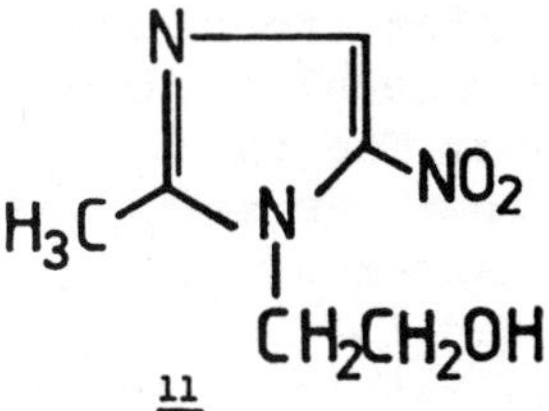

11: structure with H₃C-imidazole-NO₂, N-CH₂CH₂OH

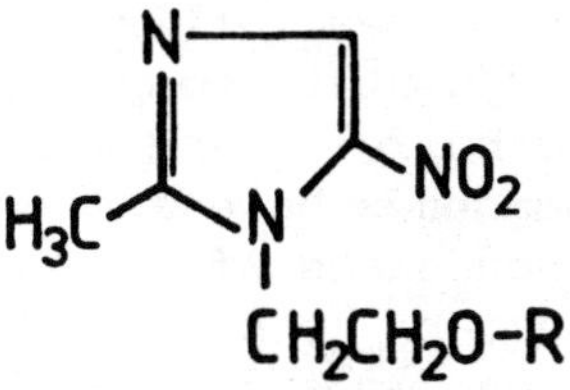

12: R = -P(=O)-(OH)₂ on CH₂CH₂O-R

13: R = -C(=O)-CH₂-N(CH₃)₂

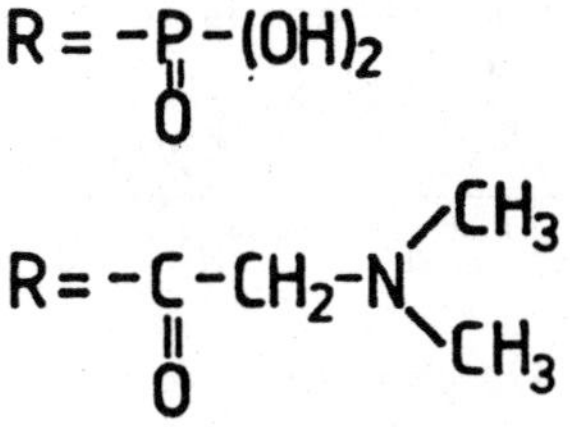

slightly lipophilic acyl group like formyl a vidarabine ester with greatly increased aqueous solubility has been obtained (55). The 5'-formate ester (15) is rapidly hydrolyzed in human blood with a half-life of about 6-8 min and it appears to be a useful parenteral delivery form of vidarabine (55). Several other examples of using this approach to increase the aqueous solubilities of drugs are given in other sections of this chapter.

Prodrugs for amides, imides and other NH-acidic compounds

N-Mannich bases

N-Mannich bases have been proposed as potentially useful prodrug candidates for NH-acidic compounds such as various amides, imides, carbamates, hydantoins and urea derivatives as well as for aliphatic or aromatic amines (7, 56-64). They are generally formed by reacting an NH-acidic compound with formaldehyde, or in very rare cases, other aldehydes and a primary or secondary aliphatic or aromatic amine. The process can be considered as an N-aminomethylation or N-amidomethylation (in the case of the NH-acidic component being an amide; Scheme 3).

$$R\text{-}CONH_2 + CH_2O + R_1R_2NH \rightleftharpoons R\text{-}CONH\text{-}CH_2\text{-}NR_1R_2 + H_2O$$

Scheme 3

Hydrolysis of N-Mannich bases. The kinetics of decomposition of a great number of N-Mannich bases in aqueous solution has been the subject of several studies (56-58, 60-64).

At constant pH and temperature, the decomposition rates of the N-Mannich bases followed strict first-order kinetics and all reactions went to completion. No general acid-base catalysis by the buffers used was apparent. The pH-rate profiles for most compounds have a sigmoidal shape as seen in Fig.2. These pH dependences of the observed apparent first-order rate constant, k_{obs}, could be accounted for by assuming spontaneous decomposition of the free Mannich bases (B) and their conjugate acids (BH^+); the expression for k_{obs} is:

$$k_{obs} = \frac{k_1 K_a}{a_H + K_a} + \frac{k_2 a_H}{a_H + K_a} \tag{1}$$

where K_a is the apparent ionization constant of the protonated N-Mannich bases, a_H is the hydrogen ion activity, and

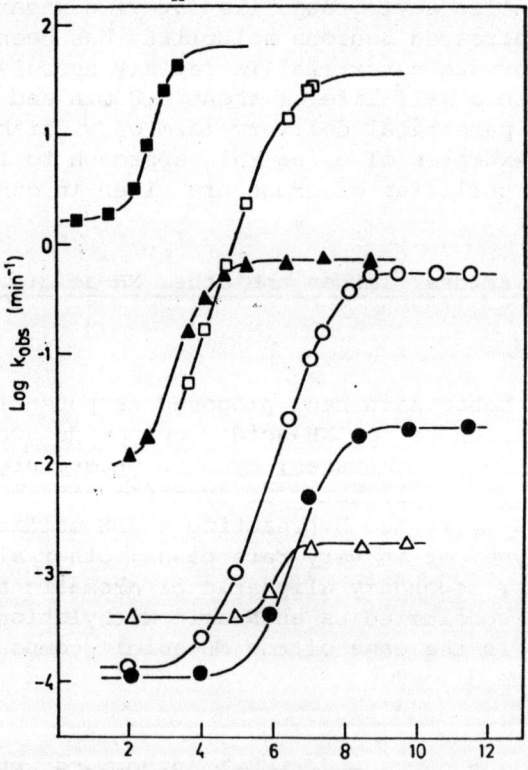

Fig. 2. The pH-rate profiles for the decomposition of various N-Mannich bases in aqueous solution at 37°C. Key: ■, N-(morpholinomethyl)-p-toluenesulphonamide; □, N-(piperidinomethyl)-trichloroacetamide; ▲, N-(morpholinomethyl)trichloroacetamide; ○, N-(diethylaminomethyl)benzamide; ●, N-(isobutylaminomethyl)-benzamide; and △, N-(benzylaminomethyl)benzamide (56, 57).

k_1 and k_2 are the apparent first-order rate constants for the spontaneous degradation of B and BH$^+$, respectively.

The reaction mechanism proposed (56, 57) for the decomposition involves as rate-determining step an unimolecular N-C bond cleavage with formation of an amide (or imide) anion and an immonium cation. In subsequent fast steps, a solvent molecule transfers a proton to the anion and a hydroxide ion to the immonium ion, giving methylolamine, which rapidly dissociates to formaldehyde and amine (Scheme 4). Loudon et al. (65) have independently proposed a similar mechanism for N-Mannich bases derived from isopropylaldehyde.

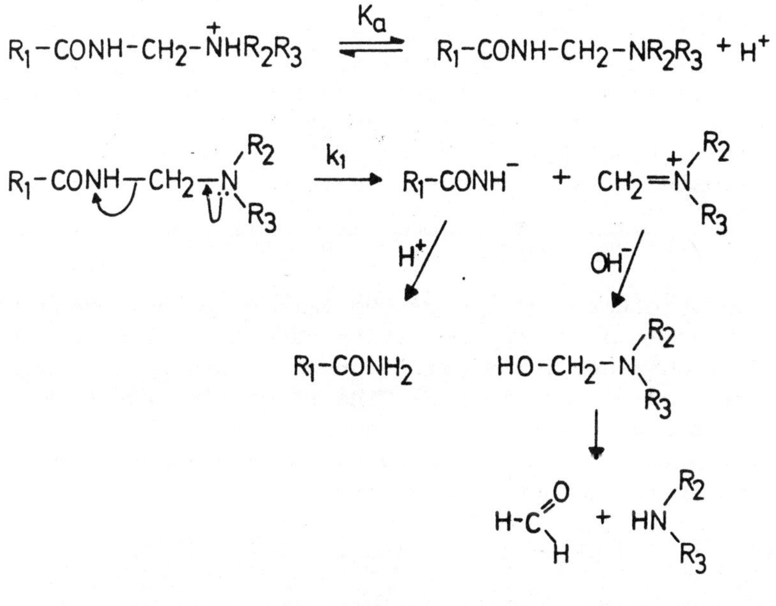

$$R_1-CONH-CH_2-\overset{+}{N}HR_2R_3 \underset{}{\overset{K_a}{\rightleftharpoons}} R_1-CONH-CH_2-NR_2R_3 + H^+$$

$$R_1-CONH-CH_2-N\begin{smallmatrix}R_2\\R_3\end{smallmatrix} \xrightarrow{k_1} R_1-CONH^- + CH_2=\overset{+}{N}\begin{smallmatrix}R_2\\R_3\end{smallmatrix}$$

$$\xrightarrow{H^+} R_1-CONH_2 \qquad \xrightarrow{OH^-} HO-CH_2-N\begin{smallmatrix}R_2\\R_3\end{smallmatrix}$$

$$\downarrow$$

$$H-C\begin{smallmatrix}=O\\H\end{smallmatrix} + HN\begin{smallmatrix}R_2\\R_3\end{smallmatrix}$$

<u>Scheme 4</u>

<u>Structural effects on decomposition rate.</u> The structural effects on the decomposition rate of N-Mannich bases derived from carboxamides, thioamides, sulphonamides or imides and aliphatic or aromatic amines involve steric effects and basicity of the amine component and acidity of the amide-type component (57, 61, 64). These factors are most pronounced with respect to the rate constant k_1 and, accordingly, to the decomposition rate in weakly acidic to basic aqueous solutions. The rates of the hydrolysis of unprotonated Mannich bases are accelerated strongly by (<u>a</u>) increasing steric effects within

the amine substituent, (b) increasing basicity of the amine component and (c) increasing acidity of the parent amide-type compound.

For some N-Mannich bases of benzamide and various amines the rate constant k_1 can be expressed by the following equation (57):

$$\log k_1 = 2.30\nu - 3.50 \quad (k_1 \text{ in min}^{-1}; 37°C) \tag{2}$$

where ν is Charton's steric substituent parameter for alkyl amino groups. The marked influence of the steric effect on k_1 can be exemplified by comparing the k_1-values for benzamide Mannich bases of diethylamine (0.52 min^{-1}) and ethylamine (0.0084 min^{-1}).

For amines with the same steric properties but differing in basicity, the rate constants k_1 for the decomposition of the respective N-Mannich bases were shown to increase almost 10-fold with an increase of unity of the pK_a of the amines. Thus, for various N-(arylaminomethyl)succinimide derivatives the following relationship was derived (61):

$$\log k_1 = 0.93 \, pK_a - 4.81 \quad (k_1 \text{ in min}^{-1}; 37°C) \tag{3}$$

The structural effect of the amide-type component in the Mannich bases on the decomposition rate was delineated from rate data obtained for several Mannich bases with either piperidine or morpholine (57). The reactivity was shown to increase strongly with increasing acidity of the parent amide-type compound. For the Mannich bases with piperidine the following relationship was derived:

$$\log k_1 = -1.42 \, pK_a + 19.3 \quad (k_1 \text{ in min}^{-1}; 37°C) \tag{4}$$

For morpholine derivatives Eq. (5) was obtained:

$$\log k_1 = -1.15 \, pK_a + 13.9 \quad (k_1 \text{ in min}^{-1}; 37°C) \tag{5}$$

Eqs. (4) and (5) in which pK_a refers to the ionization constant for the parent amide-type compounds (at 20-25°C) cover both aromatic and aliphatic carboxamides as well as a thioamide and a sulphonamide. N-Mannich bases of urea, thiourea and N-acyl thiourea derivatives were found to deviate from these relationships showing a greater reactivity than expected on the basis of their pK_a values. The N-Mannich base (16) formed between (-)-ephedrine and benzamide is also more reactive than predicted, the half-life of hydrolysis at pH 7.4 and 37°C being 2.2 min (64). A positive deviation was further observed with N-Mannich bases of salicylamide (60). Despite these exceptions the structure-reactivity relationships obtained have successfully been used to predict the reactivity of new N-Mannich bases (66, 67).

$$\underset{16}{\text{Ph-CH(OH)-CH(CH}_3\text{)-N(CH}_3\text{)-CH}_2\text{-NH-CO-Ph}}$$

Some representative rate data for the decomposition of various N-Mannich bases are given in Table 2.

The breakdown of the N-Mannich bases does not rely on enzymatic catalysis and identical decomposition rates were observed in solutions with or without addition of human plasma (66, 68).

N-Mannich bases derived from other aldehydes than formaldehyde are not readily prepared and knowledge of the reactivity of such compounds is therefore limited. Loudon et al. (65) have studied the hydrolysis of N-Mannich bases derived from some amides and isopropylaldehyde and from the data reported, it can be estimated that isopropylaldehyde Mannich bases are approximately 10 times more reactive in neutral and alkaline solutions than the corresponding N-Mannich bases with formaldehyde. Similarly, N-Mannich bases derived from amides and benzaldehyde are markedly more reactive than those prepared with formaldehyde (69).

Application of N-Mannich bases as potential prodrugs

By appropriate selection of the amine component, it should be feasible to obtain prodrugs of a given amide-type drug with varying degree of in vivo lability. Besides, other physicochemical properties such as aqueous solubility, dissolution rate and lipophilicity can be modified for the parent compounds as shown by the data in Table 3 (7, 59).

Transformation of an amide into an N-Mannich base introduces a readily ionizable amino moiety which may allow the preparation of derivatives with greatly increased water solubilities at slightly acidic pH values where, as a matter of

Table 2. Rate data for the decomposition of various N-Mannich bases in aqueous solution at 37°C [a]

Compound	k_1 (min^{-1})	$t_{1/2}$ (min)[b]
N-(Piperidinomethyl)benzamide	0.051	47
N-(Piperidinomethyl)-4-nitrobenzamide	0.17	8.0
N-(Piperidinomethyl)acetamide	0.0055	400
N-(Piperidinomethyl)dichloroacetamide	2.48	0.4
N-(Piperidinomethyl)trichloroacetamide	35	0.02
N-(Piperidinomethyl)nicotinamide	0.17	8.0
N-(Piperidinomethyl)thiobenzamide	13	0.06
N-(Morpholinomethyl)benzamide	0.0005	1400
N-(Morpholinomethyl)thiobenzamide	0.52	1.3
N-(Morpholinomethyl)-p-toluenesulphonamide	60	0.01
N-(Phenethylaminomethyl)benzamide[c]	0.0048	205
N-(Phenylpropanolaminomethyl)benzamide[c]	0.0031	225
N-(Methylaminomethyl)benzamide	0.0026	600
N-(Ethylaminomethyl)benzamide	0.0084	190
N-(Diethylaminomethyl)benzamide	0.52	4.0
N-(Dimethylaminomethyl)benzamide	0.032	58
N-(Benzylaminomethyl)benzamide	0.0020	380
N-(Morpholinomethyl)-N'-acetylthiourea	0.91	0.8
N-(Piperidinomethyl)-N'-methylurea	–	5.0
N-(Methylaminomethyl)salicylamide[d]	–	28
N-(Piperidinomethyl)salicylamide[d]	–	14
N-(Morpholinomethyl)salicylamide[d]	–	41
N-(α-Alaninomethyl)salicylamide[d]	–	17
N-(Anilinomethyl)succinimide[e]	0.36	1.9
N-(p-Toluidinomethyl)succinimide[e]	0.76	0.9

[a] From Bundgaard and Johansen (57) if not otherwise indicated. [b] At pH 7.40. [c] From Johansen and Bundgaard (64). [d] From Johansen and Bundgaard (60). [e] From Bundgaard and Johansen (61).

Table 3. Aqueous solubility and partition coefficients of various N-Mannich bases of benzamide (59).

Compound	S^a (M)	log P^b
Benzamide	0.11	0.69
N-(Ethylaminomethyl)-benzamide	0.073	0.97
- HCl salt	0.096	
N-(Isobutylaminomethyl)-benzamide, HCl salt	0.065	1.73
N-(Dimethylaminomethyl)-benzamide	2.6	0.85
- HCl salt	5.6	

^{a}The molar solubility in water at 22°C. ^{b}The partition coefficient between octanol and aqueous buffer of pH 9.2 at 22°C.

fortune, the stability may be quite high. This has been shown for various N-Mannich bases using benzamide as a model compound (59) (Table 3). Whereas N-Mannich bases prepared from secondary amines showed very high solubilities in salt form, the Mannich bases derived from primary amines did not show increased solubility even as salts. This different behaviour was attributed to the occurrence of intramolecular hydrogen bonding in the latter derivatives (17).

17

The concept of N-Mannich base formation of NH-acidic compounds to yield more soluble prodrugs has already been utilized in the case of rolitetracycline (18). This highly water-soluble N-Mannich base of tetracycline and pyrrolidine which is used clinically is decomposed quantitatively to tetracycline in neutral aqueous solution, the half-life being 40 min at pH 7.4 and 37°C (70). Similarly, various N-Mannich bases of carbamazepine (19) have been developed as water-soluble prodrugs for parenteral administration (67) (Table 4). The solubility of the hydrochloride salts of these N-Mannich bases in water was found to exceed 50% w/v, i.e. more than

10^4-fold greater solubility than the parent drug. Following intramuscular administration in rats, higher and more rapidly appearing carbamazepine plasma levels were observed from aqueous solutions of the dipropylamino N-Mannich base prodrug than from administering a suspension of the parent drug (Fig. 3) (67).

In addition, the concept may be useful for improving the dissolution behaviour of poorly soluble drugs in an effort to improve the oral bioavailability. Thus, as seen from Table 5 N-Mannich bases of various NH-acidic compounds (e.g. phthalimide, chlorzoxazone, phenytoin, barbital, p-toluenesulphonamide, acetazolamide, chlorothiazide and allopurinol) with morpholine or piperidine as the amine component were found to possess markedly greater (up to a factor of 2,000) intrinsic dissolution rates in 0.1 M hydrochloric acid in comparison with the parent compounds (58, 63). Once dissolved the

Table 4. Ionization constants and rate data for the decomposition of various N-Mannich bases of carbamazepine in aqueous solution at 37°C [a]

Compound	pK_a	k_1 (min^{-1})	k_2 (min^{-1})	$t_{1/2}$ (at pH 7.40) (min)
N-(Diethylaminomethyl)-carbamazepine	7.95	0.17	0.0017	19
N-(Dipropylaminomethyl)-carbamazepine	7.75	0.27	0.0030	7
N-(Piperidinomethyl)-carbamazepine	7.90	0.015	0.0011	165

[a] From Bundgaard et al. (67)

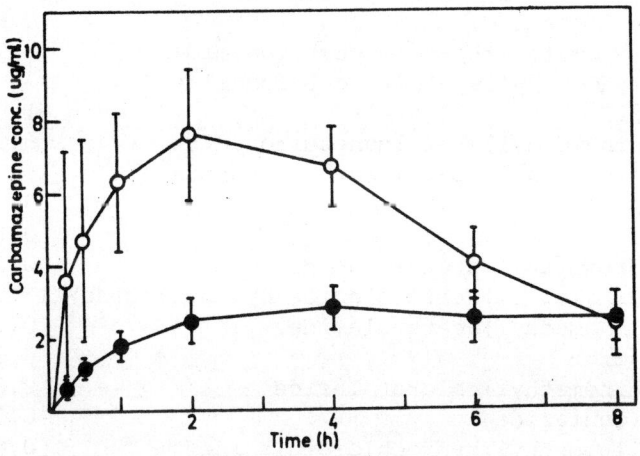

Fig. 3. Mean carbamazepine plasma levels (± S.D.) versus time plots obtained after intramuscular administration of carbamazepine (●) and N-(dipropylaminomethyl)carbamazepine hydrochloride (o) to rats at a dose of 100 mg/kg carbamazepine equivalents (67).

Table 5. Intrinsic dissolution rates (D) for various N-Mannich bases and their parent compounds in 0.1 M hydrochloric acid at 22°C[a]

Compound	D (mg cm^{-2} min^{-1})
Phthalimide	0.063
N-(Piperidinomethyl)phthalimide	7.1
N-(Piperidinomethyl)phthalimide hydrochloride	31
Barbital	0.80
N-(Piperidinomethyl)barbital	2.0
N-(Piperidinomethyl)barbital hydrochloride	>400
N-(Morpholinomethyl)barbital	1.1
N-(Morpholinomethyl)barbital hydrochloride	>400
Phenytoin	0.0050
N-(Morpholinomethyl)phenytoin	0.52
N-(Piperidinomethyl)phenytoin	1.1
N-(Piperidinomethyl)phenytoin hydrochloride	3.6
Chlorzoxazone	0.034
N-(Morpholinomethyl)chlorzoxazone	0.56
N-(Morpholinomethyl)chlorzoxazone	~120
p-Toluenesulfonamide	0.67
N-(Morpholinomethyl)-p-toluenesulfonamide	6.7
N-(Morpholinomethyl)-p-toluenesulfonamide hydrochloride	81
N-(Piperidinomethyl)-p-toluenesulfonamide	6.0
N-(Piperidinomethyl)-p-toluenesulfonamide hydrochloride	39
Acetazolamide	0.27
N-(Piperidinomethyl)acetazolamide	0.27
N-(Piperidinomethyl)acetazolamide hydrochloride	13.0
N-(Morpholinomethyl)acetazolamide	0.24
Chlorothiazide	0.062
N-(Piperidinomethyl)chlorothiazide	0.61
Hydrochlorothiazide	0.086
N-(Morpholinomethyl)hydrochlorothiazide	0.65
Allopurinol[b]	0.099
N_1-(Piperidinomethyl)allopurinol[b]	7.7
N_1-(Morpholinomethyl)allopurinol[b]	3.1
N_1-(Dimethylaminomethyl)allopurinol[b]	3.7

[a] From Bundgaard and Johansen (58), if not otherwise indicated.
[b] From Bundgaard and Johansen (63).

N-Mannich bases are cleaved very rapidly with the quantitative release of the parent compounds.

Recently, Sloan et al. (71) have prepared various N-Mannich bases of theophylline (20) and the morpholino N-Mannich base of 5-fluorouracil (21) and shown that these derivatives are effective as prodrugs for the delivery of the parent drugs through skin. The N-Mannich bases exhibit enhanced water as well as enhanced lipid solubilities as compared to the parent drugs (Table 6) and are relatively stable in aprotic solvents such as isopropyl myristate which was used as a vehicle for the diffusion experiments with hairless mouse skin. The enhanced solubilities of the derivatives relative to the parent drugs may be ascribed partly to decreased crystal lattice energy as reflected in the decreased melting points, cf. Table 6.

Various reports have indicated that the antitumor effect of hexamethylmelamine and other N-methyl-containing antineoplastic drugs possibly may be due to formaldehyde formed from N-hydroxymethylated metabolites. On this basis the hypothesis has been raised (71a) that various formaldehyde precursors may be potential antitumor agents due to liberation of the cytotoxic formaldehyde within tumor cells. Various N-Mannich bases decomposing spontaneously in aqueous solution to yield formaldehyde with half-lives of 17-47 min at physiological pH and temperature were studied on the basis of this rationale and screened in a P-388 lymphocytic leukemia tumor system. Of the compounds tested only N-(piperidinomethyl)benzamide showed a significant activity (71a).

Table 6. Solubilities and melting points of various
N-Mannich bases of theophylline and 5-fluorouracil (71)

Compound	m.p. (°C)	Solubility (mg/ml)	
		Water	Isopropyl myristate
5-Fluorouracil	282-283	26.2	0.0044
Compound 21	128-131	100	11.8
Theophylline	270-274	8.3	0.095
Compound 20:			
R = methyl	121-123	100	7.6
R = ethyl	122-124	100	32.5
R = propyl	72-73	100	27.6
R = morpholino	175-178	100	1.3
R = pyrrolidino	114-115	100	10.7

<u>N-Hydroxymethyl derivatives</u>

When an NH-acidic compound is allowed to react with formaldehyde in absence of a primary or secondary amine N-hydroxymethylation occurs (Scheme 5):

$$R-CONH_2 + CH_2O \rightleftharpoons R-CONH-CH_2OH$$

<u>Scheme 5</u>

The kinetics of decomposition of a large number of N-hydroxymethylated amides, imides, carbamates and hydantoins in aqueous solution has been studied (72, 73). It was found that the decomposition exhibited a first-order dependence on hydroxide ion concentration up to pH about 12 and that the rates increased sharply with increasing acidity of the parent compound (Fig. 4). The following linear correlation was found between log k_1 (where k_1 is the apparent hydroxide ion catalytic rate constant) and pK_a for the above-mentioned group of compounds:

$$\log k_1 = -0.77\ pK_a + 14.4 \qquad (k_1 \text{ in } M^{-1} \text{ min}^{-1};\ 37°C) \qquad (6)$$

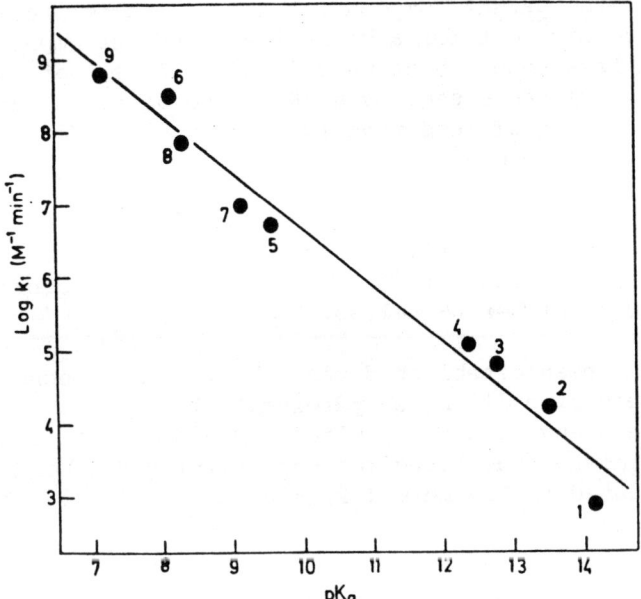

Fig. 4. Plot of the logarithm of the apparent hydroxide ion catalytic rate constant (k_1) for decomposition of various N-hydroxymethyl derivatives at 37°C against pK_a of the parent compounds. Key: 1, chloroacetamide; 2, dichloroacetamide; 3, thiobenzamide; 4, trichloroacetamide; 5, succinimide; 6, 5-chloro-2-benzoxazolinone (chlorzoxazone); 7, 5,5-dimethylhydantoin; 8, phenytoin; 9, nitrofurantoin. From Bundgaard and Johansen (73).

Eq. (6) may be expressed in a more directly useful form:

$$\log t_{\frac{1}{2}} = 0.77 \, pK_a - 8.34 \qquad (\underline{r} = 0.986; \; n = 9) \qquad (7)$$

where $t_{\frac{1}{2}}$ is the half-life for hydrolysis at pH 7.4 and 37°C (in min) and pK_a refers to the ionization constant of the parent NH-acidic compound.

This relationship allows one to predict the reactivity of an N-hydroxymethyl derivative solely from a knowledge of the pK_a of the parent compound. Thus, it can be predicted that the requirement for a half-life of the decomposition reaction of less than 1 h at pH 7.4 and 37°C is that the parent NH-acidic compound possesses a pK_a value of less than 13.1 or that a pK_a value of less than 10.8 is required for a half-life of less than one min.

A selection of half-lives for decomposition of various N-hydroxymethyl derivatives at pH 7.4 and 37°C are given in Table 7. Most values were calculated using rate constants determined at higher pH values.

It has been established that the reaction mechanism for the decomposition of the N-hydroxymethyl derivatives of amides involves a stepwise pathway with an N-hydroxymethyl anion as an intermediate undergoing rate-determining N-C bond cleavage as illustrated in Scheme 6 (72). Bansal et al. (74) have shown

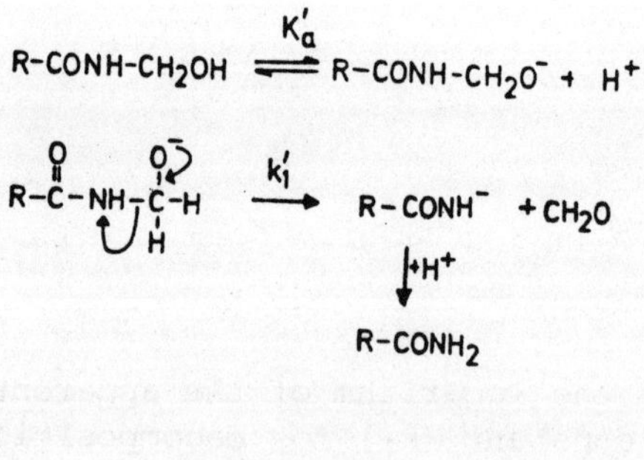

$$R-CONH-CH_2OH \;\xrightleftharpoons{K'_a}\; R-CONH-CH_2O^- + H^+$$

$$R-\overset{O}{\underset{}{C}}-NH-\overset{\overset{O^-}{|}}{\underset{H}{C}}-H \;\xrightarrow{k'_1}\; R-CONH^- + CH_2O$$

$$\downarrow +H^+$$

$$R-CONH_2$$

Scheme 6

Table 7. Apparent hydroxide ion catalytic rate constants (k_1) for the decomposition of various N-hydroxymethyl derivatives in aqueous solution at 37°C, half-lives of decomposition at pH 7.40 and 37°C and pK_a values of the parent NH-acidic compounds[a]

N-Hydroxymethyl derivative of:	k_1 ($M^{-1} min^{-1}$)	$t_{\frac{1}{2}}$	pK_a
Benzamide	1.1×10^2	183 h	14-15
4-Chlorobenzamide	2.2×10^2	88 h	
4-Nitrobenzamide	8.9×10^2	22 h	
3-Nitrobenzamide	7.4×10^2	27 h	
4-Methoxybenzamide	6.0×10^2	120 h	
3-Methoxybenzamide	1.6×10^2	317 h	
Nicotinamide	5.1×10^4	37 h	12.8
Thiobenzamide	6.3×10^2	18 min	14.2
Chloroacetamide	6.9×10^4	28 h	13.5
Dichloroacetamide	1.5×10^5	77 min	12.4
Trichloroacetamide	1.2×10^6	10 min	9.6
Succinimide	5.0×10^6	14 sec	8.3
Phthalimide	2.5×10^6	28 sec	8.2
5-Chloro-2-benzoxazolinone	3.5×10^8	0.2 sec	7.2
Nitrofurantoin	6.2×10^8	0.1 sec	8.3
Phenytoin	7.1×10^7	1.0 sec	
5,5-Dimethylhydantoin	1.0×10^7	6.9 sec	9.2

[a]From Bundgaard and Johansen (72, 73).

that similar rate-determining transition states are involved in the formation of N-hydroxymethyl derivatives of uracils. As can be expected on the basis of this reaction mechanism the rate of decomposition of N-hydroxymethyl derivatives is not catalyzed by enzymes (68).

The N-hydroxymethyl derivatives of amide- or imide-type compounds are more water-soluble than the parent compounds (59, 72-75), thus suggesting a potential area of application of N-hydroxymethyl prodrugs for nitrogenous molecules, e.g. for increasing dissolution rates and hence oral bioavailability. By replacing a proton bound to a nitrogen atom by a hydroxymethyl group intra- or inter-molecular hydrogen bonding in such molecules may be decreased, leading to a corresponding decrease in melting point and increase in water-solubility (59, 73-75). This is illustrated by the data given in Table 8.

From the structure-reactivity data given above it is readily evident that N-hydroxymethylation is not a universally applicable approach to bioreversible derivatization of NH-acidic compounds but is limited to compounds possessing a pK_a value of less than about 10.5-11 in order to provide a sufficient rate of drug regeneration at physiological pH. For example, N-hydroxymethyl derivatives of carboxamides (pK_a 14-15) are relatively stable, the half-lives for decomposition of the derivatives of e.g. benzamide and nicotinamide being 183 and 37 h, respectively, at pH 7.4 and 37°C (72). Derivatives obtained from other aldehydes than formaldehyde possess, however, a greater lability (69) but their availability is seriously restricted. Whereas N-hydroxymethyl derivatives are easily prepared by reacting formaldehyde with the NH-acidic compound in water, ethanol or other solvents most aliphatic and all aromatic aldehydes do not behave as formaldehyde does (76). The reaction with e.g. amides usually does not stop at the N-alkylol stage, RCONHCHOHR', but progresses further to yield the stable alkylidene - or arylidene-bisamide, $(RCONH)_2CHR'$. The only exceptions are the α-halogenated aldehydes such as chloral (76) and also acetaldehyde toward thiobenzamide (77). A recent study (69) on the kinetics of hydrolysis of such hydroxyalkyl compounds derived from benzamide, thiobenzamide and chloral or acetaldehyde as well as of N-(α-hydroxybenzyl)benzamide (22), the latter being obtained from hydrolysis of the N-Mannich base N-(α-morpholinobenzyl)-benzamide (69), has shown that these derivatives are much more unstable in neutral and alkaline solutions than the corresponding N-hydroxymethyl derivatives (Table 9). Thus, whereas the half-life of decomposition of N-(hydroxymethyl)benzamide is 183 h at pH 7.4 and 37°C the half-life for the benzamide compound derived from benzaldehyde (22) is only 6.5 min

Table 8. Melting points and aqueous solubilities (at 22-25°C) of various NH-acidic compounds and their N-hydroxymethyl derivatives

Compound	Melting point (°C)	Aqueous Solubility (M)	Reference
Benzamide	130	0.11	72
N-Hydroxymethylbenzamide	104-106	0.30	72
Thiobenzamide	-	0.012	72
N-Hydroxymethylthiobenzamide	64-65	0.073	72
Chlorzoxazone	191	0.0014[a]	72
N-Hydroxymethylchlorzoxazone	138-144	0.0020[a]	72
Phenytoin	295-298	0.00013[a]	73
3-Hydroxymethylphenytoin	198-199	0.0037[a]	73
Nitrofurantoin	270-272	0.00046[a]	73
3-Hydroxymethylnitrofurantoin	-	0.0012[a]	73
Uracil	340	0.03	74
1,3-Dihydroxymethyluracil	101	2.90	74
Glutethimide	85	0.005	75
N-Hydroxymethylglutethimide	82	0.022	75

[a] In 0.1 M hydrochloric acid

Table 9. Apparent hydroxide ion catalytic rate constants (k_{OH}) for the decomposition of various N-hydroxyalkyl derivatives in aqueous solution ($\mu = 0.5$; 37°C) and half-lives ($t_{\frac{1}{2}}$) of decomposition at pH 7.40 and 37°C[a]

Compound	k_{OH} (M^{-1} min^{-1})	$t_{\frac{1}{2}}$ (min)
N-(α-Hydroxybenzyl)benzamide	1.8×10^5	6.5
N-(α-Hydroxy-2,2,2-trichloroethyl)benzamide	1.7×10^3	6.9×10^2
N-(Hydroxymethyl)benzamide	1.1×10^2	1.1×10^4
N-(α-Hydroxyethyl)thiobenzamide	2.3×10^6	0.5
N-(α-Hydroxy-2,2,2-trichloroethyl)thiobenzamide	4.5×10^6	0.3
N-(Hydroxymethyl)thiobenzamide	6.3×10^4	18

[a]From Bundgaard and Johansen (69).

                    O
                    ‖
        Ph—C—NH—CHOH
                     |
                    Ph

        22

at the same conditions. The difference in reactivity was suggested to be primarily due to steric effects within the α-substituents (69). The implications of these results for the design of N-acyloxyalkyl-type prodrugs are discussed below.

Finally, it should be pointed out that although N-hydroxymethyl derivatives may be useful as such as prodrug forms the most important aspect of N-hydroxymethylation resides in the fact that the hydroxyl group introduced by this process is readily amenable to bioreversible derivatization, e.g. by esterification to produce water-soluble or lipophilic N-acyloxymethyl derivatives.

N-Acyloxyalkyl derivatives

In recent years N-acyloxyalkylation has become a commonly used approach to obtain prodrugs of various amides, imides, hydantoins, uracils, tertiary or N-heterocyclic amines, hydantoins, uracils, tertiary or N-heterocyclic amines and other NH-acidic compounds (6-9). The usefulness of this approach stems from the fact that by varying the acyl portion of the derivatives it is possible to control the rate of regeneration of the parent drug and to obtain prodrugs with varying physicochemical properties such as water-solubility or lipophilicity. Whereas the derivatives show good stability in aqueous solution in vitro similar to other esters, they are in general rapidly cleaved in vivo by virtue of enzyme-mediated hydrolysis. The regeneration of the parent NH-acidic drug takes place via a two step reaction (Scheme 7). Enzymatic cleavage of the ester grouping results in the formation of an N-hydroxyalkyl derivative which subsequently is assumed to decompose instantaneously into the corresponding aldehyde and the NH-acidic drug as described above. Thus, the rate of drug formation is solely dependent on the rate of the initial

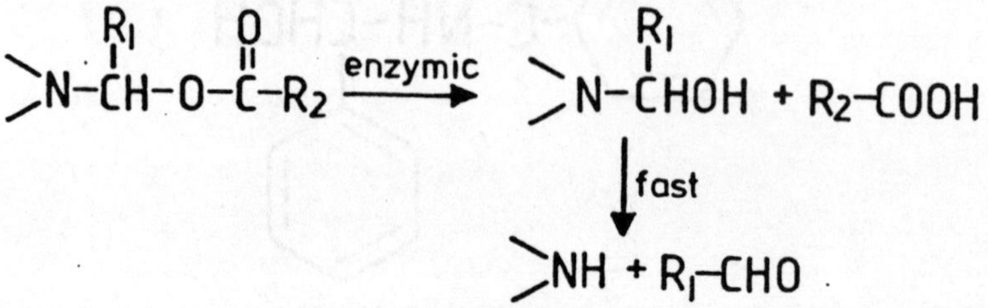

$$\begin{array}{c}\ce{>N-CH(R_1)-O-C(=O)-R_2}\end{array} \xrightarrow{\text{enzymic}} \ce{>N-CH(R_1)OH} + R_2\text{-COOH}$$

$$\downarrow \text{fast}$$

$$\ce{>NH} + R_1\text{-CHO}$$

<u>Scheme 7</u>

ester cleavage, which can be controlled by steric and electronic factors (see e.g. Table 10). It should be added that the rates of enzymatic hydrolysis of N-acyloxyalkyl derivatives of various NH-acidic compounds may also depend on the structure of the nitrogenous compound. Thus, whereas the half-life of hydrolysis of 7-pivaloyloxymethyl-theophylline in 10% human plasma at 37°C is only 3 min that of 1-pivaloyloxymethyl-5-fluorouracil is 39.5 h under the same conditions (H. Bundgaard, unpublished).

The most commonly used acyloxyalkyl derivatives are acyloxymethyl compounds, i.e. derivatives from which formaldehyde is released from an N-hydroxymethyl intermediate. As discussed above the N-acyloxymethylation approach is limited to amide-type compounds possessing a pK_a value of less than about 10.5-11 when the requirement is to be fulfilled that the intermediate N-hydroxymethyl derivative should only have a transistory existence in the overall process of drug release as outlined in Scheme 7. However, by using other aldehydes than formaldehyde, the N-α-alkylol intermediate thus formed would be more unstable than the N-methylol analogue as also discussed above, hence expanding the usefulness of N-acyloxyalkylation as a means of obtaining prodrug forms of also weakly NH-acidic drugs such as amides, carbamates and urea derivatives (pK_a >14) (69). It should be pointed out that although the availability of N-hydroxyalkyl derivatives other than those derived from formaldehyde is very limited this does not restrict a broad utility of N-acyloxyalkyl derivatives as prodrug forms. The reason is that besides being obtainable by esterification of the intermediate N-hydroxyalkyl derivative such derivatives are readily - and most often -

obtained by reacting the NH-acidic drug substance with an α-acyloxyalkyl halide (69). The latter compounds are easily available from the reaction of acid halides with a variety of aldehydes including e.g. acetaldehyde and benzaldehyde besides formaldehyde.

Several papers describing N-acyloxyalkylation as a means of obtaining prodrugs of various NH-acidic compounds have appeared in the last few years. By using this prodrug approach it has thus been possible to enhance the oral absorption of phenytoin (78) and the dermal delivery of theophylline (79), 6-mercaptopurine (80) and 5-fluorouracil (81). The increased dermal absorption observed with the prodrug derivatives is a result of the increased lipophilicity of the prodrugs along with the susceptibility of the derivatives to undergo enzymatic cleavage in the skin. In the case of 6-mercaptopurine some bioreversible S-acylaminomethyl and S-acyloxymethyl have also been prepared (80). The extent to which water-solubility can be enhanced by N-acyloxyalkylation can be illustrated with chlorzoxazone. Its solubility in water is 0.2 mg ml^{-1} while that of N-(N',N'-dimethylglycyloxymethyl)chlorzoxazone hydrochloride is about 200 ml ml^{-1} (82). Similarly, various amino group-containing N-acyloxymethyl derivatives of phenytoin have been prepared and found to possess greatly increased aqueous solubility relative to the parent drug (45, 83). Such compounds as well as the water-soluble disodium N-phosphoryl-oxymethyl-phenytoin have recently been shown to be potentially useful prodrugs of phenytoin possessing improved oral and parenteral delivery characteristics in comparison to the parent drug (45, 83).

Besides being influenced by the hydrophilic or hydrophobic properties of the acyl moiety the water-solubility and lipophilicity of N-acyloxyalkyl derivatives can be affected by the fact that the N-acyloxyalkylation may lead to decreased intermolecular hydrogen bonding in the crystal lattice. This is thus the case for the derivatives of theophylline (79), allopurinol (84, 85) and 5-fluorouracil (86). A more detailed illustration of this phenomenon is given for allopurinol (23). This compound is poorly soluble in water (0.5 mg ml^{-1}) and in various polar or apolar organic solvents. The x-ray interferogram of allopurinol shows a hydrogen bridge between the 1-NH group and 7-N of another molecule, while 2-N is bound to the hydrogen of a 5-NH group (87). The strong crystal lattice energy of allopurinol due to these intermolecular hydrogen bonds which is reflected in the high melting point of the compound (~ 365°C) is certainly responsible for the poor solubility behaviour. By blocking the 1-NH, 2-NH or 5-NH groups by N-acyloxymethylation with the formation of the corresponding acyloxymethyl derivatives (24-27) the intermolecular hydrogen bonding is decreased as reflected in decreased melting points and the water-solubility is increased. From the results given in Table 10 it can be seen that it is even feasible to obtain N-acyloxymethyl derivatives which at the same time are both more lipophilic than allopurinol and possess a higher water-solubility. The following relationship between melting points, partition coefficients (P) and water-solubilities (S, in molar concentration) for allopurinol and various N-acyloxymethyl and N_1-acyl derivatives was established (84):

Table 10. Half-times ($t_{1/2}$) of the conversion of various N-acyloxymethyl derivatives of allopurinol to the parent compound at 37°C, water-solubilities (S) and partition coefficients (P)[a]

Compound	$t_{1/2}$ pH 7.4 buffer	$t_{1/2}$ 80% human plasma (min)	S (mg/ml)	log P[b]
Allopurinol			0.50	- 0.55
1-(Acetoxymethyl)allopurinol	87 h	31	0.58	- 0.35
1-(Butyryloxymethyl)allopurinol	193 h	9	0.35	0.60
1-(Benzoyloxymethyl)allopurinol	237 h	4	0.024	1.50
1-(Nicotinoyloxymethyl)allopurinol	26 h	21	0.093	0.27
1,5-bis(Butyryloxymethyl)allopurinol	25 h	22	0.050	1.82
2,5-bis(Butyryloxymethyl)allopurinol	35 h	32	0.094	1.60
1-(N,N-Dimethylglycyloxymethyl)allopurinol, HCl	72 min	7	> 500	- 0.49[c]
1-(N,N-Diethylglycyloxymethyl)allopurinol, HCl	49 min	10	> 500	0.20[c]
1-(N,N-Dipropylglycyloxymethyl)allopurinol, HCl	50 min	12	> 400	1.27[c]
1-(DL-Phenylalanyloxymethyl)allopurinol, HBr	40 min	9	> 200	0.40[c]
1-(L-Leucyloxymethyl)allopurinol, HBr	17 min	6	> 400	0.19[c]

[a]From Bundgaard and Falch (84, 85). [b]Between octanol and water. [c]Between octanol and borate buffer pH 8.0.

$$\log S = -1.08\ (\pm\ 0.13)\ \log P\ -\ 0.0073\ (\pm\ 0.0020)\ \text{m.p.}$$
$$-\ 0.65\ (\pm\ 0.80) \tag{8}$$
$$n = 18;\ \underline{r} = 0.918$$

The data in Table 10 also demonstrate the great flexibility of the N-acyloxymethylation approach in that it is possible to greatly modify the cleavage rate, aqueous solubility and lipophilicity, and hence the delivery characteristics, by the appropriate selection of the acyl moiety of the prodrugs. The hydrolytic removal of the acyloxymethyl groups within the compounds 24-27 was shown to take place via a two-step reaction as depicted in Scheme 8 for a 1-acyloxymethyl derivative (84, 85). Rate-determining cleavage of the ester grouping results in the formation of the corresponding N-(hydroxymethyl)allopurinol which is decomposed instantaneously into formaldehyde and allopurinol.

Derivatives containing an ionizable amino group in the ester moiety appear to be particularly useful both as parenteral and rectal delivery forms of allopurinol. Such N_1-acyloxymethyl derivatives as HCl or HBr salts are highly soluble in water and show a facile enzymatic conversion in plasma (cf. Table 10). In preliminary experiments (88) it was found that intravenous administration of 1-(N,N-diethylglycyloxymethyl)allopurinol hydrochloride (28) to rabbits afforded essentially the same plasma levels of allopurinol and its major metabolite oxipurinol as those obtained by administra-

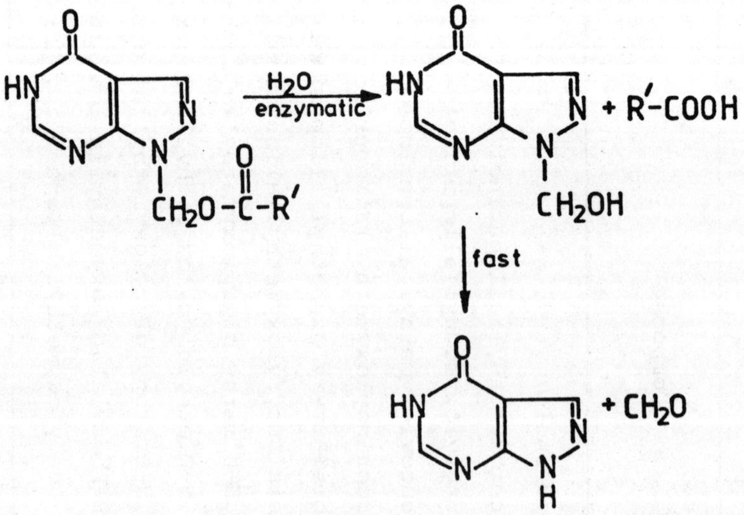

Scheme 8

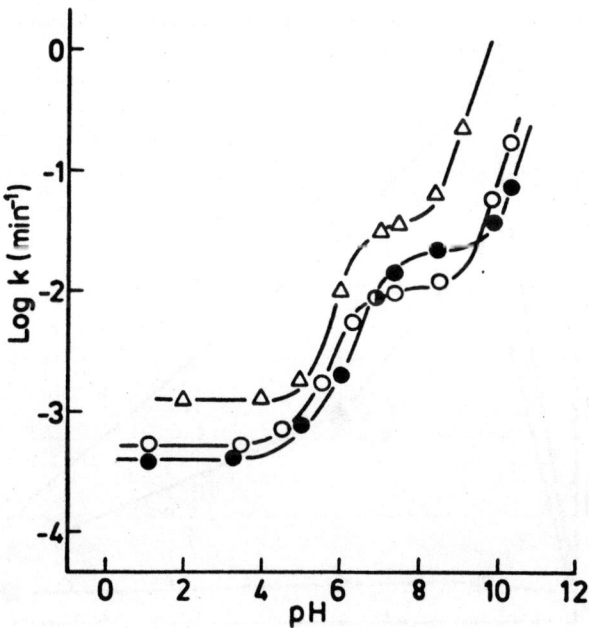

Fig. 5. The pH-rate profiles for the hydrolysis of various N-acyloxymethyl allopurinol derivatives in aqueous solution at 37°C. Key: △, 1-(DL-phenylglycyloxymethyl)allopurinol; ○, 1-(N,N-dimethylglycyloxymethyl)allopurinol; ●, 1-(N,N-diethylglycyloxymethyl)allopurinol (85).

tion of the equivalent amount of an alkaline solution of allopurinol. The compound as well as other amino acid ester derivatives are not sufficiently stable for formulation as ready-to-use solutions (pH-rate profiles for some of the compounds are shown in Fig. 5) but the stability at pH 3-5 was found to be compatible with their use as formulations to be reconstituted as solutions within several hours prior to use (85).

The results of some rectal absorption studies performed in rabbits are shown in Fig. 6 and Table 11. It is readily seen that it is feasible to select prodrug derivatives affording a greatly enhanced rectal delivery of allopurinol. The most promising prodrug candidates are N_1-acyloxymethyl derivatives containing a slightly basic amino function in the ester moiety. These derivatives combine good aqueous solubility properties with an adequate lipophilicity at pH values corresponding to those in the rectum (pH ~ 7.9). Thus, 1-(N,N-diethylglycyloxymethyl)allopurinol (28) possesses a

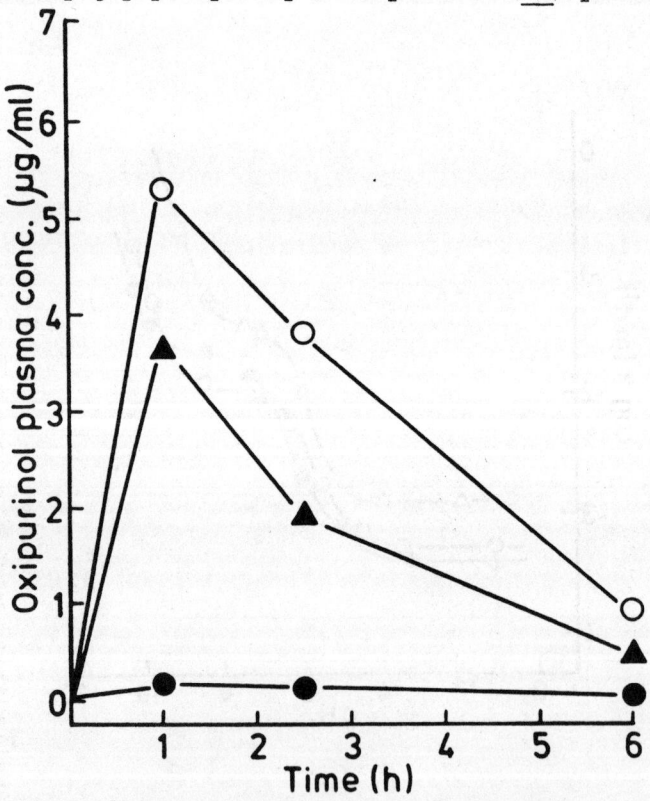

Fig. 6. Mean plasma concentrations of oxipurinol following rectal administration to rabbits of fatty acid suppositories containing allopurinol (●), 1-(butyryloxymethyl)allopurinol, (▲) or 1-(N,N-diethylglycyloxymethyl)allopurinol hydrochloride (o) in equivalent amounts (~ 25 mg allopurinol).

Table 11. Absolute bioavailability of allopurinol and various prodrugs following rectal administration to rabbits (88, 89)[a]

Compound	Bioavailability (%)	No. of rabbits
Allopurinol	< 2	3
1-(Acetyl)allopurinol	23 ± 13	2
1-(Butyryl)allopurinol	29 ± 6	2
1-(Butyryloxymethyl)allopurinol	46 ± 22	2
2,5-Bis(butyryloxymethyl)allopurinol	16 ± 13	2
1-(N,N-Dimethylglycyloxymethyl)allopurinol, HCl	34 ± 7	2
1-(N,N-Diethylglycyloxymethyl)allopurinol, HCl	57 ± 7	13
1-(N,N-Dipropylglycyloxymethyl)allopurinol, HCl	74 ± 41	4
1-(DL-Phenylglycyloxymethyl)allopurincl, HBr	30 ± 16	4
1-(DL-Phenylalanyloxymethyl)allopurinol, HBr	21 ± 10	4
1-(L-Leucyloxymethyl)allopurinol, HBr	20 ± 6	4
1-(N,N-Diethylalanyloxymethyl)allopurinol, HCl	94 ± 24	4

[a] The bioavailability was calculated from the AUC values observed after rectal administration in relation to those after intravenous administration of allopurinol in equivalent doses. All compounds were administered in the form of fatty acid suppositories (Witepsol ®), the amount of prodrug being equivalent to 25 mg of allopurinol.

pK_a value of 7.0, a log P value of 0.20 in the system octanol/ aqueous buffer pH 8.0 and a water-solubility of 4.5 mg ml^{-1} as free base form (85) which is 9 times as high as the solubility of allopurinol. In preliminary experiments in humans this compound (as free base or hydrochloride salt) has been found to be well absorbed and tolerated following rectal administration and it may hence be useful as a rectal allopurinol prodrug delivery form (88).

Similar findings have been obtained for 5-fluorouracil. A number of N-acyloxymethyl derivatives including N_1-, N_3- and N_1,N_3-substituted derivatives were shown to be promising prodrugs for enhancing the oral and rectal delivery characteristijs of the parent drug. The derivatives hydrolyzed to yield 5-fluorouracil in quantitative amounts with rates being markedly accelerated in the presence of plasma or liver enzymes (86). The derivatives have a much reduced melting point relative to that of the parent drug and this enables the preparation of N-acyloxymethyl prodrugs possessing both higher lipid solubility and higher or only slightly reduced aqueous solubilities (Table 12).

N-Acyl derivatives

N-Acylation of amide- or imide-type compounds may be a useful prodrug approach in some particular cases although this approach has received only little attention in the past (9). Its potential usefulness may be illustrated by recent studies performed in this laboratory with 5-fluorouracil (29), the aim of the studies being to improve the oral and rectal absorption characteristics of this anticancer drug by the prodrug approach. It was thought that by bioreversible derivatization it may be possible to protect the drug against first-pass metabolism and to obtain prodrugs possessing a higher lipophilicity than the parent drug. The partition coefficient of 5-fluorouracil between octanol and water is only 0.15 (90) and this low lipophilicity may be a predominant factor for the poor biomembrane permeability of the drug.

Several different derivatives have been prepared and assessed as potentially useful prodrugs for the parent compound. The chemical- and enzyme-mediated conversion of the derivatives to 5-fluorouracil was investigated and determinations of the aqueous solubility and lipophilicity of the compounds were performed. Bioavailability studies of selected derivatives are presently being performed. In the following the main findings of our studies are summarized.

Table 12. Melting points, partition coefficients (P), aqueous solubilities (S) and pK_a values of 5-fluorouracil and various prodrug derivatives (from Buur et al. (86)).

Compound	M.P. °C	log P^a	S^b (mg ml^{-1})	pK_a
5-Fluorouracil (5-FU)	280-284	-0.83	11.1	8.0, 13.0
1-Acetoxymethyl-5-FU	122-123	-0.67	43.1	7.3
1-Propionyloxymethyl-5-FU	100-102	-0.11	33.6	7.3
1-Butyryloxymethyl-5-FU	92-93	0.47	9.6	7.3
1-Pivaloyloxymethyl-5-FU	158-160	0.90	2.3	7.3
1,3-Bis(acetoxymethyl)-5-FU	105-106	-0.37	4.3	—
1,3-Bis(pivaloyloxymethyl)-5-FU	102-104	2.54	0.045	—
3-Acetoxymethyl-5-FU	158-159	-0.42	20.0	8.0

[a] Determined in octanol-acetate buffer of pH 4.0 at 22°C.

[b] Solubility in acetate buffer of pH 4.0 at 22 °C.

Various N_1-acyl (30), N_3-acyl (31) and N_1,N_3-diacyl derivatives (32) were shown to be readily hydrolyzed in aqueous buffer solutions to yield 5-fluorouracil in quantitative amounts (90). Whereas the N_1-acyl derivatives proved very

unstable N_3-acylation was suggested to be a promising means of obtaining prodrug forms of 5-fluorouracil. As seen from the data in Table 13 the rate of N_3-deacylation is markedly accelerated in human plasma. In addition to be rapidly hydrolyzed under conditions similar to those prevailing in vivo, the hydrolysis rate being controllable by the appropriate selection of the acyl group, the N_3-acyl derivatives showed improved physicochemical properties of relevance to bioavailability as compared with 5-fluorouracil. As it appears from Table 13 the derivatives are more lipophilic than 5-fluorouracil and, for som compounds, also more soluble in water. As referred to earlier this apparently anomalous behaviour can be attributed to a decreased intermolecular hydrogen bonding in the crystal lattice achieved by blocking the 3-NH group by the acylation and manifested in a pronounced melting point decrease (cf. Table 13).

In an additional study (91) various N-alkoxycarbonyl derivatives of 5-fluorouracil were examined. While the hydrolytic removal of an N_1-alkoxycarbonyl group proceeded very rapidly in aqueous buffer solutions the N_3-alkoxycarbonyl group proved highly resistant towards chemical hydrolysis. The N_3-alkoxycarbonyl derivatives (33) showed, however, enzyme-mediated cleavage in human plasma and, in particular, rat liver homogenate. Thus, N_3-phenyloxycarbonyl-5-fluorouracil was hydrolyzed to 5-fluorouracil with half-lives of 80 h at pH 7.4 and 37°C, 390 min in 80% human plasma and 20 min in 30% rat liver homogenate (91). It may be questioned whether the conversion of the N_3-alkoxycarbonyl derivatives to the parent drug is sufficiently facile in vivo.

Table 13. Rate data for the hydrolysis of N_3-acyl derivatives of 5-fluorouracil in buffer (pH 7.4) and human plasma (37°C) as well as aqueous solubilities (S), partition coefficients (P) and melting points[a]

Compound	m.p. (°C)	S^b (mg/ml)	log P^c	$t_{\frac{1}{2}}$ (min) Buffer	$t_{\frac{1}{2}}$ (min) 80% plasma
5-Fluorouracil (5-FU)	280-84	11.1	-0.83		
3-Acetyl-5-FU	116-18	42.8	-0.34	43	4.6
3-Propionyl-5-FU	113-14	35.3	0.19	50	20
3-Butyryl-5-FU	132-34	—	0.67	58	28
3-Benzoyl-5-FU	172-74	1.3	0.80	2900	110

[a]From Buur and Bundgaard (90).

[b]In acetate buffer of pH 4.0 (22°C).

[c]Partition coefficients between octanol and acetate buffer of pH 4.0.

33: R-O-C(=O)-N(uracil-5-F)

34: 1-(CONR₁R₂)-5-fluorouracil

Another potential prodrug type of 5-fluorouracil belonging to the N-acyl category is carbamoyl derivatives (34). Methyl-, ethyl-, butyryl-, phenyl- and N,N-dimethylcarbamoyl derivatives were shown to hydrolyze to yield 5-fluorouracil in quantitative amounts, the half-lives of hydrolysis at pH 7.4 and 37°C being 8-11 min for the 1-alkylcarbamoyl derivatives and 5 sec for the 1-phenylcarbamoyl derivative (92). The N,N-dimethylcarbamoyl derivative proved to be highly stable. An interesting observation of concern in prodrug design was that the hydrolysis of the derivatives was markedly inhibited by human plasma. As serum albumin produced the same effect as plasma this deceleration of the hydrolysis rate was attributed to a non-productive binding to or inclusion of the compounds by plasma proteins (92). Not all 1-carbamoyl derivatives of 5-fluorouracil behave, however, in this way. Thus, the half-life of hydrolysis of the compound 34a in rat plasma in vitro was found to be 4 min and about 3 h in buffer solution of pH 7.4 (93). The behaviour of compound 34a in human plasma has not been described.

34a: 1-[CONH(CH₂)₅CO-O-CH(CH₂OCO(CH₂)₈CH₃)₂]-5-fluorouracil

Prodrugs for amines

N-Acyl derivatives

N-Acylation of amines to give amide prodrugs has been used only to a limited extent due to the relative stability of amides in vivo. However, certain activated amides are sufficiently chemically labile and also, certain amides formed with amino acids may be susceptible to undergo enzymatic cleavage in vivo.

Thus, γ-glutamyl derivatives of dopamine, L-Dopa and sulfamethoxazole are readily hydrolyzed by γ-glutamyl transpeptidase in vivo and has been promoted as kidney-specific prodrugs because of their preferential bioactivation in the kidney (94-96). Similarly, various other amides or dipeptides of L-Dopa have been shown to be useful as prodrugs (97). Other enzymatically labile amides include various amino acid derivatives of benzocaine (98). These compounds are highly water-soluble and are cleaved rapidly in the presence of human serum.

Acylation of the pyrazole moiety in allopurinol (23) affords activated amide derivatives which may be useful as prodrugs. A series of N_1-acyl derivatives (35-41) of allopurinol have recently been synthesized and evaluated as potential prodrugs with the purpose of developing preparations suitable for rectal or parenteral administration (99). Besides being easily cleaved to allopurinol in aqueous solutions at physio-

35-41

logical pH (Fig. 7) the derivatives are susceptible to undergo a marked enzyme-catalyzed hydrolysis by human plasma (Table 14). The N-acyl derivatives were found to be more lipophilic than allopurinol but the solubility in water was even greater (for the N-acetyl derivative) or only slightly reduced as compared with allopurinol (Table 14). This behaviour was attributed to a decreased intermolecular hydrogen bonding in the crystal lattice achieved by blocking the 1-NH group by

Table 14. Half-times ($t_{1/2}$) of the conversion of various N-acyl derivatives of allopurinol to the parent compound at 37°C, water-solubilities (S) and partition coefficients (P)[a]

Compound	$t_{1/2}$ (min)		S (mg/ml at 22°C)	log P[b]
	pH 7.4 buffer	80% human plasma		
Allopurinol			0.50	-0.55
1-(Acetyl)allopurinol (35)	26	6	0.75	-0.35
1-(Propionyl)allopurinol (36)	30	4	0.30	0.30
1-(Butyryl)allopurinol (37)	36	2.5	0.11	0.85
1-(Chloroacetyl)allopurinol (38)	~ 3 sec	—	—	—
1-(Benzoyl)allopurinol (39)	20	4	0.014	1.20
1-(N,N-Dimethylglycyl)-allopurinol, HCl (40)	1.5	—	> 100	—
1-(4-N,N-dimethylaminobutyryl)-allopurinol, HCl (41)	< 3 sec	—	> 100	—

[a] From Bundgaard and Falch (99).
[b] Partition coefficients between octanol and water at 22°C

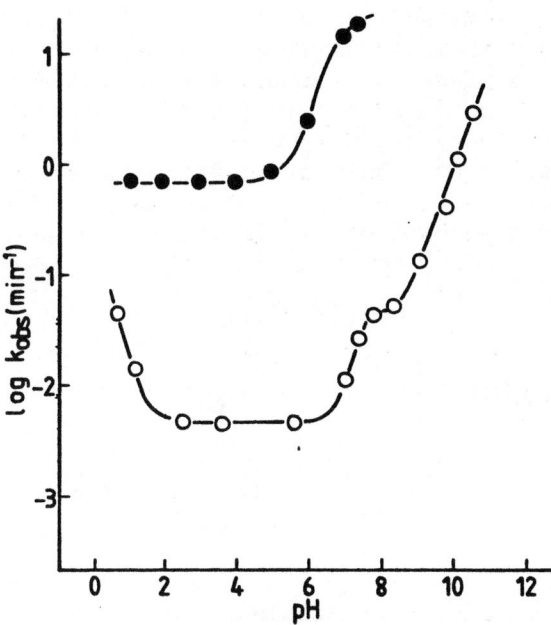

Fig. 7. The pH-rate profiles for the hydrolysis of 1-acetyl-allopurinol (o) and 1-chloroacetylallopurinol (●) in aqueous solution at 37°C (99).

acylation as supported by decreased melting points. It was suggested that N-acylation may be a promising means of obtaining prodrug forms of allopurinol with the aim of enhancing the rectal absorption of the drug (99). Allopurinol is only very slightly absorbed (< 5%) upon rectal administration (100,101) and this is most probably due to its lipophilicity and poor aqueous solubility. Preliminary experiments in rabbits showed that rectal administration of the N_1-acetyl and N_1-butyryl derivatives in the form of fatty acid suppositories resulted in a bioavailability of allopurinol of 20-30% whereas administration of allopurinol itself led to a bioavailability of less than 2% (Table 11). The N_1-acyl derivatives (40) and (41) are very soluble (> 10% w/v) in water as hydrochloride salts but due to a very limited solution stability they appear to be less suitable as parenteral prodrug delivery forms. As referred to earlier more useful allopurinol prodrugs for parenteral administration are N-acyloxymethyl derivatives in which the acyl moiety contains an ionizable amino function (85).

Various carbamate derivatives have been assessed as prodrugs for normeperidine, amphetamine, ephedrine and phenethylamine but with limited success (102-104). Unfortunately, kinetic data on their conversion in aqueous solution and in the presence of plasma or enzymes are not available. As reported by Digenis and Swintosky (1) carbamate esters of phenol are cleaved very rapidly by plasma enzymes (Scheme 9) and although these authors only classified such structures as possible prodrugs for phenols they can equally well be considered as prodrug candidates for amines. In such a case the

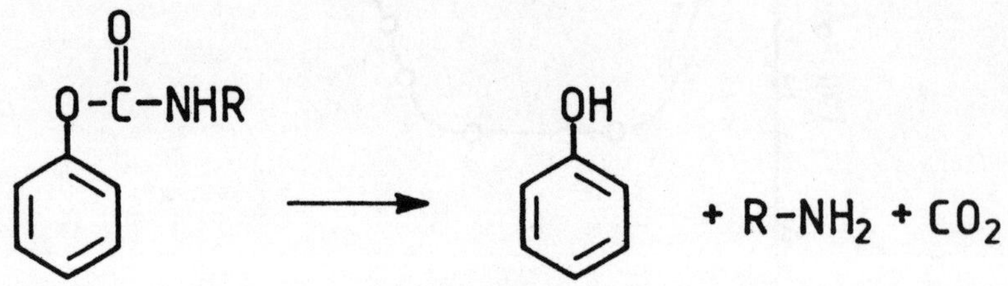

PhO-C(=O)-NHR → PhOH + R-NH$_2$ + CO$_2$

Scheme 9

phenol would be the transport group. Studies along this line are certainly warranted since there is a paucity of broadly applicable derivatives for the amino group. It is of interest that Sasaki et al. (105-107) recently showed that benzyloxycarbonyl derivatives of mitomycin C are susceptible to undergo cleavage by plasma and hepatic enzymes and more so than the corresponding amide derivatives.

N-Mannich bases

Besides being considered as a possible approach of derivatizing amide-type compounds N-Mannich base formation can also be thought of as a means of forming prodrugs of primary and secondary amines in which case the amide-type component would act as a transport group. As can be seen from Table 15, N-Mannich base formation lowers the pK_a values of the conjugate acids of amines by up to about 3 units. Therefore, a potentially useful purpose for transforming amino compounds into N-Mannich base transport forms would be to increase the lipophilicity of the parent amines at physiological pH values by depressing their protonation, resulting in enhanced biomembrane-passage properties. This expectation of increased lipophilicity has been confirmed for e.g. the N-Mannich base derived from benzamide and phenylpropanolamine. The partition coefficient of the Mannich base between octanol and phosphate

Table 15. Effect of N-Mannich base formation of amines on pK_a for the corresponding protonated species[a]

Amine	pK_a value of amine	pK_a value of N-benzamidomethylated amine
Piperidine	11.1	7.8
Methylamine	10.7	7.5
Dimethylamine	10.7	7.6
Ethylamine	10.7	7.5
Diethylamine	10.9	7.7
Isobutylamine	10.7	7.5
Cyclohexylamine	10.7	7.6
Benzylamine	9.3	6.4
Morpholine	8.3	5.6
(−)-Ephedrine	9.7	6.3
Phenylpropanolamine	9.4	6.2
Phenethylamine	9.8	7.1

[a]From Bundgaard and Johansen (56, 57, 64).

buffer pH 7.4 was found to be almost 100-times greater than that of the parent amine (64). By the benzamidomethylation the pK_a of phenylpropanolamine is decreased from 9.4 to 6.15 and the decreased extent of ionization at pH 7.4 is obviously the major contributing factor to the increased lipophilicity of the N-Mannich base derivative.

However, the selection of biologically acceptable amide-type transport groups affording an appropriate cleavage rate of a Mannich base of a given amine at pH 7.4 is restricted. In a search for generally useful candidates it was observed (60) that N-Mannich bases of salicylamide and different aliphatic amines (Scheme 10) including amino acids showed an unexpectedly high cleavage rate at neutral pH (cf. Table 2),

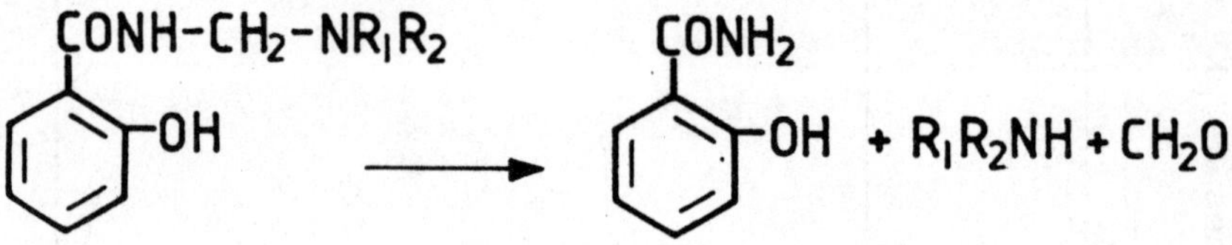

Scheme 10

thus suggesting the utility of salicylamide. The salicylamide Mannich bases possess lower pK_a values than the corresponding benzamide derivatives and the difference in reactivity may at least in part be a reflection of this difference in basicity. Interestingly, the hydrolysis of the salicylamide Mannich bases showed bell-shaped pH-rate profiles with maximum rates at pH around 7; an example is shown in Fig. 8.

For aromatic amines, more acidic amide-type transport groups such as succinimide or hydantoins have been suggested in order to ensure a rapid conversion at physiological pH (61), cf. Table 2. A potential objective for transient derivatizing aromatic amino groups in drugs may be to obtain protection against first-pass metabolism by N-acetylation (61).

Other prodrug derivatives

N-Acyloxyalkyl derivatives. N-Acyloxyalkylation of simple, acyclic primary and secondary amines does not appear to be useful because of the extreme lability of such derivatives in

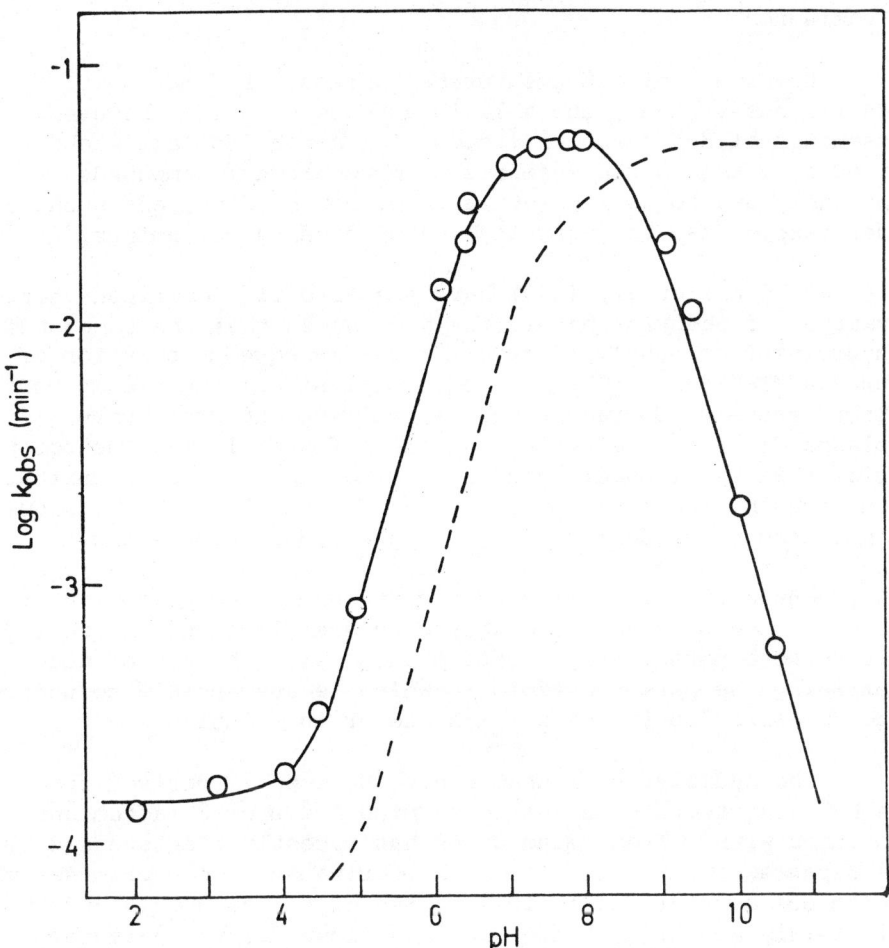

Fig. 8. The pH-rate profiles for the decomposition of N-(piperidinomethyl)salicylamide (—) and N-(piperidinomethyl)benzamide (---) in aqueous solution at 37°C (60).

aqueous solution but for tertiary amines chemically stable compounds (quaternary ammonium salts) are obtained. Due to a high susceptibility to undergo enzymatic hydrolysis (Scheme 11) these compounds are useful as prodrugs for tertiary or N-heterocyclic amines (8, 108).

$$\geq N^+ - CHR_1 - OOC-R, X^- \xrightarrow{\text{enzymic}} \geq N^+ - CHR_1 - OH, X^- + RCOOH$$
$$\downarrow \text{fast}$$
$$\geq N, HX + R_1CHO$$

Scheme 11

Enaminones

Enamines, or α,β-unsaturated amines, are like most Schiff bases highly unstable in aqueous solution. However, enamines of β-dicarbonyl compounds (enaminones) are stabilized relative to the enamines of monocarbonyl compounds, probably due to intramolecular hydrogen bonding, and such derivatives may be generally useful prodrugs of amines.

Caldwell et al. (109) have prepared five enaminone derivatives of phenylpropanolamine and showed that the compounds hydrolyzed at vastly different rates in aqueous solution of pH 7.4 (Table 16). The rate of hydrolysis of these compounds increased with decreased pH. As could be expected human plasma did not accelerate the rates of hydrolysis. The potential utility of enaminones as prodrugs for amines is further stressed by the study by Dixon and Greenhill (110) who showed that enaminones derived from various 1,3-diketones and a keto-ester had a wide range of hydrolysis rates. More recently, Jensen et al. (111) prepared an enaminone derivative of cycloserine by condensing this with acetylacetone and showed it to be a potentially useful prodrug with the aim of stabilizing the parent antibiotic which is susceptible to undergo dimerization in the solid state or in solution.

The hydrolysis of enaminones (Scheme 12) derived from ethyl acetoacetate and various amino acids or β-lactam antibiotics with a free amino group has recently been studied by a Japanese group (112, 113). The derivatives show promise as prodrugs as their half-lives of hydrolysis at pH 7.4 and 25°C is fairly short (4-98 min). As was shown for the β-lactam

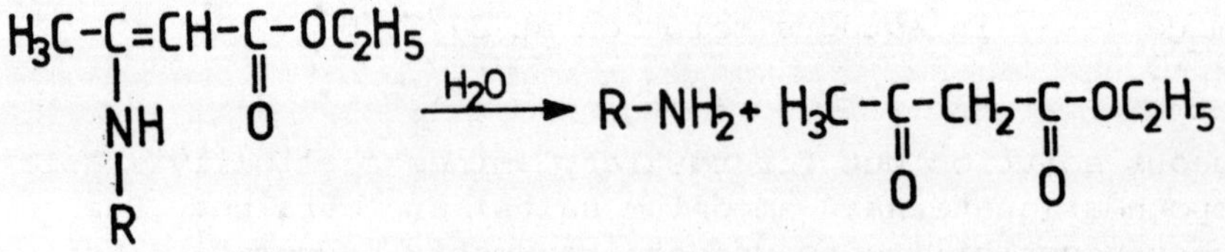

$$H_3C-\underset{\underset{R}{\overset{|}{N}H}}{\overset{|}{C}}=CH-\overset{\overset{O}{\|}}{C}-OC_2H_5 \xrightarrow{H_2O} R-NH_2 + H_3C-\overset{\overset{O}{\|}}{C}-CH_2-\overset{\overset{O}{\|}}{C}-OC_2H_5$$

Scheme 12

antibiotics the enaminone derivatives were much more lipophilic at pH 7.4 than the corresponding parent drugs (112). The use of ethyl acetoacetate as the pro-moiety of enaminone prodrugs may possibly also be attractive due to its approval as a food additive and its wide use as a flavoring agent.

Table 16. Half-lives of hydrolysis of various enaminones of phenylpropanolamine at 37°C[a]

Structure: Phenyl–CH(OH)–CH(NH-R)–CH$_3$

R	$t_{1/2}$ (min)	
	pH 7.4 buffer	2% human plasma (pH 7.4)
$-\underset{CH_3}{C} = CH - CON(C_2H_5)_2$	3.4	4.0
$-\underset{CH_3}{C} = CH - COOC(CH_3)_3$	10.3	9.8
$-\underset{CH_3}{C} = CH - COOC_2H_5$	40	36
$-CH = C(COOC_2H_5)_2$	stable	stable
$-\underset{CH_2-COOC_2H_5}{C} = CH - COOC_2H_5$	> 160	160

[a]From Caldwell et al. (109).

Enaminones certainly warrant greater attention in the future as a potentially useful bioreversible derivative type for drugs containing a free amino group. In order to be able to apply this promising prodrug approach broadly and rationally, more information is needed on the kinetics and mechanism of enaminone hydrolysis as well as on the relationship between chemical reactivity and structure, involving both the 1,3-dione component and the amino compound

Other potentially useful bioreversible derivatives of the amino group are described elsewhere (9).

Prodrugs for compounds containing carbonyl groups

Only few bioreversible derivatives have been explored of molecules containing an aldehydic or ketonic functional group but in view of the fairly large number of drugs (e.g. various steroids) containing a carbonyl group this area of prodrug chemistry is certain to attract much interest in the future. Derivatives which can be considered as prodrug candidates include Schiff bases, oximes, ketals, acetals, oxazolidines, thiazolidines and enol esters. Examples of such derivatives are given elsewhere (9) and only oxazolidines and enol esters are briefly treated here.

Oxazolidines

Oxazolidines are cyclic condensation products of β-aminoalcohols and aldehydes or ketones and they undergo a facile and complete hydrolysis in aqueous solution (Scheme 13). They have recently been proposed (114-116) as potentially useful prodrug candidates for aldehydes or ketones as well as for compounds containing a β-aminoalcohol function (e.g. β-blockers). A study (116) of the hydrolysis kinetics of several oxazolidines derived from cyclohexanone (a model of a carbonyl-containing drug) and various β-aminoalcohols has provided basic information on the structural factors within the β-aminoalcohol moiety which may influence the stability and reactivity of oxazolidines. It appears from this study that by appropriate selection of the β-aminocarbonyl moiety it is feasible to obtain oxazolidine prodrugs of carbonyl compounds with greatly varying rates of hydrolysis at physiological conditions of pH and temperature (Table 17). In addition, it is possible to confer varying degrees of lipophilicity or hydrophylicity on the oxazolidines by varying the β-aminoalcohol component. In considering oxazolidines as prodrug candidates for carbonyl-containing substances, their weakly basic character (pK_a 5-7) (115) may be advantageous in that the transformation of such substances into oxazolidines introduces a readily ionizable moiety, which may allow the preparation of derivatives with increased aqueous solubilities at acidic pH values. For example, a potentially useful purpose of transforming a carbonyl-containing drug substance into a bioreversible oxazolidine derivative could be to enhance its dissolution behaviour in an effort to improve the oral bioavailability. This aspect is currently being tested with some slightly water-soluble steroids in this laboratory.

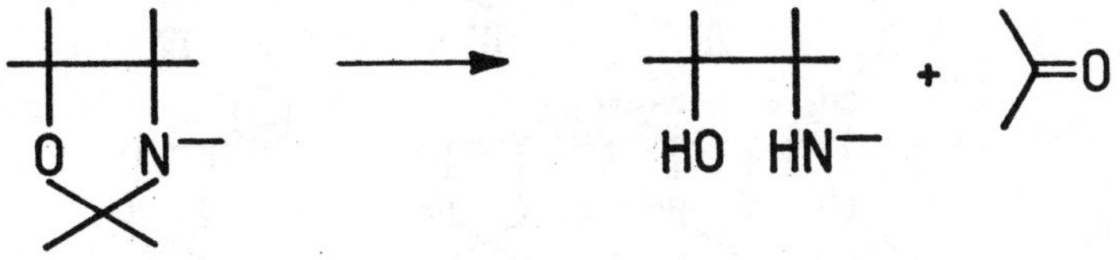

Scheme 13

A drawback of oxazolidines as prodrugs is their poor stability in aqueous solution, raising formulation-stability problems, at least for solution products. For most oxazolidines, however, the rates of decomposition are greatest at neutral and basic pH and increased stability is attained at acidic non-physiological pH values (114-116). A really effective solution of the in vitro stability problem would be further derivatization of the oxazolidines to produce compounds whose initial cleavage to oxazolidine relies on enzymatic catalysis. Studies (unpublished) in this laboratory have shown that N-acetylated or N-benzoylated oxazolidines derived from primary aminoalcohols are in fact highly stable in aqueous solution but unfortunately, they are also resistant to undergoing hydrolysis by plasma enzymes. Attempts to find more promising kinds of N-acylation or other means of derivatization of the oxazolidine nitrogen function are currently being made.

Enol esters

Several drugs contain enolizable carbonyl groups as their most prominent functional group (such as some steroids, anticoagulants and phenylbutazone). Although the keto-enol equilibrium usually lies far in favour of the keto form, the enol form can under proper conditions be trapped by alkylation or acylation of the hydroxyl (enol) group. Such enol ethers and esters may undergo ready hydrolysis with liberation of the free enol which then reverts to the keto form almost instantaneously. Using acetophenone (43) as a model for an enolizable carbonyl-containing drug substance Patel and Repta (117, 118) have demonstrated that enol esters may be quite useful

Table 17. Half-lives of overall hydrolysis of various oxazolidines of cyclohexanone in acidic and neutral aqueous solution at 37°C (116)

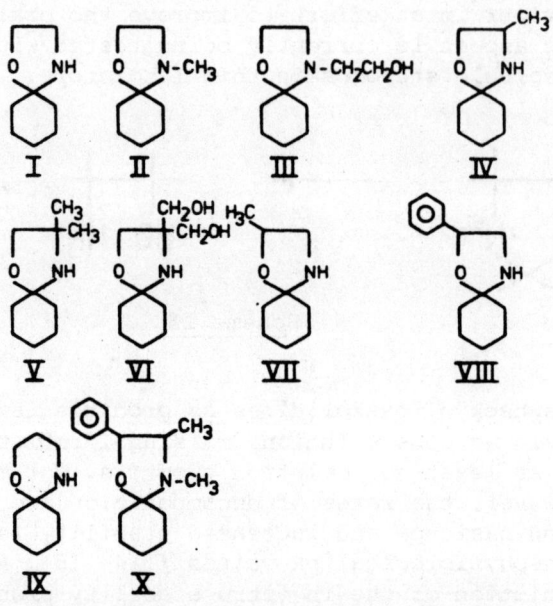

Oxazolidine	$t_{1/2}$ (min)	
	pH 2.0	pH 7.0
I	3.8	0.07
II	3.1	0.2
III	5.8	0.3
IV	14.4	0.4
V	12.6	42
VI	77.9	158
VII	6.3	0.2
VIII	5.0	0.2

as prodrugs of such agents. The stability of several enol esters of acetophenone (α-acyloxystyrenes) (42) were evaluated in aqueous buffer solutions and in human and rat plasma and liver homogenates. The derivatives behaved much as saturated esters and were relatively stable in aqueous solution with maximum stability at pH 3-5, but most derivatives hydrolyzed rapidly and completely to yield the parent acetophenone with the aid of enzymatic catalysis in plasma or liver homogenate. Some rate data are listed in Table 18. Steric and electronic effects within the acyl group are seen to have a substantial influence upon both the aqueous and enzymatic rates of hydrolysis. It is evident that by appropriate selection of the acyl group it is possible to obtain enol ester prodrugs with varying rates of hydrolysis as well as with varying lipophilicity and aqueous solubility.

Table 18. Half-lives of hydrolysis of various α-acyloxystyrenes (42) at 37°C (118)

R in 42	$t_{1/2}$ (min)		
	5% human plasma	1% rat plasma	Human liver supernatant
$-CH_3$	26	1.9	6.3
$-CH_2CH_3$	13	0.5	2.8
$-CH_2CH_2CH_3$	12	0.7	1.4
$-CH(CH_3)_2$	110	3.1	4.8
$-C(CH_3)_3$	–	2.0	11.1
$-C_6H_5$	55	1.1	2.0
$-CH_2N(CH_3)_2$	21	2.6	6.6

Prodrugs for other chemical entities

Various ring-opened derivatives of cyclic drugs have been proposed as potentially useful prodrugs with either increased water or lipid solubility (Table 19). Conversely, when a drug substance contains two or more different derivatizable functional groups or two or more of the same functional group, the formation of cyclic derivatives through bridging these groups may be an interesting and useful chemical approach to obtain prodrug forms. Some examples are shown in Table 19. A review of the properties of such derivatives is given elsewhere (9) (see also below).

The double prodrug concept

During the last decennium the prodrug approach has been generally appreciated as a most useful means to improve the delivery of various drugs and to solve various pharmaceutical formulation problems such as stability and solubility. Several drugs are now being marketed in the form of a prodrug. The application of the approach is, however, not without problems. An ideal prodrug shall satisfy several criteria (ready conversion to the parent drug, adequate in vitro stability, be nontoxic etc.) at the same time but in most cases it may be difficult to obtain a prodrug with ideal properties in all respects. For example, a prodrug designed to promote site-specific delivery through a target-specific cleavage mechanism (e.g. due to an atypical enzyme activity) may not be successful if it is not able to reach the target tissue. Both conditions should be fulfilled at the same time. Consider also a prodrug where the necessary conversion to the parent drug in vivo is triggered by the buffered and relatively constant value of the physiological pH of 7.4. A serious drawback of such prodrugs requiring chemical (non-enzymatic) release of the active drug is the inherent lability of the derivatives, raising some stability-formulation problems at least in cases of solution preparations.

A promising means of optimizing the properties of prodrugs and to overcome various drawbacks of these may involve cascade latentiation or the double prodrug concept (pro-prodrugs). Thus, it should be possible to overcome the stability problem of the prodrug considered above by derivatizing it in such a manner that an enzymatic release mechanism is required prior to the spontaneous release of the parent drug. The potential utility of such a more sophisticated approach involving prodrugs of prodrugs is discussed in the following, using a number of illustrative examples.

Table 19. Prodrug derivatives of cyclic drugs and cyclic prodrugs of acyclic parent compounds

Parent compound	Prodrug derivative	Reference
Barbituric acids	Malonuric acid esters	119, 120
Hydantoins	Hydantoic acid esters	121
Trimethadione	Isobutyric acid derivative	122
Succinimides	Succinamic acid esters	123
Glutarimides	Glutaramic acid esters	123
γ-Lactones	4-Hydroxybutyric acid esters	124
Cyclic quaternary ammonium compounds	Tertiary N-haloalkylamines	125
Benzodiazepines	2-Aminobenzophenone derivatives	126, 127
Hydroxy acids	Lactones	128, 129
4-Aminobutyric acid	2-Pyrrolidinone	130
β-Aminoalcohols	Oxazolidines	114 - 116
β-Mercapto alcohols	Thiazolidines	131
α-Aminoamides	4-Imidazolidinones	132
Catechols	Methylenedioxy derivatives	133
Acetylsalicylic acid	1,3-Benzodioxin-4-one derivatives	134, 135

Acyclovir

Acyclovir (44) is a clinically useful antiherpetic agent which exhibits great selectivity in its antiviral action through conversion to the active phosporylated species by virtue of virus-specific thymidine kinase (136,137). Acyclovir is thus a prodrug exhibiting a site-specific delivery of the active drug. It suffers, however, from poor oral bioavailability, only 10-20% of an oral dose being absorbed in humans (138-140). This can most likely be ascribed to the poor water-solubility and lipophilicity of the compound. The 6-deoxy-6-amino congener (45) of acyclovir has been studied as a prodrug in an attempt to improve the oral bioavailability (141). It is deaminated to acyclovir by adenosine deaminase (142) but oral dosing of dogs and rats with the prodrug resulted in only modest increases in acyclovir plasma levels relative to those achieved with acyclovir itself (141). A far better pro-prodrug may be 6-deoxyacyclovir (46) recently developed by Krenitsky et al. (143). This compound is 18 times more water-soluble than acyclovir and is rapidly oxidized in vivo by xanthine oxidase to 44. Studies in rats and in human volunteers showed that 6-deoxyacyclovir is readily absorbed after oral administration (5-6 times greater bioavailability relative to acyclovir) (143-145). The compound is also susceptible to undergo oxidation by aldehyde oxidase to give the inactive 8-hydroxy-6-deoxyacyclovir but this non-activating oxidation apparently plays only a minor role in comparison to the activating oxidation by xanthine oxidase (143).

Because of its far from optimal physicochemical properties acyclovir also suffers from problems concerning ocular and dermal delivery. Highly water-soluble prodrugs such as amino acid esters as recently described by Colla et al. (146) may possibly be useful for the development of e.g. an eye-drop preparation.

Terbutaline

An interesting example of the double prodrug concept is provided in the work by Olsson et al. (147, 148) on terbutaline (47). In order to achieve increased absorption, reduced first-pass metabolism and prolonged duration of action a p-pivaloyloxybenzoate double ester prodrug (48) was made. Since the pivaloyl ester group is the most susceptible to undergo enzymatic hydrolysis it was expected that the prodrug would undergo first-pass hydrolysis preferentially at the p-pivaloyloxy bond followed by conjugation reactions with sulfuric and glucuronic acid at the resulting p-hydroxybenzoyl moiety (Scheme 14). In this way the active resorcinol moiety in terbutaline would be protected during first-pass and free terbutaline may be generated from hydrolysis of the conjugated or free p-hydroxybenzoate during and after the distribution phase. Experimental support for the cascade ester to function in this way was obtained and prolonged terbutaline plasma profiles were observed in dogs with this prodrug (148).

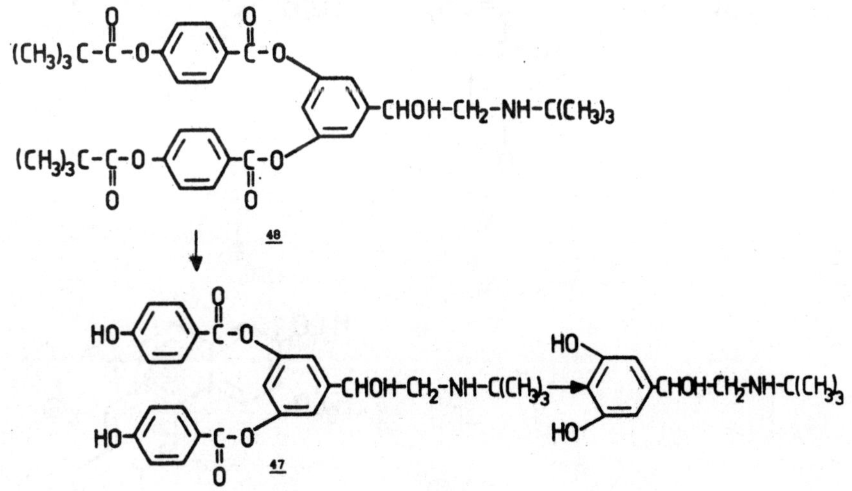

Scheme 14

Coralyne

An excellent example of the solution of delivery and formulation stability problems by using the pro-prodrug concept concerns coralyne. Repta and Patel (149) developed enol esters of 6'-acetylpapaverine as potential prodrug forms of the quaternary antitumor agent coralyne with the aim of delivering this agent to the brain. 6'-Acetylpapaverin (49) itself was previously (150) developed as a lipophilic unionized prodrug of coralyne (50) as it readily cyclizes ($t_{\frac{1}{2}} \sim$ 1 min) to coralyne at pH 7.4 and 37°C. By conversion of 6'-acetylpapaverin to an enol ester (51) cyclization is prevented. The alkyl esters prepared (51) were found to exhibit adequate stability in aqueous solutions (from a pharmaceutical standpoint) while being easily hydrolyzed in vivo to coralyne via the intermediate 6'-acetylpapaverin as a result of enzymatic catalysis by unspecific esterases (149). While the 6'-acetylpapaverin prodrug (49) was found to afford an enhanced and sustained delivery of the parent quaternary species coralyne to the brain enol esters of 6'-acetylpapaverin (51) function as pharmaceutically stable prodrug forms (151).

Pilocarpine

Although pilocarpine (52) is widely used as a topical miotic for controlling the elevated intraocular pressure associated with glaucoma the drug presents several delivery problems. Its ocular bioavailability is very low, which can be ascribed in part to resistance to corneal penetration and hence to its low lipophilicity (152-154). Besides, pilocarpine has a short duration of action, thus requiring very frequent administration. Such administration of massive amounts of the compound often results in poor patient compliance and furthermore is associated with transient peaks of high drug concentration in the eye which in turn results in undesirable side-effects such as myopia and miosis. These shortcomings of pilocarpine may probably be overcome by the prodrug approach. To be successful a pilocarpine prodrug should exhibit a high lipophilicity in order to enable an efficient penetration through the corneal membrane, should be converted to the active parent drug once the corneal barrier has been passed and finally should lead to a controlled release and hence prolonged duration of action of pilocarpine.

Pilocarpic acid esters may be promising prodrug candidates with these desirable attributes (155). A series of alkyl and aralkyl esters of pilocarpic acid (53) has been prepared and shown to function as prodrugs of pilocarpine both in vitro and in vivo (155, 156). In aqueous solution the esters undergo a quantitative and apparent specific base-catalyzed lactonization to pilocarpine (Scheme 15). As appears from the rate data obtained (Table 20) the various esters differ greatly in their rates of cyclization. Except

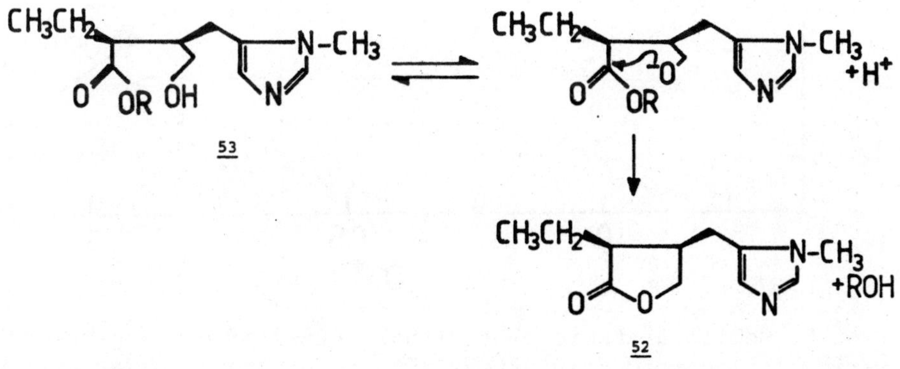

Scheme 15

for the sterically hindered 2-methylbenzyl and α-methylbenzyl esters the variation of the rates of lactonization of these ester derivatives could be fully accounted for in terms of polar effects exhibited by the alcohol portions of the esters (155, 156). The following correlation was found between the half-time (in min) of pilocarpine formation from these esters at pH 7.4 and 37°C and the Taft polar substituent parameter σ*, the latter referring to R in RCH_2OH for the alcohols (Fig. 9):

$$\log t_{\frac{1}{2}} = -1.44 \, \sigma^* + 2.73 \qquad (n = 8; \, \underline{r} = 0.998) \qquad (9)$$

It is readily evident that by appropriate variation of the alcohol portion of the esters there are ample possibilities to vary and predict the rate of ring closure and hence to

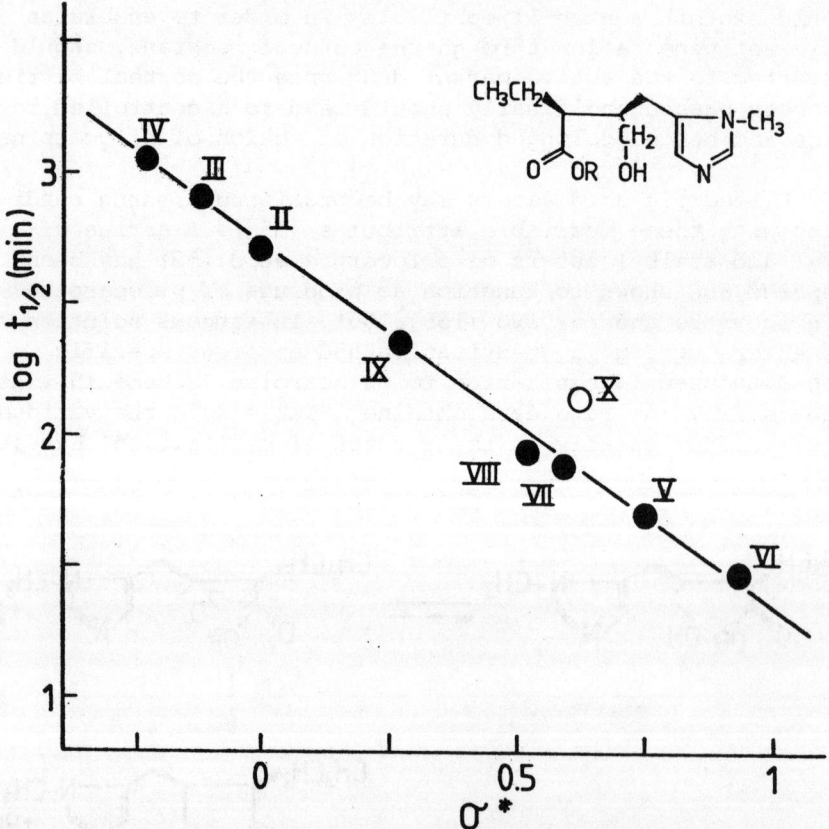

Fig. 9. Semilogarithmic plot of half-times of conversion of various pilocarpic acid esters (53) to pilocarpine (at pH 7.40 and 37°C) against the Taft polar substituent parameter σ*. The latter refers to R in RCH_2OH for the alcohol moieties in the esters. The numbers refer to the compounds in Table 20.

Table 20. Rate data for the conversion of pilocarpic acid esters to pilocarpine in aqueous solution (37°C) and partition coefficients for the compounds (155, 156)

Compound	k_{OE}^{a} (M^{-1} min^{-1})	$t_{1/2}^{b}$ (min)	log P^{c}
Pilocarpine			-0.15
Pilocarpic acid esters (53), R:			
Ethyl (II)	2.25×10^{3}	510	0.58
Butyl (III)	1.40×10^{3}	820	1.58
Hexyl (IV)	1.04×10^{3}	1105	2.56
Benzyl (V)	2.30×10^{4}	50	1.82
4-Chlorobenzyl (VI)	3.83×10^{4}	30	2.54
4-Methylbenzyl (VII)	1.49×10^{4}	77	2.31
4-tert. Butylbenzyl (VIII)	1.32×10^{4}	87	3.52
Phenethyl (IX)	5.07×10^{3}	227	2.16
2-Methylbenzyl (X)	8.28×10^{3}	139	2.27
α-Methylbenzyl (XI)	2.42×10^{3}	475	2.08

[a] Apparent specific base catalytic rate constant. [b] Half-lives of lactonization at pH 7.40. [c] Partition coefficients between octanol and 0.05 M phosphate buffer solution of pH 7.40.

control and modify the rate of pilocarpine generation. Further studies showed that even in the presence of 75% human plasma or rabbit eye tissue homogenates, the cyclization reactions predominated entirely over hydrolysis of the pilocarpic acid esters to pilocarpic acid which does not cyclize to pilocarpine at physiological pH. The lactonization rates observed in these media were identical to those in pure buffer solutions.

The pilocarpic acid esters were found to be much more lipophilic than the parent pilocarpine (Table 20). Appropriate selection of the alcohol portion of the pilocarpic acid esters enables one to confer almost any desired degree of lipophilicity on the prodrugs.

Studies in rabbits have confirmed that several of the pilocarpic acid esters give rise to improved ocular bioavailability of the parent drug and furthermore, result in a more prolonged duration of action of pilocarpine (Fig. 10).

The main drawback of these pilocarpic acid esters is their limited solution stability, making it difficult to prepare ready-to-use solutions with a not too low pH and possessing an acceptable shelf-life (156). This problem can, however, be totally overcome by blocking the free hydroxy group in the esters by esterification. The double esters (54) thus obtained are highly stable in aqueous solution even at pH 6-7 (shelf-lives exceeding 5 years at 25°C) and most significantly, are subject to facile enzymatic hydrolysis at the O-acyl bond (155, 156). It has thus been demonstrated that in the presence of human plasma or rabbit eye tissue homogenates pilocarpine is formed from these derivatives in quantitative amounts through a sequential process involving enzymatic hydrolysis of the O-acyl bond followed by the spontaneous lactonization of the intermediate pilocarpic acid ester (Scheme 16) (Fig.11). Besides solving the stability problem of the pilocarpic acid esters the cascade latentiated derivatives O-acyl pilocarpic acid esters (54) were found to possess even better ocular delivery characteristics (enhanced absorption and longer lasting pilocarpine activity) than the mono-esters (Fig. 12) (156). Furthermore, the O-acylation step gives further possibilities of varying the physicochemical properties of the prodrugs. Some properties of the derivatives are given in Table 21. It should finally be added that although the prodrugs are very lipophilic at pH 7-7.4 the basic character of the imidazole moiety in the compounds ($pK_a \sim 7.0$) allows the preparation of sufficiently water-soluble salts.

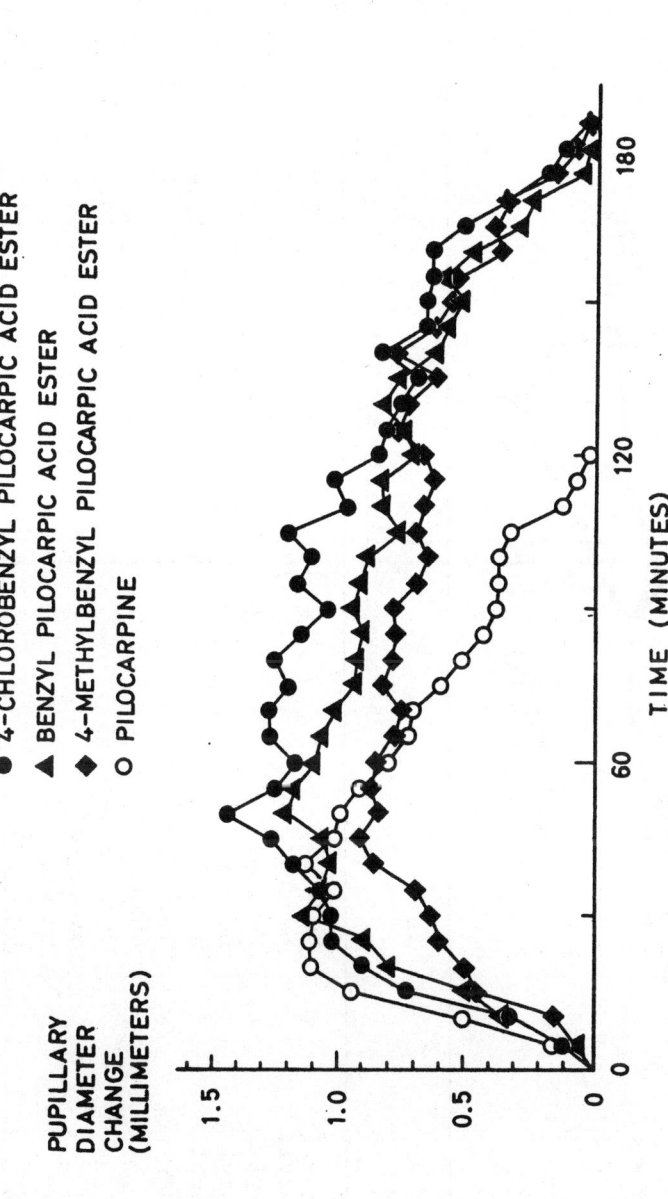

Fig. 10. Plots of the average observed changes in pupillary diameters (ΔPD, in mm) as a function of time following the instillation of 25 μℓ of isotonic aqueous solutions (pH 4.75) in equimolar concentrations (0.5% pilocarpine nitrate equivalent) of the compounds indicated. Four rabbits were used in the crossover study (155, 156).

Table 21. Rate data for the hydrolysis of O-acyl derivatives of pilocarpic acid esters (53) to the monoesters (53) at 37°C and partition coefficients for the compounds[a]

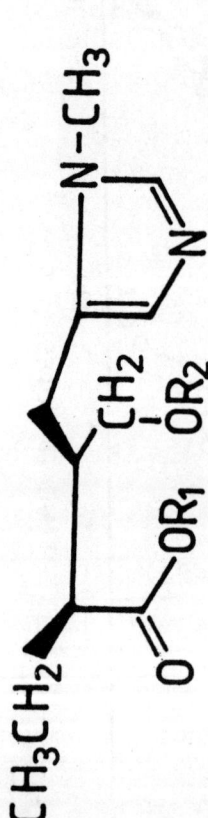

R_1	R_2	$t_{1/2}$ in 75% human plasma (min)	k_{OH}[b] (M^{-1} min^{-1})	log P[c]
Benzyl	benzoyl	12	3.8	4.22
4-Chlorobenzyl	benzoyl	17	3.4	4.75
2-Phenylethyl	benzoyl	15	3.8	4.60
4-Methylbenzyl	benzoyl	16	4.0	4.70
4-Methylbenzyl	acetyl	24	12.6	3.16
3-Methylbenzyl	butyryl	5	3.5	4.09
Benzyl	phenylacetyl	4	21.7	3.85
Benzyl	3-chlorobenzoyl	25	14.6	4.93
Benzyl	nicotinoyl	6	44.4	2.90
Benzyl	butyryl	3	3.5	3.63
Benzyl	hexanoyl	4	3.3	4.60

[a] From Bundgaard et al. (155,156). [b] Hydroxide ion catalytic rate constants for the hydrolysis.
[c] Partition coefficients between octanol and 0.05 M phosphate buffer solution of pH 7.40.

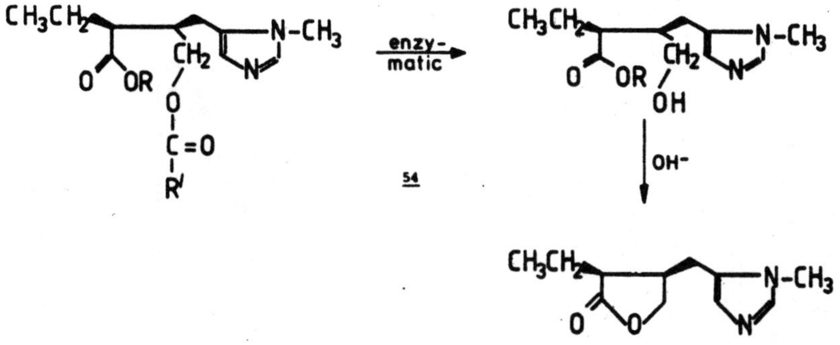

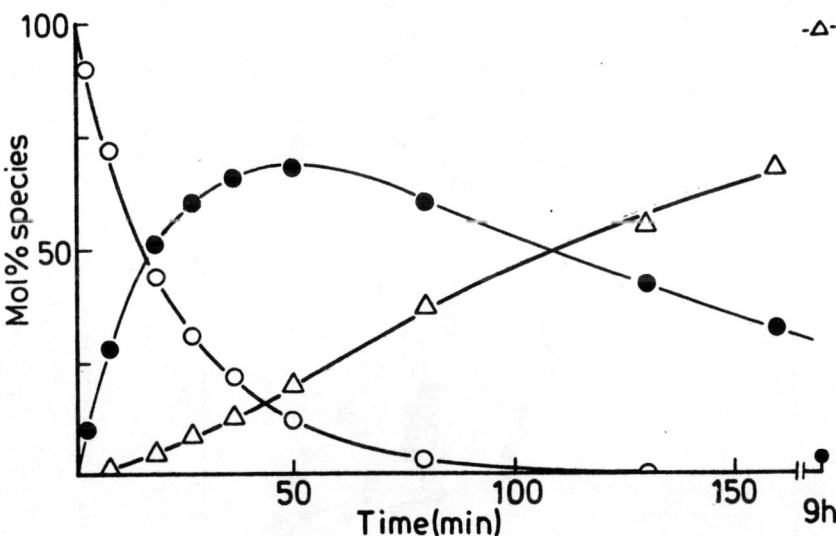

Scheme 16

Fig. 11. Time-courses for O-benzoyl pilocarpic acid 4-methyl-benzyl ester (o), pilocarpic acid 4-methylbenzyl ester (•) and pilocarpine (Δ) during incubation of the O-benzoyl derivative in 75% human plasma (pH 7.4) at 37°C. From Bundgaard et al. (155, 156).

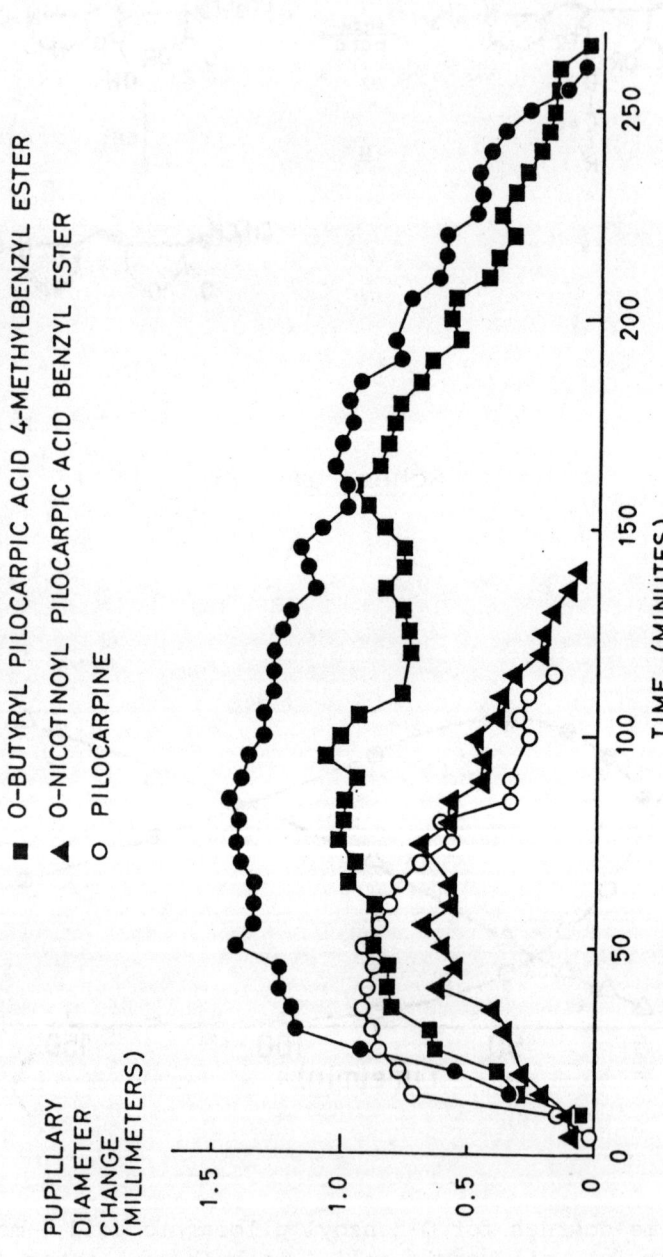

Fig. 12. Plots of the average observed changes in pupillary diameter (ΔPD, in mm) as a function of time following the instillation of 25 μℓ of isotonic aqueous solutions (pH 4.75 in equimolar concentrations (0.25% pilocarpine nitrate equivalent) of the compounds indicated. Four rabbits were used in the crossover study (155, 156).

O-Acyloxyalkyl esters

According to their cleavage mechanism acyloxyalkyl esters and ethers can be considered as double prodrugs (Schemes 1 and 2). Likewise, N-acyloxymethyl derivatives are pro-prodrugs with the unstable N-hydroxymethyl derivatives being intermediates in the overall release of the parent drugs as described earlier. An interesting variant of the acyloxyalkyl double esters is provided in the recent work of Kakeya et al. (157) on cephalosporins. They have prepared a p-glycyloxybenzoyloxymethyl ester of a cephalosporin. Due to the ionizable amino group in the pro-moiety this prodrug, as a hydrochloride salt, is highly soluble in water but because the pK_a of the glycyl amino group is relatively low the partition coefficient between octanol and water at pH 6.5 (about equal to the pH of the intestine) is sufficient to ensure good absorption. The prodrug contains three ester groupings and depending on the cleavage mechanism (Scheme 17) it may be regarded as a triple prodrug. Phenyl esters of glycine and similar amino acids are known to be rather unstable in neutral aqueous solution and the prodrug may probably undergo an initial cleavage at the glycyl ester grouping before or during the absorption from the gastrointestinal tract.

Recently, the concept of O-acyloxyalkylation has been applied to the phosphate group. Farquhar et al. (158, 159) have prepared a number of bis(acyloxymethyl) esters of phosphoric acid and model phosphomonoesters (e.g. phenyl and benzyl phosphate) and studied their degradation in aqueous

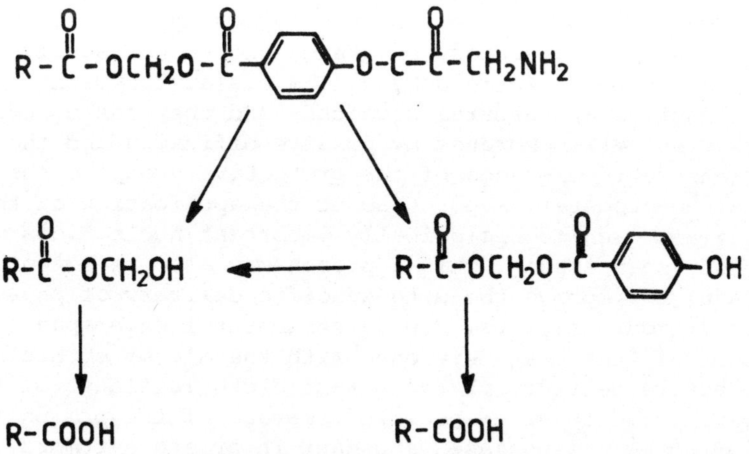

Scheme 17

buffer solutions and mice plasma or in the presence of hog liver esterase. The hydrolysis of the derivatives were subject to marked enzymatic catalysis, the effect being dependent on the nature of the acyl group. Sterically hindered groups retard the rate of hydrolysis. Both the chemical and enzyme-mediated hydrolysis take place as shown in Scheme 18 with the intermediate formation of a monoacyloxymethyl ester (159).

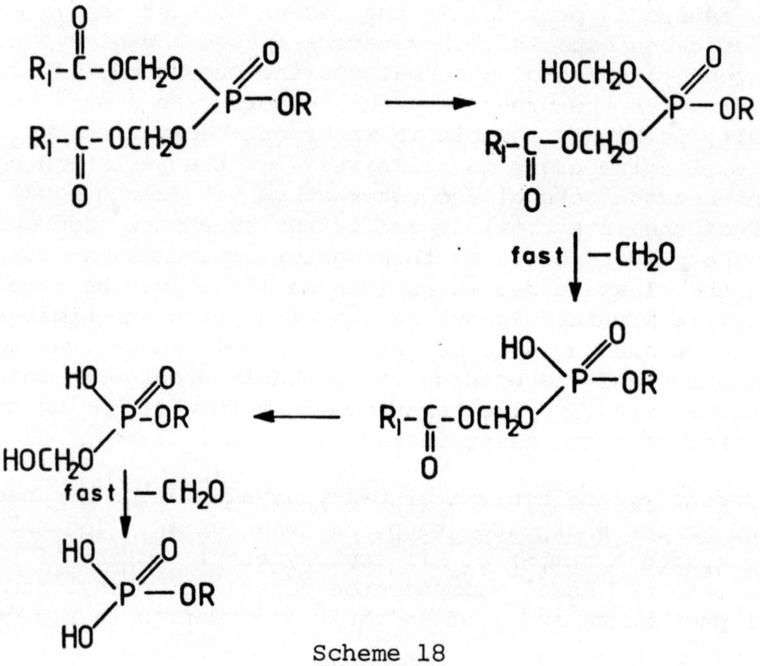

Scheme 18

The O-hydroxymethyl derivatives formed upon ester hydrolysis have only a transistory existence and spontaneously eliminate one molecule of formaldehyde. The bis(acyloxymethyl) ester derivatives are neutral compounds and they can conceivably traverse cell membranes by passive diffusion and then revert by enzymatic cleavage of the protective group to the parent phosphomonoester. Reports about the application of this prodrug approach to biologically important nucleotides may certainly soon appear. This approach may also be potentially useful to improve the site-specific delivery of phosphate ester prodrugs. Thus, diethylstilbestrol diphosphate (stilphostrol) has been developed with the aim of obtaining a selective delivery of the parent diethylstilbestrol to prostate based on site-specific cleavage of the phosphate ester prodrug by phosphatases abundant in prostate tumors. This approach has failed, however, (160), certainly because the phosphate prodrug is too polar to be able to reach the site of action. A lipophilic bis(acyloxyalkyl) ester of stilphostrol (a pro-prodrug), as well as of other phosphate ester prodrugs, may conceivably improve the transport properties.

Acylated N-Mannich bases

As described above N-Mannich bases are cleaved spontaneously (non-enzymatic) to an NH-acidic compound, formaldehyde and amine. The drawback of this type of bioreversible derivative is obviously a limited in vitro stability, raising stability-formulation problems. Appropriate acylation of the amino moiety in N-Mannich bases gives compounds which are chemically stable. In selected cases such acylated N-Mannich bases may possibly be susceptible to enzymatic hydrolysis with formation of the free N-Mannich base. This concept finds support in a recent work by Kingsbury et al. (161) on peptidyl derivatives of 5-fluorouracil. They have prepared L-alanyl-2-(5-fluorouracil-1-yl)-D,L-glycine (55) and shown that this compound is a substrate for microbial peptidases. Compound 55 is stable in water and is only cleaved slowly in the presence of human serum. However, after entry into microbial cells by a peptide carrier mechanism, the compound is enzymatically hydrolyzed by cytoplasmic peptidases, resulting in the formation of the N-Mannich base 56. This, in turn, spontaneously decomposes with the release of 5-fluorouracil, glyoxylic acid and ammonia (Scheme 19). This double prodrug concept using an α-substituted glycine peptide backbone for overcoming the permeability barrier of the microbial cytoplasmic membrane may well be of general utility for the site-specific delivery of microbial inhibitors.

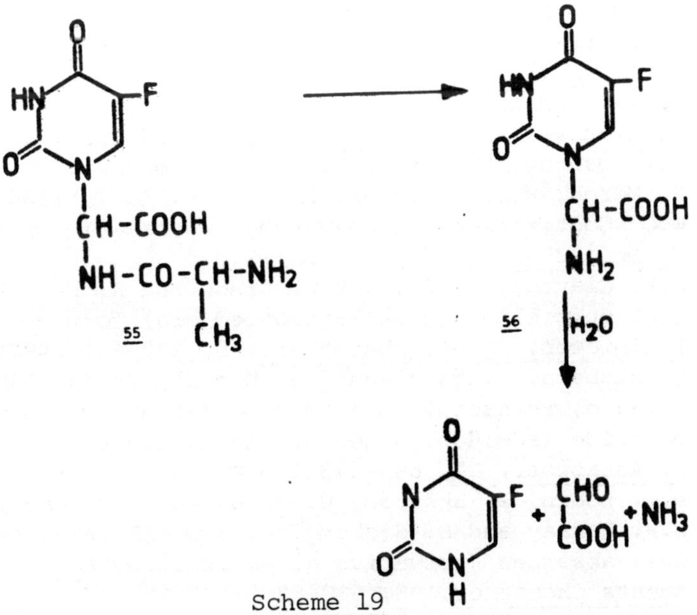

Scheme 19

References

1. G.A. Digenis and J.V. Swintosky, Drug latentiation, Handbook of Experimental Pharmacology, 28/3, 86-112 (1975).
2. A.A. Sinkula and S.H. Yalkowsky, Rationale for design of biologically reversible drug derivatives: Prodrugs, J. Pharm. Sci., 64, 181-210 (1975).
3. A.A. Sinkula, Prodrug approach in drug design, Annual Reports in Medicinal Chemistry, 10, 306-316 (1975).
4. Roche, E.B. (ed.), "Design of biopharmaceutical properties through prodrugs and analogs", American Pharmaceutical Association, Washington, D.C., 1977.
5. V. Stella, Pro-drugs: An overview and definition. In: "Pro-drugs as novel drug delivery systems", T. Higuchi and V. Stella (eds.), American Chemical Society, Washington, D.C., 1975, pp. 1-115.
6. I.H. Pitman, Prodrugs of amides, imides.and amines, Med. Res. Rev., 1, 189-214 (1981).
7. H. Bundgaard, Novel bioreversible derivatives of amides, imides, ureides, amines and other chemical entities not readily derivatizable. In: "Optimization of drug delivery", H. Bundgaard, A.B. Hansen and H. Kofod (eds.), Munksgaard, Copenhagen, 1982, pp. 178-197.
8. N. Bodor, Novel approaches in prodrug design, Drugs of the Future, 6, 165-182 (1981).
9. H. Bundgaard, Design of prodrugs: Bioreversible derivatives for various functional groups and chemical entities. In: "Design of prodrugs", H. Bundgaard (ed.), Elsevier Biomedical Press, Amsterdam, 1986, in press.
10. H. Ferres, Pro-drugs of β-lactam antibiotics, Drugs of Today, 19, 499-538 (1983).
11. A.B.A. Jansen and T.J. Russell, Some novel penicillin derivatives, J. Chem. Soc., 2127-2132 (1965).
12. W.v. Daehne, E. Frederiksen, E. Gundersen, F. Lund, P. Mørch, H.J. Petersen, K. Roholt, L. Tybring and W.O. Godtfredsen, Acyloxymethyl esters of ampicillin, J. Med. Chem., 13, 607-612 (1970).
13. J.P. Clayton, M. Cole, S.W. Elson and H. Ferres, BRL. 8988 (talampicillin), a well-absorbed oral form of ampicillin. Antimicrob. Agents Chemother., 5, 670-671 (1974.
14. Y.Shiobara, A. Tachibana, H. Sasaki, T. Watanabe and T. Sado, Phthalidyl D-α-aminobenzylpenicillinate hydrochloride (PC-183), a new orally active ampicillin ester. J. Antibiot., 27, 665-673 (1974).
15. N.O. Bodin, B. Ekström, U. Forsgren, L.P. Jalar, L. Magni, C.H. Ramsey and B. Sjöberg, Bacampicillin: A new orally well-absorbed derivative of ampicillin, Antimicrob. Agents Chemother., 8, 518-525 (1975).

16. N. Bodor, J. Zupan and S. Selk, Improved delivery through biological membranes VII. Dermal delivery of chromoglycic acid (cromolyn) via its prodrugs, Int. J. Pharm., 7, 64-75 (1980).
17. E. Falch, P. Krogsgaard-Larsen and A.V. Christensen, Esters of isoguavacine as potential prodrugs, J. Med. Chem., 24, 285-289 (1981).
18. W.S. Saari, M.B. Freedman, R.D. Hartman, S.W. King, A.W. Raab, W.C. Randall, E.L. Engelhardt, R. Hirschman, A. Rosegay, C.T. Ludden and A. Scriabine, Synthesis and antihypertensive activity of some ester progenitors of methyldopa, J. Med. Chem., 21, 746-753 (1978).
19. M.R. Dobrinska, W. Kukovetz, E. Beubler, H.L. Leidy, H.J. Gomez, J. Demetriades and J.A. Bolognese, Pharmacokinetics of the pivaloyloxyethyl (POE) ester of methyldopa, a new prodrug of methyldopa, J. Pharmacokin. Biopharm., 10, 587-600 (1982).
20. S. Vickers, C.A.H. Duncan, H.G. Ramjit, M.R. Dobrinska, C.T. Dollery, H.J. Gomez, H.L. Leidy and W.C. Vincek, Metabolism of methyldopa in man after oral administration of the pivaloyloxyethyl ester, Drug Metab. Disp., 12, 242-246 (1984).
21. J.J. Baldwin, G.H. Denny, G.S. Ponticello, C.S. Sweet and C.A. Stone, Tyrosine progenitors as antihypertensive agents, Eur. J. Med. Chem., 17, 297-300 (1982).
22. W.S. Saari, W. Halczenko, D.W. Cochran, M.R. Dobrinska, W.C. Vincek, D.C. Titus, S.L. Gaul and C.S. Sweet, 3-Hydroxy-α-methyltyrosine progenitors: Synthesis and evaluation of some (2-oxo-1,3-dioxol-4-yl)methylesters, J. Med. Chem., 27, 713-717 (1984).
23. F. Sakamoto, S. Ikeda and G. Tsukamoto, Studies on prodrugs. II. Preparation and characterization of (5-substituted 2-oxo-1,3-dioxolen-4-yl)methyl esters of ampicillin, Chem. Pharm. Bull., 32, 2241-2248 (1984).
24. T. Loftsson and N- Bodor, Synthesis and hydrolysis of some pivaloyloxymethyl and pivaloyl derivatives of phenolic compounds, Arch. Pharm. Chem., Sci. Ed., 10, 104-110 (1982).
25. N. Bodor, K.B. Sloan, J.J. Kaminski, C. Shih and S. Pogani, A convenient synthesis of (acyloxy)alkyl α-ethers of phenols, J. Org. Chem., 48., 5280-5284 (1983).
26. L.W. Ditlert and T. Higuchi, Rates of hydrolysis of carbamate and carbonate esters in alkaline solutions, J. Pharm. Sci., 55, 852-857 (1963).
27. A. Williams, Alkaline hydrolysis of substituted phenyl N-phenylcarbamates. Structure-reactivity relationships consistent with an ElcB mechanism, J. Chem. Soc. Perkin II, 808-812 (1972).

28. T. Vontor, J. Socha and M. Vecera, Kinetics and mechanism of hydrolysis of 1-naphthyl N-methyl-and N,N-dimethylcarbamates, Coll. Czech. Chem. Comm., 37, 2183-2196 (1972).
29. A.F. Hegarty and L.N. Frost, Elimination-addition mechanism for the hydrolysis of carbamates. Trapping of an isocyanate intermediate by an o-amino-group, J. Chem. Soc. Perkin II, 1719-1728 (1973).
30. A.F. Hegarty, L.N. Frost and J.H. Coy, The question of amide group participation in carbamate hydrolysis, J. Org. Chem., 39, 1089-1093 (1974).
31. H. Al-Rawi and A. Williams, Elimination-addition mechanisms of acyl-group transfer: the neutral and alkaline decomposition of 1-(N-methylcarbamoyl)imidazoles, J. Chem. Soc. Perkin II, 1064-1068 (1979).
32. U. Klixbüll and H. Bundgaard, Prodrugs as drug delivery systems. XXIX. Imidazole-1-carboxylic acid esters of hydrocortisone and testosterone, Arch. Pharm. Chem., Sci. Ed., 11, 101-110 (1983).
33. G.L. Amidon, Drug derivatization as a means of solubilization: Physicochemical and biochemical strategies. In: "Techniques of solubilization of drugs" (S.H. Yalkowsky, ed.), Marcel Dekker, Inc., New York, 1981, pp. 183-221.
34. G.L. Amidon, R.S. Pearlman and G.D. Leesman, Design of prodrugs through consideration of enzyme-substrate specificities. In: "Design of Biopharmaceutical Properties through Prodrugs and Analogs" (E.B. Roche, ed.), American Pharmaceutical Association, Washington, D.C., 1977, pp. 281-315.
35. I.C. Melby and M. St. Cyr, Comparative studies on absorption and metabolic disposal of water-soluble corticosteroid esters, Metab. Clin. Exp., 10, 75-85 (1961).
36. J.T. Burke, W.A. Wargin, R.J. Sherertz, K.L. Sanders, M.R. Blum and F.A. Sarubbi, Pharmacokinetics of intravenous chloramphenicol sodium succinate in adult patients with normal renal and hepatic function, J. Pharmacokin. Biopharm., 10, 601-614 (1982).
37. R.E. Kauffman, J.N. Miceli, L. Strebel, J.A. Buckley, A.K. Done and A.S. Dajami, Pharmacokinetics of chloramphenicol succinate in infants and children, J. Pediatr., 98, 315-320 (1981).
38. P.J. Ambrose, Clinical pharmacokinetics of chloramphenicol and chloramphenicol succinate, Clin. Pharmacokin., 9, 222-238 (1984).
39. W.G. Kramer, E.R. Rensimer, C.D. Ericsson and L.K. Pickering, Comparative bioavailability of intravenous and oral chloramphenicol in adults, J. Clin. Pharmacol., 24, 181-186 (1984).

40. B.D. Anderson and V. Taphouse, Initial rate studies of hydrolysis and acyl migration in methylprednisolone 21-hemisuccinate and 17-hemisuccinate, J. Pharm. Sci., 70, 181-186 (1981).
41. B.D. Anderson, R.A. Conradi and W.J. Lambert, Carboxyl group catalysis of acyl transfer reactions in corticosteroid 17- and 21-monoesters, J. Pharm. Sci., 73, 604-610 (1984).
42. G.L. Flynn and D.J. Lamb, Factors influencing solvolysis of corticosteroid-21-phosphate esters, J. Pharm. Sci., 59, 1433-1438 (1970).
43. K.S.L. Kwee and L.M.L. Stolk, Formulation of a stable vidarabine phosphate injection, Pharm. Weekbl. Sci. Ed., 6, 101-104 (1984).
44. W.-H. Hong and D.H. Szulczewski, Stability of vidarabine-5'-phosphate in aqueous solutions, J. Parent. Sci. Techn., 38, 60-64 (1984).
45. S.A. Varia, S. Schuller and V.J. Stella, Phenytoin prodrugs IV: Hydrolysis of various 3-(hydroxymethyl)phenytoin esters, J. Pharm. Sci., 73, 1074-1080 (1984).
46. S.A. Varia and V.J. Stella, Phenytoin prodrugs V: In vivo evaluation of some water-soluble phenytoin prodrugs in dogs, J. Pharm. Sci., 73, 1080-1087 (1984).
47. S.A. Varia and V.J. Stella, Phenytoin prodrugs VI: In vivo evaluation of a phosphate ester prodrug of phenytoin after parenteral administration to rats, J. Pharm. Sci., 73, 1087-1090 (1984).
48. S. Miyabo, T. Nakamura, S. Kuwazima and S. Kishida, A comparison of the bioavailability and potency of dexamethasone phosphate and sulphate in man, Eur. J. Clin. Pharmacol, 20, 277-282 (1981).
49. M.J. Cho, R.R. Kurtz, C. Lewis, B.M. Machkovech and D.J. Houser, Metromidazole phosphate - a water-soluble prodrug for parenteral solutions of metronidazole, J. Pharm. Sci., 71, 410-414 (1982).
50. M. Johansen and C. Larsen, Stability and kinetics of hydrolysis of metronidazole monosuccinate in aqueous solution and in plasma, Int. J. Pharm., 21, 201-209 (1984).
51. H. Bundgaard, C. Larsen and P. Thorbek, Prodrugs as drug delivery systems. XXVI. Preparation and enzymatic hydrolysis of various water-soluble amino acid esters of metronidazole, Int. J. Pharm., 18, 67-77 (1984).
52. H. Bundgaard, C. Larsen and E. Arnold, Prodrugs as drug delivery systems. XXVII. Chemical stability and bioavailability of a water-soluble prodrug of metronidazole for parenteral administration, Int. J. Pharm., 18, 79-87 (1984).
53. B.D. Anderson, see another chapter of this book.

54. D.B. Williams, S.A. Varia, V.J. Stella and I.H. Pitman, Evaluation of the prodrug potential of the sulfate esters of acetaminophen and 3-hydroxymethyl-phenytoin, Int. J. Pharm., 14, 113-120 (1983).
55. A.J. Repta, B.J. Rawson, R.D. Shaffer, K.B. Sloan, N. Bodor and T. Higuchi, Rational development of a soluble prodrug of a cytotoxic nucleoside: Preparation and properties of arabinosyladenine 5'-formate, J. Pharm. Sci., 64, 392-396 (1975).
56. H. Bundgaard and M. Johansen, Pro-drugs as drug delivery systems. IV. N-Mannich bases as potential novel pro-drugs for amides, ureides, amines, and other NH-acidic compounds, J. Pharm. Sci., 69, 44-46 (1980.
57. H. Bundgaard and M. Johansen, Pro-drugs as drug delivery systems. X. N-Mannich bases as novel pro-drug candidates for amides, imides, urea derivatives, amines and other NH-acidic compounds. Kinetics and mechanisms of decomposition and structure-reactivity relationships, Arch. Pharm., Sci. Ed., 8, 29-52 (1980).
58. H. Bundgaard and M. Johansen, Pro-drugs as drug delivery systems. XV. Bioreversible derivatization of phenytoin, acetazolamide, chlorzoxazone and various other NH-acidic compounds by N-aminomethylation to effect enhanced dissolution rates, Int. J. Pharm., 7, 129-136 (1980).
59. M. Johansen and H. Bundgaard, Pro-drugs as drug delivery systems. XII. Solubility, dissolution and partitioning behaviour of N-Mannich bases and N-hydroxymethyl derivatives, Arch. Pharm. Chem., Sci. Ed., 8, 141-151 (1980).
60. M. Johansen and H. Bundgaard, Pro-drugs as drug delivery systems. XIII. Kinetics of decomposition of N-Mannich bases of salicylamide and assessment of their suitability as possible pro-drugs for amines. Int. J. Pharm., 7, 119-127 (1980).
61. H. Bundgaard and M. Johansen, Prodrugs as drug delivery systems. XIX. Bioreversible derivatization of aromatic amines by formation of N-Mannich bases with succinimide, Int. J. Pharm., 8, 183-192 (1982).
62. H. Bundgaard and M. Johansen, Hydrolysis of N-Mannich bases and its consequences for the biological testing of such agents, Int. J. Pharm., 9, 7-16 (1981).
63. H. Bundgaard and M. Johansen, Pro-drugs as drug delivery systems. XVIII. Bioreversible derivatization of allopurinol by N-aminomethylation to effect enhanced dissolution rates, Acta Pharm. Suec., 18, 129-134 (1981).
64. M. Johansen and H. Bundgaard, Pro-drugs as drug delivery systems. XXIV. N-Mannich bases as bioreversible lipophilic transport forms of ephedrine, phenethylamine and other amines, Arch. Pharm. Chem., Sci. Ed., 10, 111-121 (1982).

65. G.M. Loudon, M.R. Almond and J.N. Jacob, Mechanism of hydrolysis of N-(1-aminoalkyl)amides, J. Am. Chem. Soc., 103, 4508-4515 (1981).
66. H. Bundgaard and M. Johansen, Kinetics of hydrolysis of plafibride (an ureide N-Mannich base with platelet anti-aggregant activity) in aqueous solution and in plasma, Arch. Pharm. Chem., Sci. Ed., 10, 139-145 (1982).
67. H. Bundgaard, M. Johansen, V. Stella and M. Cortese, Pro-drugs as drug delivery systems. XXI. Preparation, physicochemical properties and bioavailability of a novel water-soluble pro-drug type for carbamazepine, Int. J. Pharm., 10, 181-192 (1982).
68. M. Johansen and H. Bundgaard, Decomposition of rolitetracycline and other N-Mannich bases and of N-hydroxymethyl derivatives in the presence of plasma, Arch. Pharm. Chem., Sci. Ed., 9, 40-42 (1981).
69. H. Bundgaard and M. Johansen, Hydrolysis of N-(α-hydroxyalkyl)benzamide and other N-(α-hydroxyalkyl)amide derivatives: implications for the design of N-acyloxyalkyl-type prodrugs, Int. J. Pharm., 22, 45-56 (1984).
70. B. Vej-Hansen and H. Bundgaard, Kinetics of degradation of rolitetracycline in aqueous solutions and reconstituted formulation, Arch. Pharm. Chem., Sci. Ed., 7, 65-77 (1979).
71. K.B. Sloan, S.A.M. Koch and K.G. Siver, Mannich base derivatives of theophylline and 5-fluorouracil: syntheses, properties and topical delivery characteristics, Int. J. Pharm., 21, 251-264 (1984).
71a. H. Bundgaard, Formaldehyde pro-drugs as potential antitumor agents, Arch. Pharm. Chem., Sci. Ed., 9, 133-136 (1981).
72. M. Johansen and H. Bundgaard, Pro-drugs as drug delivery systems. VI. Kinetics and mechanism of the decomposition of N-hydroxymethylated amides and imides in aqueous solution and assessment of their suitability as possible pro-drugs, Arch. Pharm. Chem., Sci. Ed., 7, 175-192 (1979).
73. H. Bundgaard and M. Johansen, Pro-drugs as drug delivery systems. VIII. Bioreversible derivatization of hydantoins by N-hydroxymethylation, Int. J. Pharm., 5, 67-77 (1980).
74. P.C. Bansal, I.H. Pitman, J.N.S. Tam, M. Mertes and J.J. Kaminski, N-Hydroxymethyl derivatives of nitrogen heterocycles as possible prodrugs I: N-Hydroxymethylation of uracils, J. Pharm. Sci., 70, 850-854 (1981).
75. P.C. Bansal, I.H. Pitman and T. Higuchi, N-Hydroxymethyl derivatives of nitrogen heterocycles as possible prodrugs II: Possible prodrugs of allopurinol, glutethimide and phenobarbital, J. Pharm. Sci., 70, 855-857 (1981).

76. H.E. Zaugg and W.B. Martin, α-Amidoalkylations at carbon, Organic Reactions, 14, 52-269 (1965).
77. H. Böhme, K.H. Ahrens and H.-H. Hotzel, Eigenschaften und Umsetzugen von N-[α-Hydroxyalkyl]-thiocarbonsäureamiden, Arch. Pharm., 307, 748-755 (1974).
78. Y. Yamaoka, R.D. Roberts and V.J. Stella, Low-melting phenytoin prodrugs as alternative oral delivery modes of phenytoin: A model for other high-melting sparingly water-soluble drugs, J. Pharm. Sci., 72, 400-405 (1983).
79. K.B. Sloan and N. Bodor, Hydroxymethyl and acyloxymethyl prodrugs of theophylline: enhanced delivery of polar drugs through the skin, Int. J. Pharm., 12, 299-313 (1982).
80. K.B. Sloan, M. Hashida, J. Alexander, N. Bodor and T. Higuchi, Prodrugs of 5-thiopurines: enhanced delivery through the skin, J. Pharm. Sci., 72, 372-378 (1983).
81. B. Møllgaard, A. Hoelgaard and H. Bundgaard, Pro-drugs as drug delivery systems. XXIII. Improved dermal delivery of 5-fluorouracil through human skin via N-acyloxymethyl pro-drug derivatives, Int. J. Pharm., 12, 153-162 (1982).
82. M. Johansen and H. Bundgaard, Pro-drugs as drug delivery systems. KVI. Novel water-soluble pro-drug types for chlorzoxazone by esterification of the N-hydroxymethyl derivative, Arch. Pharm. Chem., Sci. Ed., 9, 43-54 (1981).
83. S. Varia, S. Schuller, K.B. Sloan and V.J. Stella, Phenytoin prodrugs III: Water-soluble prodrugs for oral and/or parenteral use, J. Pharm. Sci., 73, 1068-1073 (1984).
84. H. Bundgaard and E. Falch, Allopurinol prodrugs. II. Synthesis, hydrolysis kinetics and physicochemical properties of various N-acyloxymethyl allopurinol derivatives, Int. J. Pharm., 1985, in press.
85. H. Bundgaard and E. Falch, Allopurinol prodrugs. III. Water-soluble N-acyloxymethyl allopurinol derivatives for rectal or parenteral use, Int. J. Pharm., 1985, in press.
86. A. Buur, H. Bundgaard and E. Falch, Prodrugs of 5-fluorouracil. IV. Hydrolysis kinetics, bioactivation and physicochemical properties of various N-acyloxymethyl derivatives of 5-fluorouracil, Int. J. Pharm., in press.
87. P. Prusiner and M. Sundaralingam, Stereochemistry of nucleic acids and their constituents XXIX. Crystal and molecular structure of allopurinol, a potent inhibitor of xanthine oxidase, Acta Cryst., B28, 2148-2152 (1972).
88. H. Bundgaard and E. Falch, Improved rectal and parenteral delivery of allopurinol using the prodrug approach, Arch. Pharm. Chem., Sci., Ed., 13, 39-48 (1985).

89. H. Bundgaard, E. Falch, S.B. Pedersen and G.H. Nielsen Allopurinol prodrugs. IV. Improved rectal and parenteral delivery of allopurinol using the prodrug approach as evaluated in rabbits, Int. J. Pharm., in press.
90. A. Buur and H. Bundgaard, Prodrugs of 5-fluorouracil. I. Hydrolysis kinetics and physicochemical properties of various N-acyl derivatives of 5-fluorouracil, Int. J. Pharm., 21, 349-364 (1984).
91. A. Buur and H. Bundgaard, Prodrugs of 5-fluorouracil. II. Hydrolysis kinetics, bioactivation, solubility and lipophilicity of N-alkoxycarbonyl derivatives of 5-fluorouracil, Arch. Pharm. Chem., Sci. Ed., 12, 37-44 (1984).
92. A. Buur and H. Bundgaard, Prodrugs of 5-fluorouracil. III. Hydrolysis kinetics in aqueous solution and biological media, lipophilicity and solubility of various 1-carbamoyl derivatives of 5-fluorouracil, Int. J. Pharm., 23, 209-222 (1985).
93. K. Takada, H. Yoshikawa and S. Muranishi, Conversion of a novel 5-fluorouracil (5-FU) derivative to 5-FU in rats, Research Comm. Chem. Path. Pharmacol., 40, 99-108 (1983).
94. S. Wilk, H. Mizoguchi and M. Orlowski, γ-Glutamyl Dopa: A kidney-specific dopamine precursor, J. Pharmacol. Exp. Ther., 206, 227-232 (1978).
95. M. Orlowski, H. Mizoguchi and S. Wilk, N-Acyl-γ-glutamyl derivatives of sulfamethoxazole as models of kidney-selective prodrugs, J. Pharmacol. Exp. Ther., 212, 167-172 (1979).
96. J.J. Kyncl, F.N. Minard and P.H. Jones, L-γ-Glutamyl dopamine, an oral dopamine prodrug with renal selectivity, Adv. Biosci., 20, 369-380 (1979).
97. N. Bodor, K.B. Sloan, T. Higuchi and K. Sasahara, Improved delivery through biological membranes. 4. Prodrugs of L-Dopa, J. Med. Chem., 20, 1435-1445 (1977).
98. Z. Zlojkowska, H.J. Krasuka and J. Pachecka, Enzymatic hydrolysis of amino acid derivatives of benzocaine, Xenobiotica, 12, 359-364 (1982).
99. H. Bundgaard and E. Falch, Allopurinol prodrugs. I. Synthesis, stability and physicochemical properties of various N_1-acyl allopurinol derivatives, Int. J. Pharm., 23, 223-237 (1985).
100. S.-L. Chang, W.G. Kramer, S. Feldman, R. Ballentine and L.S. Frankel, Bioavailability of allopurinol from oral and rectal dosage forms, Am. J. Hosp. Pharm., 38, 365-368 (1981).
101. S.J. Appelbaum, M. Mayersohn, R.T. Dorr and D. Perrier, Allopurinol kinetics and bioavailability. Intravenous, oral and rectal administration, Cancer Chemother. Pharmacol., 8, 93-98 (1982.

102. A.J. Verbiscar and L.G. Abood, Carbamate ester latentiation of physiologically active amines, J. Med. Chem., 13, 176-179 (1070).
103. S.M. Kupchan and A.C. Isenberg, Drug latentiation. III. Labile amide derivatives of normeperidine, J. Med. Chem., 10, 960-961 (1967).
104. G.B. Baker, R.T. Coutts, A.J. Nazarali, T.J. Danielson and M. Rubens, Proc. West. Pharmacol. Soc., 27, 523-525 (1984).
105. H. Sasaki, E. Mukai, M. Hashida, T. Kimura and H. Sezaki, Development of lipophilic prodrugs of mitomycin C. I. Synthesis and antitumor activity of la-N-substituted derivatives with aromatic pro-moiety, Int. J. Pharm., 15, 49-59 (1983).
106. H. Sasaki, E. Mukai, M. Hashida, T. Kimura and H. Sezaki, Development of lipophilic prodrugs of mitomycin C. II. Stability and bioactivation of la-N-substituted derivatives with aromatic pro-moiety, Int. J. Pharm., 15, 61-71 (1983).
107. H. Sasaki, M. Fukumoto, M. Hashida, T. Kimura and H. Sezaki, Development of lipophilic prodrugs of mitomycin C. III. Physicochemical and biological properties of newly synthesized alkoxycarbonyl derivatives, Chem. Pharm. Bull., 31, 4083-4090 (1983).
108. N.S. Bodor, Labile, non-heterocyclic quaternary ammonium salts/esters as transient derivatives, U.S. Patent 4,160,099 (1979).
109. H.C. Caldwell, H.J. Adams, R.G. Jones, W.A. Mann, L.W. Dittert, C.W. Chong and J.V. Swintosky, Enamine prodrugs, J. Pharm. Sci., 60, 1810-1812 (1971).
110. K. Dixon and J.V. Greenhill, A study of the rates of hydrolysis of certain enaminones, J. Chem. Soc. Perkin II, 164-168 (1974).
111. N.P. Jensen, J.J. Friedman, H. Kropp and F.M. Kahan, Use of acetylacetone to prepare a prodrug of cycloserine, J. Med. Chem., 23, 6-8 (1980).
112. T. Murakami, H. Tamauchi, M. Yamazaki, K. Kubo, A. Kamada and N. Yata, Biopharmaceutical study on the oral and rectal administrations of enamine prodrugs of amino acid-like β-lactam antibiotics in rabbits, Chem. Pharm. Bull., 29, 1986-1997 (1981).
113. T. Murakami, N. Yata, H. Tamauchi, J. Nakai, M. Yamazaki and A Kamada, Studies on absorption promoters for rectal delivery preparations. I. Promoting efficacy of enamine derivatives of amino acids for the rectal absorption of β-lactam antibiotics in rabbits, Chem. Pharm., Bull., 29, 1998-2004 (1981).

114. H. Bundgaard and M. Johansen, Pro-drugs as drug delivery systems. XX. Oxazolidines as potential pro-drug types for β-aminoalcohols, aldehydes or ketones, Int. J. Pharm., 10, 165-175 (1982).
115. M. Johansen and H. Bundgaard, Prodrugs as drug delivery systems. XXV. Hydrolysis of oxazolidines - a potential new prodrug type, J. Pharm. Sci., 72, 1294-1298 (1983).
116. A. Buur and H. Bundgaard, Prodrugs as drug delivery systems. XXVIII. Structural factors influencing the rate of hydrolysis of oxazolidines - a potential prodrug type, Int. J. Pharm., 18, 325-334 (1984).
117. J.P. Patel and A.J. Repta, Enol esters as potential prodrugs I. Stability and enzyme-mediated hydrolysis of α-acetoxystyrene, Int. J. Pharm., 5, 329-333 (1980).
118. J.P. Patel and A.J. Repta, Enol esters as potential pro-drugs II. In vitro aqueous stability and enzyme-mediated hydrolysis of several enol esters of acetophenone, Int. J. Pharm., 9, 29-47 (1981).
119. H. Bundgaard, A.B. Hansen and C. Larsen, Pro-drugs as drug delivery systems. III. Esters of malonuric acids as novel pro-drug types for barbituric acids, Int. J. Pharm., 3, 341-353 (1979).
120. H. Bundgaard, E. Falch and C. Larsen, Pro-drugs as drug delivery systems. XI. Preparation and characterization of a novel water-soluble pro-drug type for barbituric acids, Int. J. Pharm., 6, 19-27 (1980).
121. V. Stella and T. Higuchi, Esters of hydantoic acids as prodrugs of hydantoins, J. Pharm. Sci., 62, 962-967 (1973).
122. H. Bundgaard and C. Larsen, Pro-drugs as drug delivery systems. II. Open-ring ester derivatives as novel pro-drug candidates for trimethadione, Arch. Pharm. Chem., Sci. Ed., 7, 41-50 (1979).
123. H. Bundgaard and C. Larsen, Pro-drugs as drug delivery systems. V. Cyclization of methyl esters of succinamic and glutaramic acids to the corresponding imides (phensuximide and glutethimide) in aqueous solution, Acta Pharm. Suec., 16, 309-318 (1979).
124. H. Bundgaard and C. Larsen, Pro-drugs as drug delivery systems. XVII. Esters of 4-hydroxybutyric acids as potential pro-drug types for γ-lactones, Int. J. Pharm., 7, 169-176 (1980).
125. B. Holmberg, B. Lindberg, R. Dahlbom and S.B. Ross, Cyclizing compounds. V. Tertiary haloalkylamine derivatives related to the tricyclic psychopharmacological agents promazine, imipramine and amitriptyline, Acta Pharm. Suec., 21, 31-42 (1984).

126. H. Bundgaard, Pro-drugs as drug delivery systems. IX. Reversible cyclization kinetics of 2-aminoacetamido-5-chlorobenzophenone to demethyldiazepam, in aqueous solution, Arch. Pharm. Chem., Sci. Ed., 8, 15-28 (1980).
127. K. Hirai, T. Ishiba, H. Sugimoto, T. Fujishita, Y. Tsukinoki and K. Hirose, Novel peptidoaminobenzophenones, and N-(acylglycyl)aminobenzophenones as open-ring derivatives of benzodiazepines, J. Med. Chem., 24, 20-27 (1981).
128. G.L. Bundy, D.C. Peterson, J.C. Cornette, W.L. Miller, C.H. Spilman and J.W. Wilks, Synthesis and biological activity of prostaglandin lactones, J. Med. Chem., 26, 1089-1099 (1983).
129. J. Lettieri and H.-L. Fung, Improved pharmacological activity via pro-drug modification: Comparative pharmacokinetics of sodium γ-hydroxybutyrate and γ-butyrolactone, Research Comm. Chem. Path. Pharmacol., 22, 107-118 (1978).
130. P.S. Callery, M. Stogniew and L.A. Geelhar, Detection of the in vivo conversion of 2-pyrrolidinone to γ-aminobutyric acid in mouse brain, Biomed. Mass Spectr., 6, 23-26 (1979).
131. H.T. Nagasawa, D.J.W. Goon, W.P. Muldoon and R.T. Zera, 2-Substituted thiazolidine-4(R)-carboxylic acids as prodrugs of L-cysteine. Protection of mice against acetaminophen hepatotoxicity, J. Med. Chem., 27, 591-596 (1984).
132. U. Klixbüll and H. Bundgaard, Prodrugs as drug delivery systems. XXX. 4-Imidazolidinones as potential bioreversible derivatives for the α-aminoamide moiety in peptides, Int. J. Pharm., 20, 273-284 (1984).
133. A. Campbell, R.J. Baldessarini, V.J. Ram and J.L. Neumeyer, Behavioral effects of (-) 1,11-methylenedioxy-N-n-propylnoraporphine, an orally effective long-acting agent active at central dopamine receptors, and analogous aporphines, Neuropharmacol., 21, 953-961 (1982).
134. G.Y. Paris, D.L. Garmaise, D.G. Cimon, L. Swelt, G.W. Carter and P. Young, Glycerides as prodrugs. 2. 1,3-Dialkanoyl-2-(2-methyl-4-oxo-1,3-benzodioxan-2-yl)-glycerides (Cyclic aspirin triglycerides) as antiinflammatory agents, J. Med. Chem., 23, 79-82 (1980).
135. A.B. Hansen and A. Senning, Chemical feasibility studies concerning potential prodrugs of acetylsalicylic acid, Acta Chem. Scand., B37, 351-359 (1983).
136. G.B. Elion, P.A. Furman, J.A. Fyfe, P. De Miranda, L. Beauchamp and H.J. Schaeffer, Selectivity of action of an antiherpetic agent, 9-(2-hydroxyethoxymethyl)guanine, Proc. Natl. Acad. Sci. U.S.A., 74, 5716-5720 (1977).

137. H.J. Schaeffer, L. Beauchamp, P. De Miranda, G.B. Elion, D.J. Bauer and P. Collins, 9-(2-Hydroxyethoxymethyl)guanine activity against viruses of the herpes group, Nature, 272, 583-585 (1978).
138. P. De Miranda, H.C. Krasny, D.A. Page and G.B. Elion, The disposition of acyclovir in different species, J. Pharmacol. Exp. Ther., 219, 309-315 (1981).
139. P. De Miranda and M.R. Blum, Pharmacokinetics of acyclovir after intravenous and oral administration. J. Antimicrob. Chemother., 12 (Suppl. B), 29-37 (1983).
140. R.B. Van Dyke, J.D. Connor, C. Wyborny, M. Hintz and R.E. Keeney, Pharmacokinetics of orally administered acyclovir in patients with herpes progenitalis, Am. J. Med., 73, (1A), 172-175 (1982).
141. S.S. Good, H.C. Krasny, G.B. Elion and P. De Miranda, Disposition in the dog and the rat of 2,6-diamino-9-(2-hydroxyethoxymethyl)purine (A134U), a potential prodrug of acyclovir, J. Pharmacol. Exp. Therap., 227, 644-651 (1983).
142. T. Spector, T.E. Jones and L.M. Beacham, III, Conversion of 2,6-diamino-9-(2-hydroxyethoxymethyl)purine to acyclovir as catalyzed by adenosine deaminase, Biochem. Pharmacol., 32, 2505-2509 (1983).
143. T.A. Krenitsky, W.W. Hall, P. De Miranda, L.M. Beauchamp, H.J. Schaeffer and P.D. Whiteman, 6-Deoxyacyclovir: A xanthine oxidase-activated prodrug of acyclovir, Proc. Natl. Acad. Sci. U.S.A., 81, 3209-3213 (1984).
144. P. Selby, S. Blake, E.K. Mbidde, E. Hickmott, R.L. Powles, K. Stolle, T.J. McElwain, P.D. Whiteman and A.P. Fiddian, Amino(hydroxyethoxymethyl)purine: a new well-absorbed prodrug of acyclovir, Lancet, ii, 1428 - 1430 (1984).
145. P.D. Whiteman, A. Bye, A.S.E. Fowle, S. Jeal, G. Land and J. Posner, Tolerance and pharmacokinetics of A515U, an acyclovir analogue, in healthy volunteers, Eur. J. Clin. Pharmacol., 27, 471-475 (1984).
146. L. Colla, E. De Clercq, R. Busson and H. Vanderhaeghe, Synthesis and antiviral activity of water-soluble esters of acyclovir [9-[(2-hydroxyethoxy)methyl]guanine], J. Med. Chem., 26, 602-604 (1983).
147. O.A.T. Olsson, L.Å. Svensson and K.I.L. Wetterlin, Therapeutically active derivatives of phenylethanol amines, Eur. Pat. Appl. 46144 (1981).
148. O.A.T. Olsson and L.Å Svensson, New lipophilic terbutaline ester prodrugs with long effect duration, Pharm. Research, 1, 19-23 (1984).
149. A.J. Repta and J.P. Patel, Enol esters as potential prodrugs. III. Stability and enzyme-mediated hydrolysis of enol esters of 6'-acetylpapaverin, Int. J. Pharm., 10, 29-42 (1982).

150. M.J. Cho, A.J. Repta, C.C. Cheng, K.Y. Zee-Cheng, T. Higuchi and I.H. Pitamn, Solubilization and stabilization of the cytotoxic agent coralyne, J. Pharm. Sci., 64, 1825-1830 (1975).
151. A.J. Repta, M.J. Hageman and J.P. Patel, Enol esters as potential prodrugs. IV. Enhanced delivery of the quaternary species coralyne to rat brain using 6'-acetylpapaverin and its enol esters as prodrugs, Int. J. Pharm., 10, 239-248 (1982).
152. C.F. Asseff, R.L. Weisman, S.M. Podos and B. Becker, Ocular penetration of pilocarpine in primates, Am. J. Ophthalmol., 75, 212-215 (1973).
153. T.F. Patton, Pharmacokinetic evidence for improved ophthalmic drug delivery by reduction of instilled volume, J. Pharm. Sci., 66, 1058-1059 (1977).
154. V.H.-L. Lee and J.R. Robinson, Mechanistic and quantitative evaluation of precorneal pilocarpine disposition in albino rabbits, J. Pharm. Sci., 68, 673-684 (1979).
155. H. Bundgaard, E. Falch, C. Larsen and T.J. Mikkelson, Pilocarpine prodrugs, Eur. Patent Appl. 106,541 (1984).
156. H. Bundgaard, E. Falch, C. Larsen, G.L. Mosher and T.J. Mikkelson, Pilocarpic acid esters as novel sequentially labile pilocarpine prodrugs for improved ocular delivery, J. Med. Chem., 1985, in press.
157. N. Kakeya, K.-I. Nishimura, A. Yoshimi, S. Nakamura, S. Nishizawa, S. Tamaki, H. Matsui, T. Kawamura, M. Kasai and K. Kitae, Studies on prodrugs of cephalosporins. I. Synthesis and biological properties of glycyloxybenzoyloxymethyl and glycylaminobenzoyloxymethyl esters of 7β-[2-(2-aminothiazol-4-yl)-(Z)-2-methoxyiminoacetamido]-3-methyl-3-cephem-4-carboxylic acid, Chem. Pharm. Bull., 32, 692-698 (1984).
158. D. Farquhar, D.N. Srivastva, N.J. Kuttesch and P.P. Saunders, Biologically reversible phosphate-protective groups, J. Pharm. Sci., 72, 324-325 (1983).
159. D.N. Srivastva and D. Farquhar, Bioreversible phosphate protective groups: Syntehsis and stability of model acyloxymethyl phosphates, Bioorg. Chem., 12, 118-129 (1984).
160. F.P. Abramson and H.C. Miller, Jr., Bioavailability, distribution and pharmacokinetics of diethylstilbestrol produced from stilphostrol, J. Urol., 128, 1336-1339 (1982).
161. W.D. Kingsbury, J.C. Boehm, R.J. Mehta, S.F. Grappel and C. Gilvarg, A novel peptide delivery system involving peptidase activated prodrugs as antimicrobial agents. Synthesis and biological activity of peptidyl derivatives of 5-fluorouracil, J. Med. Chem., 27, 1447-1451 (1984).

Chapter 3
Chemical Drug Delivery Systems

Nicholas Bodor

Department of Medicinal Chemistry
College of Pharmacy
J. Hillis Miller Health Center, Box J-4
University of Florida
Gainesville, Florida 32610

Introduction

The importance of the therapeutic index (TI) of a drug, as the prime objective of the drug design, has been emphasized recently (1, 2). As the TI represents a ratio between the efficacy and the toxicity of a drug, it can be improved as much by reducing drug toxicity (T[D]) as by enhancing its activity. Drug toxicity is, however, a rather complex property; it is actually the sum of the toxicities of the structurally close analog metabolites ($D_1...D_n$), having similar activity, of the toxicity of different metabolites ($M_1...M_n$) and of the toxicity of the reactive intermediates ($I_1^*...I_n^*$). One important, last term in this sum is the <u>intrinsic toxicity</u> (T_i) of the drug, which is basically a molecular property and it represents mainly the <u>drug selectivity</u>.

$$T(D) = T_i + T(D_1...D_n) + T(M_1...M_n) + T(I_1^*...I_n^*)$$

The drug selectivity is, however, a complex term. It can be improved by molecular manipulations, that is, by enhancing the receptor specificity of the drug, but since most receptors are not localized exclusively in target organs, the <u>site specificity</u> is a major component of the drug selectivity. Site specific drug delivery has been one of the most pursued goals in therapeutics, originating with Paul Ehrich's vision of targeted drugs as "magic bullets" for the eradication of diseases. While this objective was also named "guided missiles," "toxic warheads," "smart bombs," etc., these new names represent more the advancement of the military arsenal than any real progress in drug targeting. The simplest way to achieve drug targeting is to limit its access to a specific site by physical means, such as localized devices. Unfortunately, this approach is rather limited, and formulation can improve the therapeutic index more by achieving controlled drug release than by site or organ targeting. Another way, which is much talked about, is biological targeting. This theoretically attractive approach, which includes drug-monoclonal antibody conjugates, or drugs combined with other macromolecular ligands with specific affinity or transport properties, suffers from a number of problems. The first problem is stoichiometry: a very limited number of drug molecules can be transported by the relatively large carriers, without affecting their important properties. Other problems relate to in vivo transport, as well as stability and drug release. Thus, the probability of achieving therapeutic drug levels at specific targets in vivo is rather low.

Chemical modifications of the drug structure in order to improve its therapeutic index provides the most versatile approach. The classical way is to design the molecule to have the best fit to the target receptor. Since the structure of receptor site is generally not known in detail, this is an iterative process: We learn the structure of the receptor from the various substrates. This approach, however, cannot generally lead to the elusive "magic bullet," not only because of the limitations of the receptor specificity, but also due to the distribution of the receptors. These facts require additional chemical modifications to be considered. It was suggested that prodrugs (PD), the inactive chemical precursors of the active drugs, can improve drug specificity. Essentially, prodrugs are designed in such a way that their major or preferably single metabolic pathway is the one leading to the active drug ($k_3 \gg k_1 + k_2$; $k_2 \approx 0$).

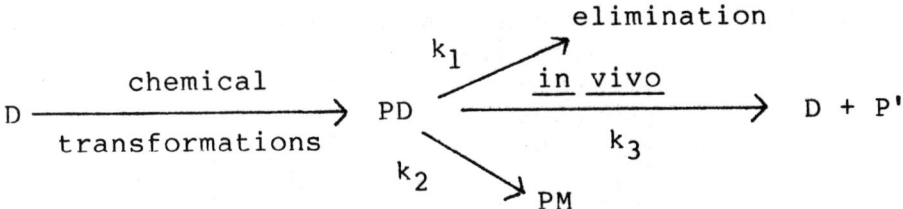

Prodrugs might effectively reduce some toxicities by protecting the drug from unwanted degradations, particularly those occurring in the gastrointestinal tract prior and during absorption or possibly during the first passage through the liver. Several reviews discuss these aspects (3-5). It was, however, found that simple prodrug manipulations cannot, in most cases, affect site specificity of the drugs (1, 6-8). In general, the prodrug approach can improve drug delivery or can provide delivery to sites inaccessible to the drug. For example, pralidoxime (**1**), the drug of choice for reactivating inhibited acetylcholine esterase (AchE), is ineffective in the brain since as a charged, quaternary pyridinium salt, it cannot pass the blood-brain barrier (BBB). It could, however, be delivered to the brain in its lipophilic, dihydropyridine prodrug form (**2**), which then <u>in situ</u> is oxidized to the active form **1** (9). The overall result was a dramatic improvement in the reactivation <u>in vivo</u> of the phosphorylated AchE. It should be emphasized, however, that this is not a site-specific delivery; the drug was delivered to the brain <u>in addition</u> to the rest of the body.

There are a few cases where simple prodrugs lead to organ- and/or site-enhanced delivery. An extension of the above approach (**1⇌2**) to a larger quaternary salt, berberine (**3**), leads to its specific accumulation and retention in the brain (10) as the BBB hinders the efflux of large quaternary salts, contrary to the facile elimination of small charged species like **2**, which presumably is done by an active transport system (11). Thus, **3** was found in high and sustained concentrations in brain following administration of **4**.

There are a few other examples for limited site-enhanced drug delivery using prodrugs (8), primarily based on differential and selective enzyme distributions.

Drug targeting can, however, be accomplished by using site-specific chemical delivery systems or simply "chemical delivery systems" (CDS's). The term CDS was previously used for describing prodrugs (4). It is, however, suggested that these two terms be separated. As compared to prodrugs, chemical delivery systems (12) actually represent a more advanced step. A CDS is formed by transforming a drug to a more removed, inactive form which will undergo several predictable transformations ultimately resulting in the delivery of the drug at the site of action. The emphasis is on the several, successive steps which will result in the optimization not only of the drug delivery, but of the therapeutic index, by effectively separating the site of action from the rest of the body. This can be achieved by physical and affinity based separations of the intermediate delivery forms, which are also inactive. The final step, the activation of the last intermediate (which could be called a prodrug formed in situ) to the active species, takes place preferentially at the site of action due to the specific accumulation of the direct precursor (DP) at the site, or by specific affinity or enzyme distribution differences. One could also call a CDS a pro-pro-pro-...drug or in a simple form a $(pro)_n$-drug, but it is believed that the CDS is a simple and descriptive term. A CDS can be illustrated as shown in Scheme 1.

$$[D] + \begin{Bmatrix} CS_1 \\ CS_2 \\ \vdots \\ CS_n \end{Bmatrix} \xrightarrow{\text{chemical transformations}} [CDS] \xrightarrow{\text{delivery to body}} [CDS] \xrightarrow{p^E}$$

$$\underset{\text{at site}}{[D] + p^1} \xleftarrow{\underset{\text{activation}}{\text{final}}} [DP] \xleftarrow{\underset{\text{reaction(n)}}{\text{enzymatic}}} [CDS]_2 \xleftarrow{\underset{\text{reaction(2)}}{\text{enzymatic}}} [CDS]_1 \xleftarrow{\underset{\text{reaction (1)}}{\text{enzymatic}}}$$

with p^E partial elimination at each enzymatic step.

p^E - partial elimination
$CS_1...CS_n$ - labile moities

Use of the Chemical Delivery Systems for Site-Specific Drug Delivery

A good example for site-specific delivery of a natural endogenous compound, epinephrine (5), is provided by the CDS based on diesters of adrenalone, for example, the diisovaleryl derivative (6). It was found some years ago (13), that adrenalone diesters have a high level of ocular sympathomimetic activity. Both mydriactic response and reduction of intraocular pressure were observed using these compounds at a low concentration of 0.04%. This finding is more surprising in view of the lack of sympathomimetic activity of adrenalone (7) itself, even at a high 2% concentration. It is remarkable that some of the esters (6) are more potent than the highly active prodrug form (14) of adrenalin, dipivalyl adrenaline (8). The pharmacological basis for the observed activity was unclear, but it was assumed that 6 is somehow transformed into the active adrenaline (5) in the eye via a combined reduction-hydrolysis process while adrenalone (7) is not reduced to 5.

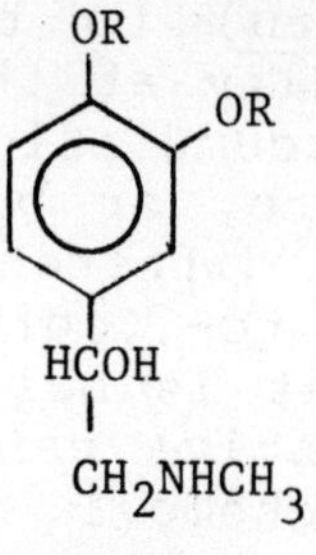

	Nr	
	5	R = H
	8	R = $-CO-C(CH_3)_3$
	9	R = $-CO-CH_3CH(CH_3)_2$
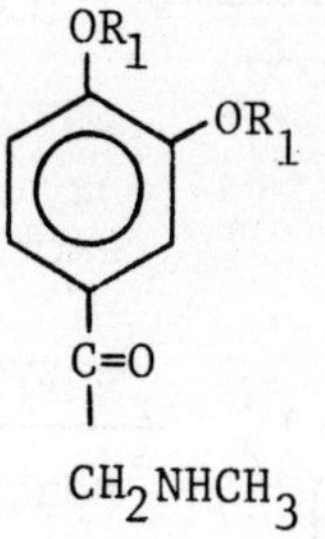	7	R_1 = H
	6	R_1 = $-CO-CH_2CH(CH_3)_2$

Structures shown:
- Compounds 5, 8, 9: benzene ring with two OR groups, HCOH–CH$_2$NHCH$_3$ side chain.
- Compounds 7, 6: benzene ring with two OR_1 groups, C=O–CH$_2$NHCH$_3$ side chain.

In most of the studies dealing with the transport and the disposition of topically applied ophthalmic agents, the anterior segment has been considered to be the target area. Few of these studies, however, consider the quantitative distribution and metabolism of the drug in ocular tissues and structures. In many instances only drug levels in aqueous humor are determined, and from these data conclusions are often made concerning transport efficiency and bioavailability. In the case of the delivery system of the type **6**, the analysis of tissue concentrations within the eye and the determination of the major site of biotransformation of these compounds are critical to the evaluation of the drug of action. Analysis of the aqueous humor alone would not accurately reflect the various processes that determine adrenalone activity. Thus, the concentration of both the inactive **7** and that of epinephrine (**5**) were determined in various compartments of the eye (15), following administration of one of the more potent diesters of adrenalone, **6**. The results are shown in Table 1.

Table 1. Tissue Concentration of Adrenalone (7) and Adrenaline (5) Following Topical Administration of Diisovaleryl Adrenalone (6)

	Concentration of adrenalone, 7		
	15 min ($\mu g\ g^{-1}$)	30 min ($\mu g\ g^{-1}$)	60 min ($\mu g\ g^{-1}$)
Cornea	4.47±1.14	7.75±1.92	2.72±0.84
Aqueous humor	0.33±0.09	0.87±0.27	0.52±0.12
Iris/ciliary body	0.42±0.14	2.61±0.72	1.11±0.86

	Concentration of adrenalin, 5		
	15 min ($\mu g\ g^{-1}$)	30 min ($\mu g\ g^{-1}$)	60 min ($\mu g\ g^{-1}$)
Cornea	--[b]	--[b]	--
Aqueous humor	--[b]	--[b]	--
Iris/ciliary body	0.09±0.05	0.58±0.35	0.04±0.01

[a]Dose equivalent to 0.05% adrenaline.

[b]Below detection limit for adrenaline of 0.035 µg/g tissue. HPLC with EC detector was used (potential 0.7V).

Comparable results following administration of the prodrug diisovaleryl adrenaline (9) and adrenalone (7), respectively, are shown in Tables 2 and 3.

Table 2. Tissue Concentrations of Adrenalin (5) Following Topical Administration of Diisovaleryl Adrenaline (9).[a]

Cornea	5.72±0.50 µg g^{-1}
Aqueous humor	0.14±0.04 µg g^{-1}
Iris/ciliary body	0.29±0.09 µg g^{-1}

[a]Determined at 30 min after administration. Dose equivalent to 0.05% of parent compound (adrenalin).

Table 3. Tissue Concentration of Adrenalone Following Its Topical Administration (30 Min)[a]

Cornea	0.52±0.13 µg g^{-1}
Aqueous humor	0.04±0.03 µg g^{-1}
Iris/ciliary body	0.13±0.09 µg g^{-1}

[a]Determined at 30 min after administration. A solution of 2% adrenalone-HCl was used. <u>No</u> adrenalin could be detected.

Following administration of the diester **6**, tissue concentrations of adrenalone can be seen to increase and decrease quite rapidly. The highest levels were found in the cornea, and this is characteristic of its role as both the major barrier to penetration and its capacity to act as a drug reservoir. The concentration of adrenalone in the aqueous humor follows the same time course as that determined in other tissues, but the levels are significantly lower. The iris/ciliary body tissues were found to have a fairly large concentration of adrenalone, with peak levels coinciding with those of the aqueous humor and the cornea. The most interesting and significant finding of these experiments was the detection and quantitation of the potent adrenergic agonist, adrenalin, in the uveal tissues. The presence of a significant quantity of adrenalin exclusively in the iris/ciliary body tissue in the same time frame as the peak levels of adrenalone is indicative of drug biotransformation. The bioactivation of adrenalone esters, either the diester or the monoester forms, by a reduction process appears to account for the detection of adrenalin as a metabolite of adrenalone. Control animals did not have any detectable quantities of endogenous adrenalin present (detection limit = 200 pg). Based on evidence reported in the literature and on our own experiments, the iris/ciliary body tissue appears to be one of the major sites of drug metabolism in the eye. It is not surprising, therefore, that adrenalin is found there and only there. On the other hand, the rapid disappearance of the adrenalin produced is probably related to significant levels of monoamine oxidase (MAO) and catechol O-methyltransferase (COMT) activity in these tissues. The role of COMT and MAO in the inactivation of catecholamines is well known, and the presence of these enzyme systems may limit the amount of detectable adrenalin due to rapid metabolism before the tissue can be extracted. The question of stereospecificity of the adrenalone reductase and its specificity for the diester form or the catecholamine itself is unclear. However, the low intrinsic activity of the D-enantiomer implies that a considerable proportion (and maybe all) of the adrenalin was produced in the L-form. In an important supportive experiment, a 2% concentration of adrenalone was studied; this is 40 times higher than the dose equivalent used when testing the diester. Tissue concentrations were determined, as in the case of **6**, indicating high levels in the cornea and significant concentrations in the iris/ciliary body (Table 3). However, no activity was observed, supporting again the assumption that adrenalone is not a good substrate for the reductive enzyme. In addition, when a 0.05% solution of the diisovaleryl adrenalin (**3**) was administered, adrenalin (**7**) concentrations were comparable in the iris/ciliary body, but much higher in the cornea and the aqueous humor (compare Tables 2 and 4). Thus, it appears that the diester and the monoesters of adrenalone may be the preferred substrates for the reductase as shown in Scheme 2, summarizing the bioactivation of 6.

Scheme 2

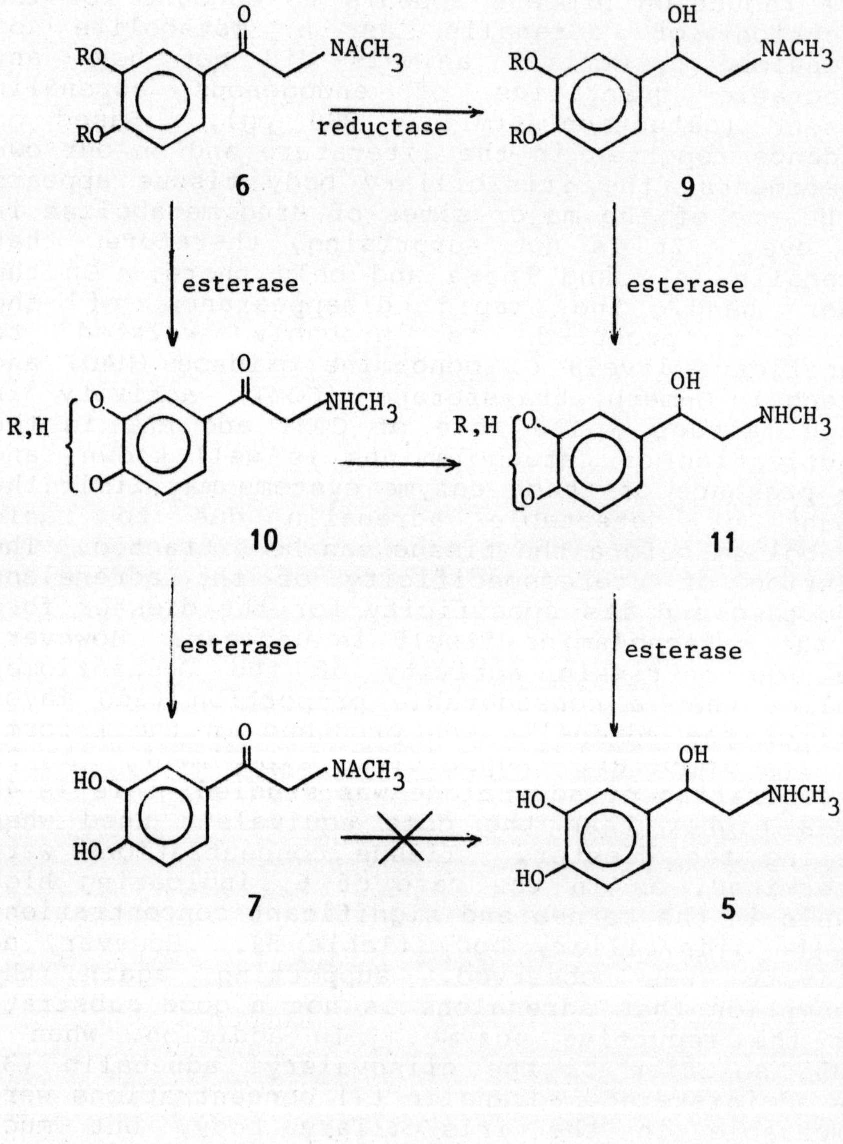

According to this, the diisovaleryl adrenalone undergoes two major transformations: either (1) direct or sequential hydrolysis by esterases of the esterified catechols to the inactive adrenalone, or (2) reduction of the ketone to the alcohol followed by esterase cleavage of the esters eventually leading to the active adrenaline.

These investigations clearly indicate that the diester derivatives of adrenalone are not simply prodrugs, but rather comprise efficient chemical delivery systems, that is, site-specifically activated. This type of system is superior to other chemical approaches, for example, adrenalin prodrugs (14) because of fast and predictable metabolism of the transport form, formation of the active component only at the site of action and, thus, avoidance of toxic effects resulting from nontarget tissue exposure. An adrenalin prodrug such as 9 delivers the drug to all compartments of the eye, and, due to substantial drainage, it will also deliver it sytemically.

The detection of significant quantities of adrenalin as a major metabolite of the CDS 6 implies that enzymatic carbonyl reduction occurs in the eye and this activity can be useful in the design of other bioreversible transport systems.

It is evident that the concept of developing methods for site-specific delivery of biologically active agents is highly desirable to improve efficacy and decrease toxicity. The site-specific and sustained release of drugs to the brain is even more difficult. The delivery of drugs to the brain is often seriously limited by transport and metabolism factors and, more specifically, by the functional barrier of the endothelial brain capillary wall called the blood-brain barrier (BBB). It is generally accepted that the ability of the molecule to cross the blood-brain barrier is a function of its partition coefficient between lipid and water. Lipid-insoluble or highly ionized compounds fail to achieve a cerebrospinal fluid (CSF) over plasma distribution ratio of 1, unless they are actively transported. This is due to the 8act that the rate of entry is much slower than the rate of exit from the CSF. The approach of derivatizing the compound and forming a prodrug that exhibits improved physicochemical properties for the transport through the blood-brain barrier should be treated with caution. Indeed, while one can improve delivery of the drug to the brain, the prodrug may simultaneously exhibit improved transport to other tissues and depots, thus increasing the incidence of systemic side effects. In addition, one has to keep in mind that these prodrugs, in analogy with lipidic compounds which do pass the blood-brain barrier, can be kept at <u>therapeutically useful levels in the brain only if there is sufficient circulating concentration</u>. In other words, one has to keep the whole body loaded with the compound, and generally at relatively high concentrations. This is a serious limitation in many cases due to peripheral toxicity. Delivering drugs exclusively or preferentially to the brain is very difficult, and, until recently, no simple and general method to achieve this goal had been known. A general method based on a dihydropyridine⇌pyridinium-type redox delivery system for brain-specific sustained release of the drugs was recently developed (16) which can be summarized as shown in Scheme 3.

According to this scheme (17), a drug [D] is either coupled to a tertiary amino heteroaromatic carrier [C] and then quaternized, or coupled to a quaternary pyridinium carrier [QC]$^+$ directly, and the obtained [D-QC]$^+$ is reduced chemically to the lipophilic dihydro form [D-DHC]. After <u>in vivo</u> administration of this [D-DHC] compound, it is quickly distributed (k_o) throughout the body, including the brain. The dihydro form [D-DHC] is then oxidized in the brain (k_1^1) and in the body (k_1^2) (e.g., by NAD/NADH systems) to the original [D-QC]$^+$ (ideally inactive) quaternary salt. (Superscript 1 refers to processes in the brain, while superscript 2 indicates similar process in the body. These latter processes are assigned an overall rate, e.g., k_1^2, for oxidation, although the actual process takes place with different rates in the various organs.) Due to its ionic hydrophilic character, [D-QC]$^+$ should be eliminated rapidly from the brain ($k_2 \gg k_3$; $k_2 \gg k_7$). Enzymatic cleavage of the [D-QC]$^+$ that <u>is trapped in the brain</u> will result in a sustained delivery of the drug species [D], followed by its normal elimination (k_5^1) and metabolism. A properly selected carrier, [QC]$^+$, will also be easily eliminated rapidly from the brain ($k_6^1 \gg k_3$). Due to the facile elimination of $[D-QC]^+$ from the general circulation, only small amounts of the drug are released in the body ($k_2 \gg k_4^2$), hence D will be released primarily in the brain ($k_4^1 > k_3$). The overall result, ideally, will be a <u>brain-specific</u> <u>sustained</u> <u>release</u> <u>of</u> <u>the</u> <u>target</u> <u>drug</u>.

A quick analysis of the concept indicates that this is not a simple prodrug type design, but again, a "chemical delivery system." That is, the final $[D-QC]^+$ species can be considered a prodrug of [D], but the reduced [D-DHC] form, which is actually delivered, is not a prodrug; rather, it is a special pro-prodrug with additional properties resulting in a site-specific and sustained release. In practice, in many instances, additional derivatization of other hydrophilic functions in the molecule is necessary. Thus, following "lock-in" of the changed species, a number of enzymatic reactions (see Scheme 1) are required to release the active drug.

One additional, very significant aspect of the present redox delivery system relates to toxicity: It is expected to significantly reduce systemic toxicity by accelerating the elimination of the drug-quaternary carrier system from the general circulation. On the other hand, even the central toxicity should be reduced by providing a low-level sustained release of the active species in the brain. One main factor in this whole picture is the <u>choice</u> <u>of</u> <u>the</u> <u>quaternary</u> <u>carrier</u>, which must be of <u>low toxicity</u> alone and in combination with the drug.

It is important to note that this method will provide the desired level of a drug in the CNS without requiring high circulatory concentrations. The drug blood level has virtually no effect on the brain levels, once the last oxidation step and the "lock-in" process have taken place.

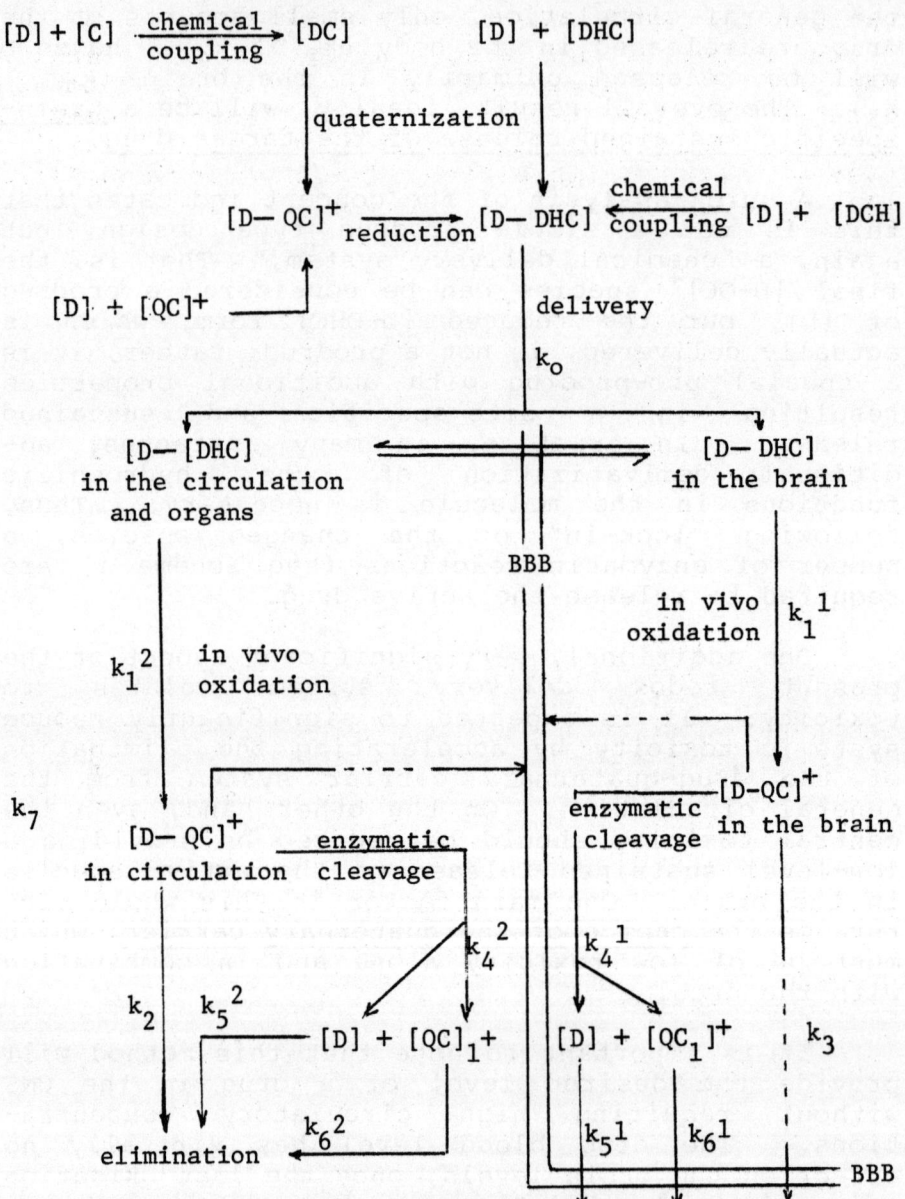

This general approach was applied in the past several years to the brain-specific delivery of a variety of CNS agents and centrally acting endogenous compounds and drugs. Particular attention was paid to the redox carrier system, trying to use analogs of the ubiquitous $NAD^+ \rightleftarrows NADH$ coenzyme system. Thus, the first and most studied carrier system is the trigonelline (2) $\rightleftarrows$ dihydrotrigonelline (13)-type:

$$R = -\overset{O}{\underset{}{C}}- \quad ; \quad -\overset{O}{\underset{}{C}}-CH_2- \quad ;$$

This redox delivery system was successfully applied for the brain delivery of phenylethylamine (12), testosterone (18), and for the more complex case of dopamine (19, 20). The case of dopamine (14) demonstrates the complexity of multiple hydrophilic groups in a molecule, and ultimately the redox carrier (see 13) was placed on the amino function, while the catechol system was protected by acylation.

It was shown (19) that following administration of the CDS **15**, the direct precursor (**16**) was "locked in" the brain at high and sustained concentrations, while it was quickly eliminated from the general circulatory system, indicating successful brain-specific delivery. The locked in precursor **16** then slowly releases dopamine (**14**), as first demonstrated by a substantial and prolonged inhibition of prolaction. Thus a small 1 mg/kg dose of **15** produces a 65-80% reduction in prolactin levels in male rats for at least 12 hours. The effect is clearly due to the release of dopamine, since the locked in precursor **16**, the CDS **15**, or other intermediates are completely void of intrinsic dopaminergic activity (lack of activity <u>in vitro</u> pituitary preparations). However, we did not detect stereotypic activity at any of these times in response to the drug. Thus, **14** may be selectively formed and released in the hypothalamus at a rate which suppresses pituitary prolactin release but does not induce stereotypy. This is not surprising, since prolactin inhibition is detected at doses of dopaminergic drugs which are 10 to 30 times lower than that needed to induce stereotypic behavior.

To document formation of dopamine from the delivery system, we treated animals intravenously with two of the CDS's, R = pivalyl **15a** or isovaleryl **15b**, or **14** itself and 30 minutes later administered the aromatic amino acid decarboxylase inhibitor m-hydroxybenzylhydrazine (NSD 1015) to block formation of endogenous **14**. While administration of dopamine did not alter the concentrations of dopamine (**14**) and its major metabolites, DOPAC (dihydroxyphenylacetic acid, **17**) and HVA (homovanillic acid, **18**) in the striatum or hypothalamus, **15a** and **15b** caused a 17 to 20% increase in striatal levels of **14** and a 4- to 5-fold increase in hypothalamic levels of **14** as shown in Table 4.

Table 4. Influence of the dopamine CDS's **15a** and **15b** and dopamine **14** on the brain dopamine concentration and metabolism in rats[a]

Compound tested	N	Dopamine 14 pmol/mg ±S.D.	DOPAC 17 pmol/mg ±S.D.	HVA 18 pmol/mg ±S.D.
		Striatum[b]		
Placebo	13	64.4±4.78	2.39±0.72	4.19±0.73
Dopamine[c] 14	7	62.1±3.20	1.90±0.31	3.96±0.42
15a	7	75.5±5.87*	12.3±1.18*	1.87±0.24*
15b	7	81.5±2.94	9.15±1.16	1.52±0.18*
		Hypothalamus[b]		
Placebo	13	2.27±0.25	0.18±0.04	0.25±0.04
Dopamine[c] 14	7	2.27±0.31	0.19±0.02	0.28±0.04
15a	7	9.83±3.71*	1.09±0.22*	0.31±0.04
15b	7	10.40±5.45	0.82±0.18	0.33±0.03

[a]Male rats were given i.v. **15a** and **15b** at 30 mg/kg (68 and 72 pmol/kg, respectively) in 60% DMSO-water; 30 min later, 100 mg/kg of NSD 1015, m-hydroxybenzylhydrazine was given i.p.
[b]One hour following administration.
[c]Dopamine was given at only 17.5 μmol/kg dose due to its toxicity.
*$p<0.05$.

As expected, concentrations of **17** were increased in both the striatum and hypothalamus after **15a** or **15b**, and levels of **18** were increased in the hypothalamus but decreased in the striatum. These data (24) demonstrate that inhibition of endogenous synthesis of **14** is required to document the delivery of dopamine by our redox system and suggest that **14** formed from **15a** and **15b** competes with newly synthesized **14** for available storage vesicles. Since newly synthesized **14** is preferentially released from dopaminergic neurons, the amount of **14** formed from **15a** and **15b** would appear to replete a functional, releasable pool of dopamine.

Recently, the effectiveness of the CDS **15** in the treatment of prolactin releasing tumors was demonstrated (22). When prolactin releasing tumors were implanted s.c. in rats, as expected, significant reduction in their brain dopamine levels were observed. However, the brain levels of **14** could be restored to the normal level following treatment with the CDS **15**.

The redox delivery system of the type **12**⇌**13** was also employed for the delivery of other neurotransmitters and their natural precursors. Thus, significant brain-specific delivery for tryptamine (**19**) and tryptophan (**20**) was demonstrated (23).

The redox delivery system for dopamine exerted differential metabolic and pharmacologic effects in the hypothalamus and striatum. In normal rats, the delivery system reduced serum prolactin in association with increased hypothalamic concentrations of both **17** and **18**, while in the striatum, the increase in levels of **17** was consistently associated with a reduction in concentrations of **18** and an absence of stereotypy. Compound **18** is formed by the sequential 3-O-methyltyramine. The increase in hypothalamic **18** following **15a** or **15b** may indicate enhanced release of dopamine, since, among other neuronal sites, COMT is located on the postsynaptic membranes. This interpretation is consistent with the reduction in serum prolactin associated with <u>in vivo</u> administration of **15a** and provides evidence for the relative absence of auto-receptors for **14** or an effective dopamine reuptake system for **14** in tuberoinfundibular neurons. Thus, in the hypothalamus and, in particular, the tuberoinfundibular dopamine system, this compound is formed from this chemical delivery system and appears to be released from nerve terminals and delivered to the pituitary to inhibit prolactin secretion.

Although **14** is formed from **15a** or **15b** in the striatum, we did not observe stereotypy and consistently found reduced concentrations of **18**. Collectively, these observations indicate that concentrations of striatal **14** achieved by the drug are not sufficient to cause the profound stimulation of striatal dopamine receptors needed to induce stereotypy.

GABA (γ-aminobutyric acid, **21**) is another important neurotransmitter implicated particularly in epilepsy. It does not penetrate the BBB. It was converted to various redox CDS's (24), among which the benzyl ester **22** was particularly effective. It was found that after administration of **22** to rats, **22** and the corresponding oxidized **23** disappear quickly (detectable only for a maximum of 1 hour) from the blood and the various organs (liver, kidney, lung, heart), except the brain. In the brain, significant concentrations of **23** can be found for over 8 hours (25).

More importantly, very significant anti-convulsant activity for **22** was found (25) in the bicuculline induced convulsion. The CDS **22** was more effective (ED_{50} = 23 mg/kg) than the known progabide (ED_{50} = 50 mg/kg) or its acid metabolite, SL75102 (ED_{50} = 75 mg/kg).

The above examples illustrate brain-specific delivery of compounds which cannot otherwise be delivered to the brain: Circulating neurotransmitters generally do not penetrate the BBB, except some of their precursors like L-DOPA or tryptophan, which are actively transported.

The brain-specific redox delivery system, however, is very useful for drugs which do penetrate the BBB. While most steroid hormones readily pass into and out of the brain due to their lipophilic nature, the necessary blood-brain equilibrium has limited their usefulness in treating brain-specific, steroid-deprivation syndromes, such as hot flushes. Also, the use of steroidal hormones to achieve reduction in gonadotropin secretion for contraception and the treatment of steroid-dependent diseases such as endometriosis and prostatic hypertrophy, is limited by the unwanted peripheral side effects of these hormones.

For these reasons, this redox system for the specific delivery of steroids to the CNS was evaluated. Application of the redox system to testosterone resulted in the accumulation of the ionized form of the chemical delivery system in the brain and persistent, local release of the active steroid (26). Both the brain-blood concentration ration and the brain-elimination half-life were dramatically changed (26).

In a very important, recent development, it was shown that the sustained brain-specifc delivery of the natural estrogen, estradiol (24), can also be accomplished. First, it was established (27) that when the CDS 25 was administered to male rats, the corresponding charged precursor 26 was essentially cleared from the liver by 6 hours and from the lung and kidney by 24 hours, while brain levels of 26 remained elevated.

To evaluate the response of luteinizing hormone (LH) to this chemical delivery system, the CDS **25** (3.0 mg/kg), an equimolar dose of estradiol (2.1 mg/kg), or the dimethylsulfoxide (DMSO) vehicle were administered to male rats at 2 weeks after orchidectomy. Both estradiol and **25** reduced serum LH concentrations equivalently by 68 to 79% from 4 to 48 hours. From 4 to 12 days after drug administration, the LH levels in estradiol-treated animals increased progressively to levels equivalent to those in DMSO-treated rats. By contrast, LH concentrations in animals treated with **25** continued to be suppressed by 82, 88, and 90% when compared to control (DMSO) values at 4, 8, and 12 days after treatment, respectively.

To better define the time-course of the suppression of LH by **25**, the aforementioned study was repeated and animals sampled for serum LH and estradiol concentrations at 12 to 24 days after administration of **25**, estradiol, or DMSO. While estradiol did not suppress serum LH from 12 to 24 days after a single intravenous injection, compound **25** reduced LH concentrations by 88, 86, and 66% relative to the DMSO controls at 12, 18, and 24 days, respectively (Table 5). It is important to note that serum concentrations of estradiol were not different among treatment groups and were undetectable in most samples. Thus, a persistent elevation in circulating concentrations of estradiol subsequent to the administration of compound **25** was not responsible for the observed, chronic suppression of LH release. Rather, <u>local release of estradiol in the brain</u>, and in particular the hypothalamus, would appear to be responsible for the sustained suppression of LH release (28).

Table 5. Serum Concentrations of LH and Estradiol After Intravenous Administration of DMSO, Estradiol, or Compound 25 in Orchidectomized Rats

	Days After Administration		
	12	18	24
	Serum LH (ng/ml)		
DMSO	6.8±0.8(7)[a]	12.4±2.5(7)	8.6±1.7(7)
Estradiol (2.1 mg/kg)	12.9±1.7(6)*	12.1±0.9(6)	11.6±1.4(7)
Compound 25 (3.0.mg/kg)	0.8±0.4(7)*	1.7±0.7(7)	2.9±1.1(7)
	Serum Estradiol (pg/ml)		
DMSO	27.5±3.8(4/7)[b]	<20(7/7)	24.4±3.3(4/7)
Estradiol (2.1 mg/kg)	29.3±5.9(4/6)	<20(6/6)	31.2±8.6(3/6)
Compound 25 (3.0 mg/kg)	25.9±3.9(5/7)	<20(7/7)	24.1±3.2(5.7)

Serum was assayed for LH and estradiol by radioimmunoassay in duplicate. a = mean ± SEM (number of animals per group). b = mean ± SEM (number of samples which were below the sensitivity limit of the assay (20 pg/ml)/number of animals per group). * = significantly ($p<0.05$) different from both other groups.

In these experiments the effect of the delivered estradiol on LHRH containing neurons directly could not be dissociated from effects which may be mediated by an action of estradiol on the anterior pituitary gland subsequent to estradiol release from median eminence into the hypophyseal portal system. However, the observation of (1) the accumulation in the brain of the ionized, hydrophilic quaternary pyridinium salt-type ester of estradiol (26), (2) chronic (at least 24 days) suppression in LH secretion in rats following a single intravenous injection of **25**, d (3) low circulating concentrations of estradiol at 12 to 24 days after **25** administration strongly support a local action of the drug in the CNS, presumably on hypothalamic LHRH-containing neurons. The "lock-in" to the brain of the pyridinium salt, compound **26**, and the sustained local release of estradiol may provide a useful tool for the determination of the central versus peripheral site of action of this gonadal steroid in behavioral and physiological processes for which the locus of estradiol's site of action is uncertain. This chemical delivery system for estradiol may be useful clinically (1) in the treatment of vasomotor instability associated with ovariectomy or the menopause, particularly in women for whom peripheral estrogen activity is contraindicated, and (2) in the chronic reduction of gonadotropin secretion for fertility regulation or for the treatment of gonadal steroid-dependent disease, such as endometriosis and prostatic hypertrophy. Since gonadal steroids are believed to influence a variety of functions of the CNS, the presently described steroid delivery system may have uses beyond those related to regulation of gonadotropin secretion.

The use of the above redox brain delivery system was recently extended (29) to a variety of other important drug classes, including antiviral agents, antitumor drugs, analgesics, antiinflammatory and antibacterial agents, etc.

Conclusions

The concept of site-specific chemical delivery systems, or simply <u>chemical delivery systems (CDS's)</u>, provides an essentially unlimited opportunity to achieve the most pursued goal in therapeutics: drug targeting. The use of CDS's was exemplified in the present paper by specific delivery of epinephrine to the iris/ciliary body in the eye and by a variety of applications of a redox system to deliver in a specific and sustained way drugs to the brain. There are many other useful systems which allow drug targeting to other organs. Novel CDS's are currently investigated for drug targeting to the lung, liver, and heart.

Acknowledgements

Acknowledgement is made to the the National Institutes of Health (GM27167 and EYO5800-01) and to Pharmatec, Inc., for support of the research described. Special thanks are extended to Mss. Laurie Johnston, Joan Martignago, and Julie Driggers for preparation of the manuscript.

References

1. N. Bodor, Novel approaches to the design of safe drugs: soft drugs and site-specific chemical delivery systems. In: "Advances in Drug Research," Academic Press, London, 1984, pp. 255-331.
2. N. Bodor, Soft drugs: principles and methods for the design of safe drugs, Med. Res. Reviews, 4, 449 (1984).
3. A. Sinkula and S. Yalkowsky, Rationale for design of biologically reversible drug derivatives: prodrugs, J. Pharm. Sci., 64, 181 (1975).
4. T. Higuchi and V. Stella (Eds.), "Prodrugs as Novel Drug Delivery Systems," American Chemical Society, Washington, D.C., 1975.
5. N. Bodor, Novel approaches in prodrug design. In: "Optimization of Drug Delivery," Munksgaard, Copenhagen, 1982, pp. 156-177.
6. N. Bodor, Prodrugs vs. soft drugs, In: "Prodrugs," Elsevier, Amsterdam, 1985, pp. 331-352.
7. V.J. Stella and K.J. Himmelstein, Critique of prodrugs and site specific delivery. In: "Optimization of Drug Delivery," Munksgaard, Copenhagen, 1982, pp. 134-155.
8. V. Stella and K.T. Himmelstein, Prodrugs: A chemical approach to targeted drug delivery. In: "Directed Drug Delivery," Humana Press, Clifton, New Jersey, 1985, pp. 247-267.
9. N. Bodor, E. Shek and T. Higuchi, Delivery of a quaternary pyridinium salt across the blood brain barrier by its dihydropyridine derivative, Science, 190, 155 (1975).
10. N. Bodor and M.E. Brewster, Improved delivery through biological membranes XV. Sustained brain delivery of berberine, Eur. J. Med. Chem., 18, 235 (1983).

11. N. Bodor, R.G. Roller and S.H. Selk, Elimination of a quaternary salt delivered as its derivative from the brain of mice, J. Pharm. Sci., 67, 685 (1978).
12. N. Bodor and H.H. Farag, A redox chemical drug delivery system as its use for brain-specific delivery of phenylethylamine, J. Med. Chem., 26, 313 (1983).
13. N. Bodor, J.J. Kaminski and R.G. Roller, Improved delivery through biological membranes VI. Potent sympathomimetic adrenalone derivatives, Int. J. Pharm., 1, 189 (1976).
14. A. Hussain and J. Truelove, Prodrug aproaches to enhancement of physicochemical properties of drugs IV: novel epinephrine prodrug, J. Pharm. Sci., 65, 1510 (1976).
15. N. Bodor and G. Visor, Formation of adrenaline in the iris-ciliary body from adrenalone diester, Exp. Eye Res., 38, 621 (1984).
16. N. Bodor, H.H. Farag and M.E. Brewster, Site specific and sustained release of drugs to the brain, Science, 214, 1370 (1981).
17. N. Bodor and M.E. Brewster, Problems of delivery of drugs to the brain, Pharm. & Ther., 19, 337 (1983).
18. N. Bodor and H.H. Farag, Brain-specific, sustained delivery of testosterone using a redox chemical delivery system, J. Pharm. Sci., 73, 385 (1986).
19. N. Bodor and H.H. Farag, Brain-specific delivery of dopamine with a dihydropyridine⇌pyridinium salt type redox delivery system, J. Med. Chem., 26, 528 (1983).
20. N. Bodor and J.W. Simpkins, Redox delivery system for brain-specific, sustained release of dopamine, Science, 221, 65 (1983).
21. J.W. Simpkins, N. Bodor and A. Enz, Direct evidence for brain-specific release of dopamine from a redox delivery system, J. Pharm. Sci., 74, 1033 (1985).
22. J.W. Simpkins, W. Anderson and N. Bodor, unpublished results.
23. N. Bodor, T. Nakamura and M.E. Brewster, unpublished results.
24. P.A. Woodard, "Delivery of potential antiepileptics to the brain utilizing a dihydropyridine⇌pyridinium salt redox system," Ph.D. thesis, University of Florida, 1985.

25. P.A. Woodard, D. Winwood, M.E. Brewster, and N. Bodor, Improved delivery through biological membranes XI. Design, synthesis and anti- agents. (Submitted for publication.)
26. N. Bodor and H.H. Farag, Improved delivery through biological membranes XIV. Brain-specific, sustained delivery of testosterone using a redox chemical delivery system, J. Pharm. Sci., 73, 385 (1984).
27. J. McCornack. The application of dihydropyridine⇌pyridinium salt redox system to brain-specific delivery of estradiol, M.S. thesis, University of Florida, 1983.
28. J.W. Simpkins, J. McCornack, K.S. Estes, M.E. Brewster, E. Shek and N. Bodor, Sustained brain-specific delivery of estradiol causes long-term suppression of LH secretion. (Submitted for publication, 1985.)
29. N. Bodor, "Brain-specific drug delivery," U.S. Patent 4,540,564/Sept. 10, 1985.

Chapter 4
Application of Physical Organic Concepts to In Vitro and In Vivo Lability Design of Water Soluble Prodrugs

Bradley D. Anderson and Robert A. Conradi

Department of Pharmaceutics
College of Pharmacy
University of Utah
Salt Lake City, UT 84112

Introduction

The synthesis of a prodrug to increase the aqueous solubility of a poorly soluble drug to allow for intravenous or intramuscular injection or opthalmic delivery would appear to be a relatively trivial undertaking. Naively, we might assume that the only requirement is that the parent compound have a suitable functional group to serve as a "handle" to which one could attach an ionizable pro-moiety. Given recent advances in derivatization techniques for various functional groups as discussed by Hans Bundgaard in this book, the availability of a suitable "handle" is no longer the constraint it once was. It would seem, therefore, that water soluble prodrug formation is now a part of the classical armamentarium, and the chemist synthesizing the parent drug could just as easily supply a water soluble prodrug for use in injectable solution dosage forms.

As drug delivery system design has become more sophisticated and controlled, however, it has become increasingly apparent that while the coupling of a drug and a solubilizing moiety in a bioreversible manner may indeed constitute the synthesis of a water soluble prodrug, this is not prodrug design. Prodrug design entails the optimization of the physical and chemical properties of the prodrug so that its effectiveness as a delivery system for the parent drug is also optimized. This chapter will address the many factors which must be considered in water soluble prodrug design with particular emphasis on the control of lability in the formulation and in vivo.

Much of this discussion will center around a case history involving a specific prodrug design problem - the development of a solution stable, water soluble prodrug of a corticosteroid. However, the considerations addressed in this problem are sufficiently general that this example will hopefully serve as a prototype in prodrug optimization.

The design of a solution stable, water soluble prodrug for use in an injectable formulation poses to the researcher seemingly conflicting demands on lability. In vitro, the prodrug should be sufficiently stable to allow for the development of a ready-to-inject solution. Water soluble prodrugs which are unstable in solution may be lyophilized and reconstituted before use but this adds significantly to the cost of the product and to the inconvenience in their use. Ideally, therefore, a water soluble prodrug should have a shelf-life of two years or more at room temperature (15-30 °C). Assuming that the shelf-life is determined by the time required for 10% degradation, the prodrug's half-life in vitro should be $\simeq$ 13 years. If the only purpose of prodrug formation is solubilization of the parent compound, then bioconversion of the prodrug to parent drug in vivo should be rapid to closely mimic the properties of the parent compound. For purposes of this discussion, we may reasonably assume that >90% of the prodrug should be converted to the parent compound within 30 minutes after injection. For this ideal case the half-life in vivo should therefore be 10 minutes or less. Ideal water soluble prodrug design therefore requires an in vivo/in vitro lability ratio of nearly 10^6. Ratios of this order of magnitude or higher are readily achievable if the bioconversion is enzyme catalyzed. In the absence of enzyme mediated bioconversion such ratios would be extremely difficult to achieve.

This discussion will address the design of carboxylic acid esters as prodrugs. For such compounds, we can rely on enzyme catalyzed hydrolysis to achieve the desired lability in vivo. However, it will become increasingly apparent in the ensuing discussion that while the attainment of adequate formulation stability is a major problem for water soluble ester prodrugs, accomplishing this without sacrificing in vivo lability is significantly more challenging.

For convenience, this treatment is divided into two main sections. The first addresses those physical organic considerations which are important in determining the in vitro stability of esters. The second will focus on in vivo lability and the splitting of in vitro and in vivo reaction rates. We will demonstrate that formulation stability can be systematically designed into a prodrug molecule. While it would be presumptuous to make the same claim for in vivo lability, it will be shown that the ideal of achieving solution stability without sacrificing in vivo lability is realizable.

The specific objective which will serve as a basis for this discussion involved the design of a solution stable, water soluble derivative of the corticosteroid methylprednisolone (MP) for use in a ready-to-inject solution formulation[1-3] to replace the currently marketed succinate ester (1a). The structures of various esters of methylprednisolone which were examined in the pursuit of this goal are shown in Scheme I.

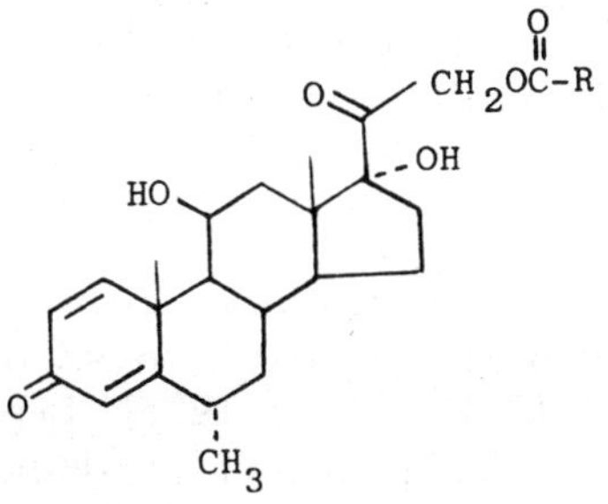

1a-u

a: R = -(CH$_2$)$_2$COOH
b: R = -CH$_3$
c: R = -CH$_2$COOH
d: R = -(CH$_2$)$_4$COOH
e: R = -(CH$_2$)$_6$COOH
f: R = -(CH$_2$)$_2$SO$_3$H
g: R = -(CH$_2$)$_5$SO$_3$H
h: R = -(CH$_2$)$_{10}$SO$_3$H
i: R = -(CH$_2$)$_2$CONHCH$_2$COOH
j: R = -(CH$_2$)$_2$(CONHCH$_2$)$_2$COOH
k: R = -(CH$_2$)$_5$SCH$_2$COOH

l: R = -(CH$_2$)$_5$SOCH$_2$COOH
m: R = -(CH$_2$)$_5$SO$_2$CH$_2$COOH
n: R = -(CH$_2$)$_2$CONH(CH$_2$)$_2$SO$_3$H
o: R = -(CH$_2$)$_2$CON(CH$_3$)CH$_2$CH$_2$SO$_3$H
p: R = -(CH$_2$)$_2$CONH(CH$_2$)$_2$N(CH$_3$)$_2$
q: R = -(CH$_2$)$_2$CON(CH$_3$)CH$_2$CH$_2$N(CH$_3$)$_2$
r: R = -(CH$_2$)$_5$N(CH$_3$)$_2$
s: R = -(CH$_2$)$_6$CON(CH$_3$)CH$_2$CH$_2$N(CH$_3$)$_2$
t: R = -(CH$_2$)$_6$CON(Et)CH$_2$CH$_2$N(Et)$_2$
u: R = -(CH$_2$)$_6$CON(CH$_3$)CH$_2$CH$_2$SO$_3$H

Scheme I

Succinate esters of corticosteroids, which are marketed by several manufacturers in lyophilized form,[4] provide a typical example of many of the shortcomings in current prodrug technology. Lyophilization is necessary due to the inadequate solution stability of succinate esters. Upon reconstitution, aqueous solutions of succinate esters of corticosteroids may exhibit shelf-lives of 48 hours or less at room temperature due to ester hydrolysis and precipitation of the hydrolysis product, the free corticosteroid.[5-7]

At the same time, the bioconversion of succinate ester prodrugs appears to be too slow relative to competing processes in some cases. Thus, free corticoid concentrations in plasma after intravenous or intramuscular injections of phosphate esters of corticosteroids were found to be significantly higher than the corresponding plasma levels after injections of equivalent amounts of the succinate esters.[8] The lower bioavailability of succinate esters was attributed to metabolism of the intact ester prior to hydrolysis. The succinate ester of chloramphenicol also appears to undergo slow, variable hydrolysis, adding an additional and unpredictable element to chloramphenicol dosing.[9,10] Clearly, succinate esters as prodrugs represent suboptimal design and thus will be a useful point of reference.

Design of Solution Stability

We will discuss three general principles which have proven valuable in the design of solution stable prodrugs. They are: (a) pH-solubility behavior is an important determinant of solution stability; (b) pH-degradation rate profiles can be optimized by considering the effects of neighboring substituents on ester hydrolysis; and (c) building micelle-forming properties into a prodrug can be advantageous in improving stability and solubilizing otherwise insoluble degradation products. Many prodrug design problems may require the application of all of the above principles simultaneously to achieve the necessary degree of stability improvement. This was the case in the design problem of interest.

pH-Solubility Profile Design

Since ester hydrolysis is both specific acid and specific base catalyzed, ester hydrolysis rates are pH-dependent generally exhibiting V-shaped pH-hydrolysis rate profiles in accordance with equation [1]:[11]

$$k_{obs} = k_{H^+}[H^+] + k_{H_2O} + k_{OH^-}[OH^-] \quad [1]$$

where the three terms represent acid catalysis, neutral water attack, and hydroxide ion attack, respectively. The pH of optimum stability for such compounds can be estimated by setting the derivative of equation [1] with respect to hydrogen ion equal to zero and solving for H^+_{min} to give equation [2]:

$$H^+_{min} = (K_w \cdot k_{OH^-}/k_{H^+})^{1/2} \qquad [2]$$

Since k_{OH^-} is generally much larger than k_{H^+}, the pH of optimum stability is typically between 3.5 and 5. For example, MP succinate's pH_{min} is 3.6[6] while that of MP acetate (1b) is 4.4.[12] This is the pH at which an ester in a solution formulation would exhibit greatest stability and it would therefore be advantageous to formulate at this pH. Injection of solutions at pH's of 3.5-5 should not pose a significant problem providing that the buffer capacity of such solutions is minimized.

In this treatment we are assuming that the ester linkage is the only reactive bond in the prodrug molecule. Other points of lability may exist which exhibit a significantly different pH dependence. These factors must be considered in the overall design. In the case of 21-esters of corticosteroids, ester hydrolysis was shown to be the major reaction limiting shelf-life.[1]

Derivatives which are made water soluble by the incorporation of an ionizable acidic or basic functional group into the pro-moiety exhibit pH-dependent solubilities which may or may not be compatible with the pH-stability constraints outlined above. Monoprotic acids, for example, exhibit solubilities, S, which have the following dependency on pH:[13]

$$S = C_o (1 + K_a/H^+) \qquad [3]$$

where C_o is the intrinsic solubility of the unionized species and K_a is the acid ionization constant. The ionized species is assumed in the above equation to have unlimited water solubility. Similar considerations apply for monobasic prodrugs where the pH dependence of the solubility would follow equation [4].

$$S = C_o (1 + H^+/K_a) \qquad [4]$$

C_o in this case would be the intrinsic solubility of the free base and the protonated species is assumed to have infinite solubility.

Assume for the sake of illustration that a 0.1 M solution formulation is desired. Rearranging equation [3] and solving for the pH required to achieve this solubility for the succinate ester of methylprednisolone which has an intrinsic solubility of 6×10^{-5} M[1] and a pKa of 4.54[6] gives a pH of 7.8 - far above the pH of optimum stability of 3.6. (Due to self-micellization of water soluble corticoid esters,[14] the actual pH required to attain a given solubility is somewhat lower. This example nevertheless illustrates the more general case where micelle formation does not occur.)

Ionizable derivatives having the requisite solubility at the pH-stability optimum can, in theory, be designed either by increasing the intrinsic solubility of the unionized species or altering the acidity or basicity of the solubilizing moiety.

Shown in Table I are several carboxylic acid containing esters of methylprednisolone in which two basic concepts were applied to increase water solubility. To increase intrinsic solubility additional polar functional groups were incorporated into the pro-moiety thus increasing the overall hydrophilicity of the molecule. To decrease the carboxylic acid's pKa electronegative substituents were attached to the carbon alpha to the carboxyl functionality. The relative solubilities of the compounds in this limited series allows us to assess the utility of these approaches.

Pro-Moiety Hydrophilicity and Intrinsic Solubility. The influence of polar functional groups on overall hydrophilicity is most clearly seen in their effects on oil/water partition coefficients. Functional group contributions to partitioning properties, though well documented, are not well understood at the molecular level.[15-16] Nevertheless, these empirical relationships are extremely useful in building into a molecule the desired hydrophilicity.

The relationship between hydrophilicity as measured by oil/water partition coefficients and aqueous solubility is more complex, requiring in addition an understanding of functional group effects on solid-state properties. This issue has been addressed elsewhere.[17] While a quantitative understanding of functional group contributions to aqueous solubility is lacking, it is frequently assumed that increasingly hydrophilic solutes have correspondingly higher water solubilities. However, some studies have shown that a correlation between aqueous solubility and hydrophilicity may not always exist. For example, the incorporation of polar, hydrogen bonding substituents into a series of prostaglandin derivatives resulted in an increase in both crystalline interaction energies and hydration energies and therefore aqueous solubility did not increase.[18]

Examining Table I, the more hydrophilic compounds in this series did exhibit higher intrinsic solubilities. However, the magnitudes of solubility increase were less than

Table I. Physicochemical Properties Relating to the Solubility of Various Carboxylic Acid Containing Prodrugs of Methylprednisolone

Cmpd No.	R (Scheme I)	P.C.[a]	Co (M x 10^4)	Taft σ^*[d]	pKa[e]	pH Required for 0.1 M Solubility[f]
1a	$-(CH_2)_2COOH$	240	0.60[c]	0.82	4.2(4.5)	7.8
1i	$-(CH_2)_2CONHCH_2COOH$	34	2.4[b]	1.56	3.7	6.3
1j	$-(CH_2)_2(CONHCH_2)_2COOH$	2.8	7.4[b]	1.56	3.7	5.8
1k	$-(CH_2)_5SCH_2COOH$	---	0.14[c]	1.44	3.8(4.1)	8.0
1l	$-(CH_2)_5SOCH_2COOH$	---	2.3[c]	2.88	2.8(2.6)	5.2
1m	$-(CH_2)_5SO_2CH_2COOH$	---	0.86[c]	3.68	2.3(2.7)	5.8

[a] Partition coefficients between ethyl acetate and water were determined at pH 2.5 and 25°C.
[b] Intrinsic solubilities determined in water at pH 2.5 and 25°C.
[c] Intrinsic solubilities obtained by least squares curve fitting of equation [3] to solubility data versus pH at 25°C.
[d] Constants are for substituents attached to the α-carbon atoms; from Ref. 21.
[e] predictions are from equation [5]. Values in parentheses were experimentally determined from solubility data at 25°C.
[f] Estimated from equation [3] (neglecting micelle formation).

might have been expected. Compare, for example, the ethyl acetate/water partition coefficients and intrinsic solubilities of methylprednisolone 21-hemisuccinate (1a), its glycine amide (1i), and the glycylglycine amide (1j). Whereas the ethyl acetate/water partition coefficient decreased by a factor of about 10 per additional $-CONHCH_2-$ group, the aqueous solubility increased by factors of only 3-4 within this series. Coupling these data with previous observations suggests that strategies to increase water solubility by increasing the hydrophilicity of a prodrug are unreliable.

<u>Modification of Pro-Moiety pKa</u>. Predictive relationships such as the Taft[19] and Hammett[20] equations enable one to use substituent effects to modify pKa. The Taft relationship for the pKa's of α-substituted carboxylic acids, RCH_2COOH, is:

$$pKa = 4.76 - 0.67 \; \sigma^* \qquad [5]$$

where σ^* is the Taft aliphatic substituent constant.

In Table I are listed the σ^* values for the substituents attached to the α-carbon adjacent to the carboxylic acid functionality and the estimated and experimental (when available) pKa's of each derivative. The -SOR and $-SO_2R$ groups were chosen for this comparison because they are strongly electron withdrawing, as evident in their σ^* values. The α-sulfinyl and α-sulfonyl substituted carboxylic acid promoieties therefore provide a means of obtaining carboxylic acid derivatives with pKa's of 2-3. These compounds are water soluble at a lower pH due largely to their lower pKa's. Also listed in Table 1 are the pH's at which 0.1 M solution formulations could be prepared based on the intrinsic solubilities and pKa's of each compound (neglecting micelle formation). Since ester stability increases by 10-fold per unit decrease in pH in the base catalyzed region, this comparison shows that increases in formulation stability of several orders of magnitude are possible by careful design of the pH-solubility profile, such that the prodrug is soluble at or near the pH-degradation rate minimum.

A simpler method of modifying pro-moiety acidity or basicity is to select other more acidic or basic ionizable functional groups. Convenient solubilizing moieties for ester prodrugs where the formulation pH should be between 3.5-5 would be those containing either sulfonic acid (pKa<2) or tertiary amine (pKa>8) functionalities. Quaternary ammonium containing moieties would also be obvious choices for water soluble derivatives if solubility were the only consideration. Most of the discussion which follows will focus on sulfonate or amine containing prodrugs due to their advantageous solubility-pH profiles.

pH-Hydrolysis Rate Profile Design

A wealth of literature on the influence of structure on ester reactivity[11,19,22] should enable the pharmaceutical chemist to predict lability of various ester prodrugs within a series after a limited number of baseline experiments. It is therefore feasible, within the constraints imposed by the inherent reactivity of the ester linkage, to design ester prodrugs with a desired pH-hydrolysis rate profile.

We will consider the influence of substituents acting as direct participants in the degradation reaction through intramolecular catalysis as well as the electronic and steric effects of substituents in the vicinity of the ester linkage.

Intramolecular Catalysis by Substituents. Succinate esters serve as examples of derivatives which exhibit less than optimal pH-hydrolysis rate behavior due to their increased reactivity in water as a result of intramolecular catalysis of hydrolysis by the terminal carboxylic acid functionality.[6,12] Intramolecular catalysis of the hydrolysis of MP 21-succinate by the terminal carboxyl group results in a rate enhancement of nearly 100-fold.

Acyl migration of the succinate moiety from the 21- to the 17-OH, shown in Scheme II, is also catalyzed intramolecularly. Intramolecular catalysis brings about a reversal in the relative rates of the 21->17 migration and 21-ester hydrolysis. In solutions of pH>7.4 hydrolysis dominates while acyl migration is dominant in the intramolecularly catalyzed region between pH 3.6 and 7.4.

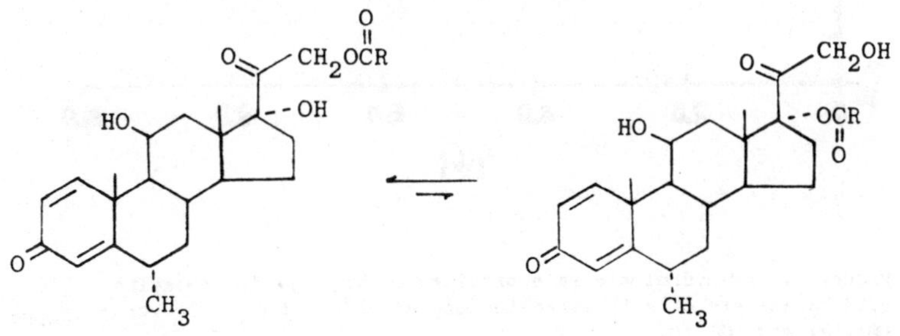

Scheme II

Since intramolecular catalytic effects are quite sensitive to geometric factors and distances separating the interactive groups,[23] intramolecular catalysis by a terminal ionizable group should be easily controlled by varying chain length. Plots of the pH-hydrolysis rate profiles of the 21-malonate (1c), succinate (1a), and adipate (1d) esters of methylprednisolone are shown in Figure 1 to illustrate the sensitivity of intramolecular catalysis to chain length. With 4 methylene groups separating the terminal carboxyl from the ester linkage, no intramolecular catalysis is observed. Decreasing chain length by 2 or 3 methylene groups resulted in rate enhancements in the catalyzed region of 100- and 7700-fold, respectively, in comparison to the rate constants for base catalyzed hydrolysis of the anions.

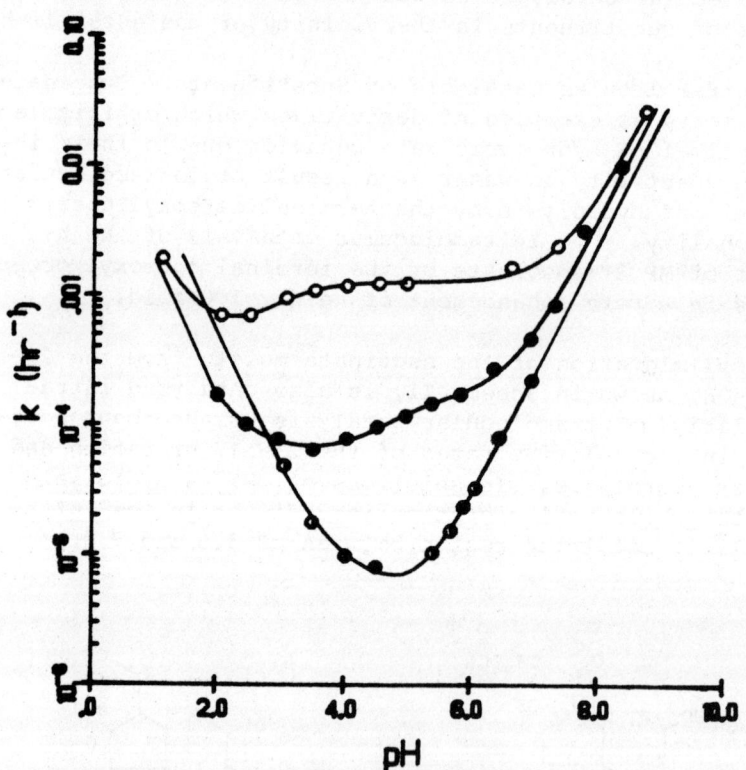

Figure 1. pH-hydrolysis rate profiles of various dicarboxylic acid hemiesters of methylprednisolone at $25°C$. Key: (O) 1c; (●) 1a; and (◐) 1d.

Similar chain length effects were seen in the intramolecular catalysis of acyl migration as shown in Figure 2. Again, increasing chain length from succinate to adipate completely eliminated catalysis by the terminal carboxylic acid group. Additional examples of the sensitivity of intramolecular catalysis to carboxyl group proximity have been reported previously.[23]

One approach taken to vary the solubilizing moiety in prodrugs of methylprednisolone utilized dicarboxylic acids as spacers, the desired terminal group being attached to the spacer via an amide linkage. Rate constants for acid and base catalyzed hydrolysis of several such amides of MP

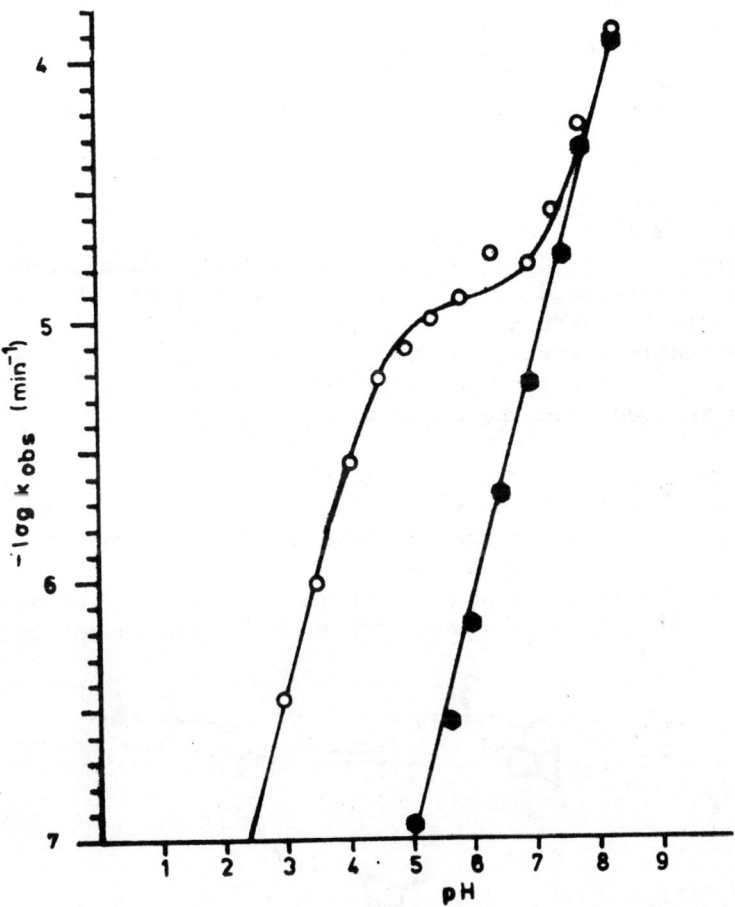

Figure 2. Profiles of 21->17 acyl migration rates versus pH for dicarboxylic acid hemiesters of methylprednisolone at 25°C. Key: (O) 1a and (●) 1d.

Table II. Relative Rate Constants (Acetate = 1.0) for Acid and Base Catalyzed Hydrolysis of Various Amide Containing Esters of Methylprednisolone at 25°C.

Cmpd. No.	R	Relative k_{H^+}	Relative k_{OH^-}
1i	$-(CH_2)_2CONHCH_2COOH$	0.42	2.6
1j	$-(CH_2)_2CONHCH_2CONHCH_2COOH$	0.38	90
1n	$-(CH_2)_2CONHCH_2CH_2SO_3H$	0.47	4.9
1o	$-(CH_2)_2CON(CH)_3CH_2CH_2SO_3H$	0.46	0.33
1p	$-(CH_2)_2CONHCH_2CH_2N(CH_3)_2$	0.13	226
1q	$-(CH_2)_2CON(CH_3)CH_2CH_2N(CH_3)_2$	0.12	1.81

21-succinate, in relation to those of the 21-acetate (1b) (k_{H^+} = .085 $l\ mol^{-1}\ hr^{-1}$ and k_{OH^-} = 1.45 x $10^4\ l\ mol^{-1}\ hr^{-1}$) are compared in Table II. While differences in rate constants for acid catalyzed hydrolysis are unremarkable, the rate constants for hydroxide ion catalyzed hydrolysis fluctuate dramatically - particularly noteworthy considering the fact that in most cases structural variations were at least six bonds removed from the ester linkage.

The unusual variability in reactivity of the succinamides under basic conditions is attributed to intramolecular catalysis. Previous studies have established that the succinamide anion may act as an intramolecular nucleophilic catalyst as shown in Scheme III generating the free alcohol and a cyclic imide.[24] N-methyl amides which cannot undergo

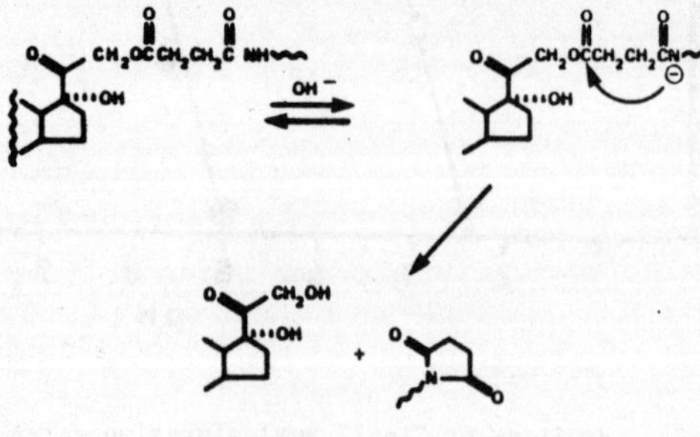

Scheme III

Reproduced with permission of the copyright owner, the American Pharmaceutical Association.

ionization are much less reactive, differing only modestly from the acetate. In addition, k_{OH^-} correlates with the Taft σ^* parameters for substituents attached to the α-carbon adjacent to the amide nitrogen as shown in Figure 3. This inverse relationship between reactivity and the amide anion pKa further supports the hypothesis that the amide anion is the reactive species.

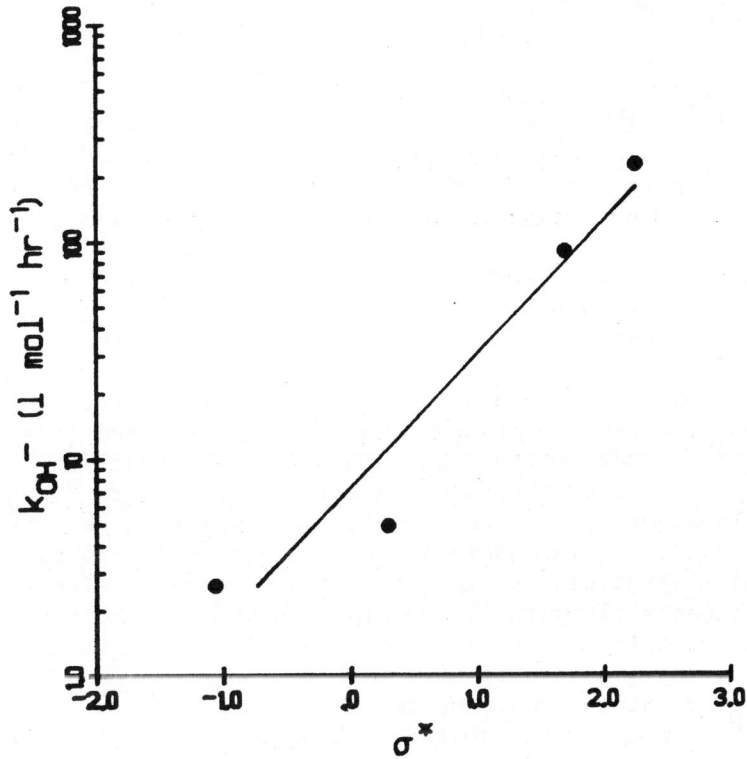

Figure 3. Semilogarithmic plot of the base catalyzed ester hydrolysis rate constants, k_{OH^-}, of various succinamide esters versus the Taft σ^* values for the substituents on the α-carbon adjacent to the amide nitrogen.

Polar and Steric Substituent Effects. Apart from intramolecular catalytic effects, ester hydrolysis in vitro is governed largely by the steric bulk of substituents in the vicinity of the ester linkage and the electron withdrawing or donating effects of these groups. A separation of the total effect of a substituent into a steric term and a polar term was accomplished by Taft[19] following a suggestion by Ingold.[25] The basis of the method is that acid catalyzed ester hydrolysis appears to be insensitive to electronic effects of substituents presumably because it is a multistep reaction, with the effect of substituents in some steps cancelling that in others. Thus relative rates of acid-catalyzed hydrolysis reflect largely steric effects. It is further assumed that steric effects are similar for acid and base catalyzed reactons so the sum of the steric and polar effects are obtained fom the relative rates of the base catalyzed hydrolyses. The linear free energy relationship developed by Taft is shown in Equation [6]:

$$\log (k/k_o) = \rho^* \sigma^* + \delta \cdot E_s \qquad [6]$$

where E_s is the steric parameter, a property of the substituent and δ (= 1.0) reflects the sensitivity of ester hydrolysis to steric effects of substituents on the acyl portion. The σ^* values represent substituent polar parameters and ρ^* for aliphatic ester hydrolyses is 2.48. Others have extended the above approach and have demonstrated its applicability to prodrug design. Tables of σ^* and E_s or related parameters can be found in several references.[21,22]

Rarely would prodrug lability in vitro be increased unless this were necessary to achieve the desired in vivo lability. More often, the objective is to increase stability. Since the polar substituent constants for most functional groups are positive or only slightly negative, however, little improvement can be achieved in stability beyond that gained by minimizing the electronic effects of substituents altogether. Nothing can be done about electron withdrawing (activating) substituents in the parent compound. Indeed, the presence of an α-carbonyl makes 21-esters of corticosteroids already quite activated toward nucleophilic attack. From the standpoint of prodrug stability, it is important to avoid further activation of the bioreversible linkage by substituents in the pro-moiety. This is quite easily done, as illustrated in Table III.

Shown in Table III are the relative rates of base catalyzed hydrolysis for three series of ω-substituted alkanoates of corticosteroids varying in the terminal solubilizing moiety. Estimated σ^* values for $-NH(CH_3)_2^+$, $-SO_3^-$ and $-COO^-$ are +4.36, +0.81, and -1.06, respectively. These values decrease with distance by a multiplying factor of approximately 0.36 per methylene group.[21] As seen in Table III, k_{OH^-} is highly sensitive to solubilizing moiety at a short chain length, becoming relatively insensitive with increasing distance between the activating substituent and the ester linkage.

These data show that pro-moieties such as N,N-dimethyl

Table III. Relative rates of base-catalyzed hydrolysis (k_{OH^-}/k_{OH^-} (acetate)) for various ω-substituted alkanoates of corticosteroids.

Compound No.	Pro-Moiety	Relative k_{OH^-}
1e	$-COCH_2COO^-$	0.39^b
1a	$-CO(CH_2)_2COO^-$	$0.31^b (0.25^a)$
1d	$-CO(CH_2)_4COO^-$	0.21^b
--	$-COCH_2NH(CH_3)_2^+$	1376^a
--	$-CO(CH_2)_2NH(CH_3)_2^+$	350^a
1r	$-CO(CH_2)_5NH(CH_3)_2$	0.86^b
1f	$-CO(CH_2)_2SO_3^-$	1.5^b
1g	$-CO(CH_2)_5SO_3^-$	0.20^b
1h	$-CO(CH_2)_{10}SO_3^-$	0.18^b

^{a}Estimates obtained from hydrocortisone ester data[27,28].

^{b}Estimates obtained from methylprednisolone ester data[1].

glycine, glycine, and lysine, which are frequently explored as solubilizing moieties(though such derivatives are seldom marketed) have a major disadvantage due to their tendency to activate the resulting ester toward base catalyzed hydrolysis. Longer chain sulfonate or amine containing pro-moieties therefore appear to be superior to their short chain length homologues on this basis. Long chain carboxylate containing pro-moieties are also preferred over the succinate or malonate but this is due to their decreased ability to catalyze hydrolysis intramolecularly rather than to electronic effects. We have already shown that carboxylate containing prodrugs also suffer from low solubility at the pH of optimum ester stability.

Marked increases in solution stability can be realized by increasing steric bulk in the pro-moiety. E_s values range from 0 for methyl to as low as -3 to -4 for highly hindered groups, suggesting that theoretical improvements of 3- 4 orders of magnitude are possible through steric effects. This approach was employed successfully by Garrett in the early 60's to improve the stability of soluble steroid hemiesters.[29] He demonstrated that the hydroxyl ion catalyzed hydrolysis of the hindered methylprednisolone hemi-β,β'-dimethylglutarate was approximately 30-fold slower than that of the corresponding acetate but bioconversion data were not reported.

While substituent effects on ester lability in vivo will be discussed in a later section, it is essential that substituent effects in enzyme catalyzed hydrolysis be considered simultaneously with their effects on lability in aqueous solution. Consider steric hindrance, for example, which has been shown to be quite effective in improving aqueous stability. Several studies indicate that enzyme catalyzed hydrolyses are also subject to steric effects with varying degrees of sensitivity.[22] Charton, using ν as the steric parameter, has developed linear free energy relationships for the hydrolysis of acyl-substituted para-nitrophenyl esters, $4\text{-}O_2NC_6H_4O_2CR$, in a number of different systems. The relative rates of enzyme catalyzed hydrolysis of these compounds by human serum are given by equation [7]:[30]

$$\log k_{rel,R} = -6.53 \nu_R + 5.86 \quad [7]$$

On the other hand, the rate constants for acid catalyzed hydrolysis of 4-nitrophenyl carboxylates in water are correlated by equation [8]:[31]

$$\log k_R = -1.25 \nu_R + 1.54 \quad [8]$$

suggesting that serum esterase catalyzed hydrolysis is much more sensitive than solution reactions to steric effects.

Increasing steric bulk may therefore decrease the in vivo/in vitro prodrug lability ratio. Only if this lability ratio for a given series of prodrugs is sufficiently large that one can afford to decrease the rate of prodrug bioconversion in an attempt to improve solution stability will increasing steric hindrance be beneficial.

Solution Stable, Water Soluble Prodrugs of Methylprednisolone

The prodrugs 1t and 1u (Scheme I) have incorporated into their pro-moieties those features discussed in the preceding sections as necessary to achieve water solubility and formulation stability. The compounds both possess solubilizing moieties which are fully ionized at the pH of optimum stability, there are no functional groups capable of catalyzing hydrolysis intramolecularly in close proximity to the ester linkage, and the electron withdrawing nature of the substituents is minimized by using a hydrocarbon chain spacer. In Figure 4 are the pH-hydrolysis rate profiles at 25°C for dilute solutions of 1t and 1u superimposed on that of MP 21-succinate. At the pH of optimum stability, both 1t and 1u exhibit 10% degradation or less in two years.

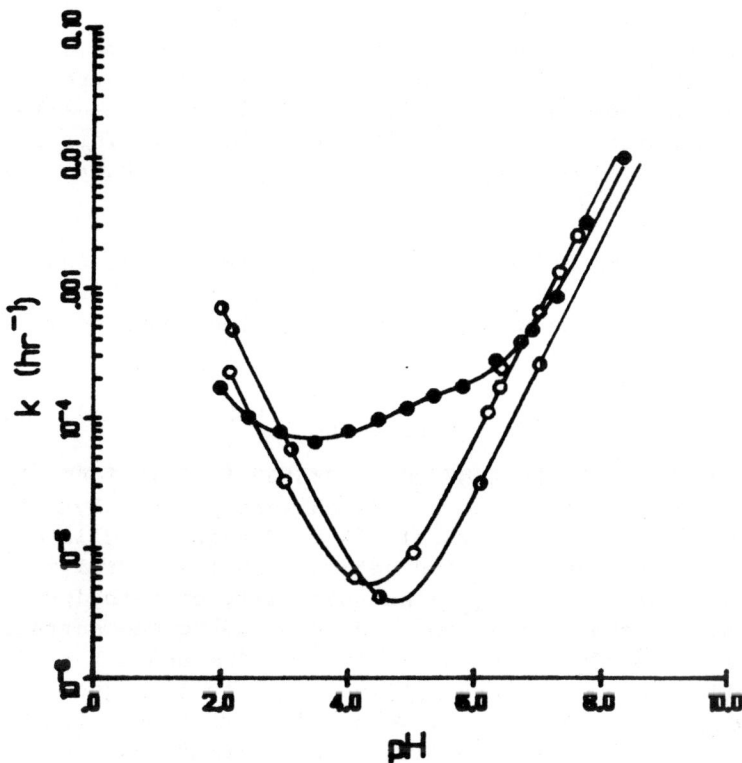

Figure 4. Dilute solution pH-hydrolysis rate profiles at 25°C for the solution stable prodrugs 1t(O) and 1u(◐) superimposed on that of the succinate ester, 1a(●).

Thus far, however, only a few factors have been taken into account in the design problem. Several critical factors have yet to be addressed. Among these are the difficult problem of solubilizing the small percentage of insoluble parent drug which forms during storage of the product due to hydrolysis of the prodrug, the dependence of bioconversion rates on pro-moiety structure, and the influence of pro-moiety structure on prodrug safety. We will explore these phenomena in the sections that follow.

Micellar Prodrugs

The water soluble prodrug approach is often considered a last resort in the development of a solution formulation of a drug candidate. It is usually applied to a compound which cannot be solubilized by cosolvents or other formulation additives because its solubility may be orders-of-magnitude lower than the desired formulation concentration. If the parent compound is very insoluble, the shelf-life of a water soluble prodrug may not be determined by the time required for 10% loss of the prodrug but by the time required to reach saturation with respect to the parent drug -- usually a major degradation product in the formulation. This situation has been discussed previously with regard to other water soluble prodrugs.[32,33]

If the parent drug has a solubility of less than 10% of the formulation concentration of the prodrug, the theoretical shelf-life will be determined by the time required for precipitate formation as given in Equation [9]:

$$\text{Shelf-life} = S_{\text{parent drug}}/(k_{obs}[\text{Prodrug}]) \quad [9]$$

The actual shelf-lives of concentrated formulations of the example compounds 1t and 1u, which were previously shown to exhibit less than 10% hydrolysis in 2 years in dilute solutions, therefore depend not only on the hydrolysis rate constant but also on both the solubility of methylprednisolone in the formulation and the prodrug concentration. Assuming a prodrug concentration of 0.1 M and a formulation solubility of methylprednisolone equal to its aqueous solubility of 2.5×10^{-4} M, we conclude that only 0.25 % hydrolysis would lead to precipitate formation. This would occur in less than 3 weeks.

The only "solution" to this problem is to somehow solubilize the parent drug. The micellar prodrug approach may have general applicability in such cases.

Self-association of water soluble corticosteroid derivatives has been observed in several studies.[2,14,34] Flynn and Lamb, for example, found that hydrocortisone 21-phosphate formed micelles above concentrations of 0.01-0.02 M resulting in an increase in the degradation rate of this compound.[34] In the same study, the solubility of methylprednisolone in solutions of MP 21-phosphate was found to increase sharply above the CMC.

In view of the known tendency for water soluble corticosteroid derivatives to self-associate, several studies have been conducted by the authors to evaluate the use of micelle-forming prodrugs to achieve two basic purposes: (1) solubilize insoluble, hydrophobic degradation products which would otherwise precipitate in the formulation; and (2) provide added stability to the prodrug. The few studies which exist in the literature suggest that reactivity can be significantly altered either favorably or unfavorably by substrate self-aggregation into micelles.[35,36]

The above objectives could perhaps be accomplished by the addition of surfactants to a formulation of a water soluble prodrug without relying on the micellization of the prodrug itself. Numerous examples of classical micellar solubilization with surfactants have been reported. However, the use of the prodrug itself as the surfactant affords several potential advantages over the classical micellar solubilization approach. One of these is that micellar prodrugs may be converted in vivo to fragments which are no longer surfactants. The toxic effects frequently associated with surfactants[37-39] would be minimized in these compounds due to the short lifetimes of the micellar prodrug in vivo. Other advantages of the micellar prodrug approach are discussed below.

<u>Parent Drug Solubilization.</u> Most simplistically, micelle formation is viewed as a process similar to phase separation and micellar solubilization as a partitioning phenomenon above the critical micelle concentration (CMC).[40] Thus, the solubility of parent drug in a solution containing micellar prodrug may be expressed by Equation [10]

$$S_{parent\ drug} = Cs + K \cdot [Cs] \cdot [C_T - CMC] \quad [10]$$

where Cs is the saturation solubility of parent drug in water, C_T-CMC is the concentration of micellized prodrug, and K is a constant proportional to the partition coefficient of the parent compound between water and the micellar pseudophase. Equation [10] predicts that the solubility of parent drug should be linearly related to the prodrug concentration above the CMC.

Shown in Figure 5 is such a plot of solubility of methylprednisolone versus the concentration of several of its prodrugs on a % weight/volume basis. The micellar prodrug solubilization data represent methylprednisolone solubilities at 30°C and pH 4.5 in 0.1 M and 0.2 M solution formulations of six amine containing derivatives varying in pro-moiety chain length and amine substitution. A similar solubilization capacity was seen for the sulfonate containing compound 1u. Thus, within this series the solubilization capacities of the micellar prodrugs are not highly sensitive to pro-moiety structure when prodrug concentration is expressed on a % weight/volume basis. At high prodrug concentrations the amount of methylprednisolone solubilized is approximately 3.5-4% of the ester concentration thus increasing the percent hydrolysis allowable in a 0.1 M formulation by a factor of about 15.

Also illustrated in Figure 5 is the increase in methylprednisolone solubility in solutions of the nonionic surfactants Triton WR-1339[41] and Polysorbate 80[42] as reported in the literature. Clearly the solubilizing power of the micellar prodrugs is superior to that of these surfactants. This is not unexpected since mixing of methylprednisolone

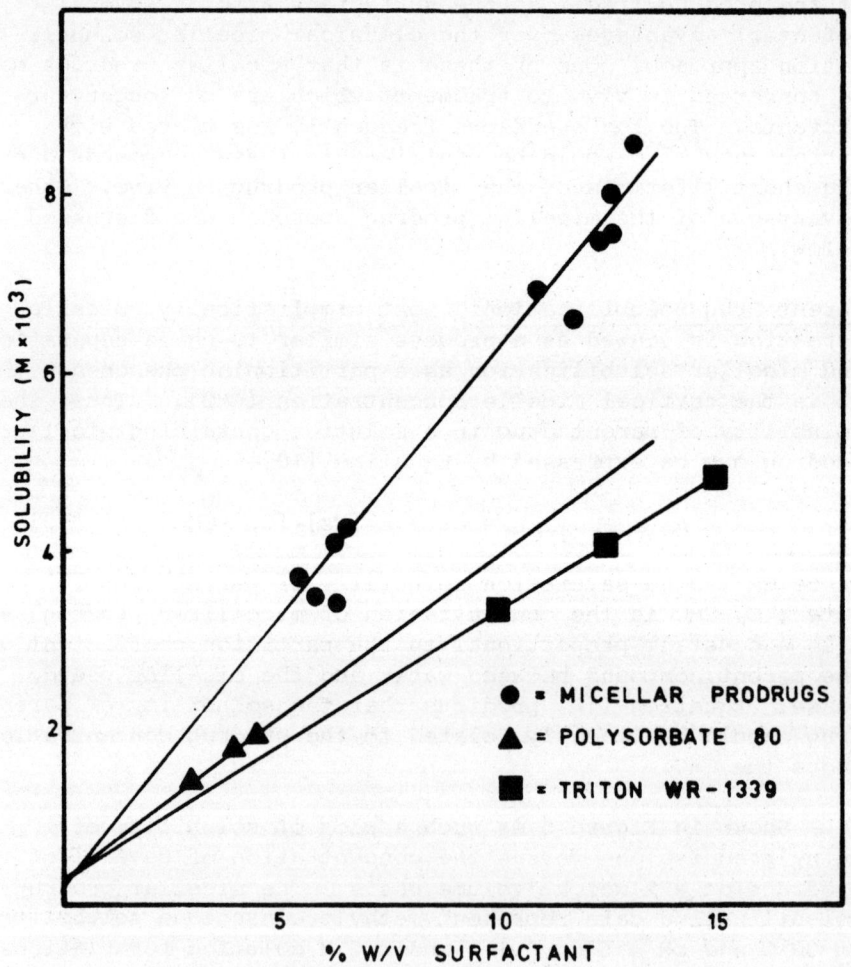

Figure 5. Solubility of methylprednisolone versus the concentration of several micellar prodrugs(●) and the nonionic surfactants Polysorbate 80(▲) and Triton WR-1339(■).

with micellar prodrug may be a more ideal process than the
mixing of MP with the structurally dissimilar nonionic
surfactant micelles. Micellar prodrugs may therefore be
preferred surfactants for the solubilization of parent drug.

The micellar prodrug approach may have broad applicability. Recent studies of phenytoin phosphate have shown
that its associated solutions increase the aqueous solubility
of phenytoin and provide increased stability.[33] Similar
observations have been made in other prodrug systems[43] but
generally there has been no attempt to design self-
associative tendencies into water soluble prodrugs.

Stabilization in Micellar Prodrug Systems. Of primary
concern in the design of a micellar prodrug, in addition to
the degree of solubilization of free parent drug, is the
effect of association on prodrug lability. Micellar
catalysis, for example, would be counterproductive to the
overall objectives of this approach. We have conducted
several studies of micellar prodrugs of corticosteroids to
ascertain the effect of molecular modification in the
pro-moiety on both aggregation and kinetics. Two variables
which were specifically explored were the effect of
increasing prodrug hydrophobicity through increases in
pro-moiety chain length and the effect of ionic charge on the
aggregation and solution kinetics.

Intuitively, stabilization through self-micellization
would appear to offer several advantages over the classical
micellar solublization approach. Drug present in micellar
form and therefore in a more hydrophobic environment may
exhibit enhanced stability over that in pure aqueous media.
By varying the chain length of the pro-moiety the CMC can be
lowered thus forcing more drug into the micelle. Traditional
micellar solubilization relies on the partition coefficient
of the drug between water and the micelle which cannot be
readily manipulated. Also, in a micelle forming prodrug the
reactive portion of the molecule may on average spend more
time in a more hydrophobic environment due to the constraints
in its location within the micelle resulting from its attachment to other groups. The added stabilization brought about
by self-micellization would be in effect only at concentrations above the CMC of the derivative. Therefore,
dilution upon injection would remove this added protection
allowing rapid bioconversion of the prodrug back to the
active parent compound.

The effect of pro-moiety chain length on the kinetics of
hydrolysis and acyl migration in aggregated corticosteroid
systems was studied in a series of dicarboxylic acid hemi-

esters of methylprednisolone.[14] Shown in Figure 6 are the absolute hydrolysis rates of these compounds as a function of total concentration at pH 8.47 and 25°C. CMC's indicated by break points in the plots and determined independently in partitioning studies, decreased with pro-moiety chain length from 0.02 M for the 21-succinate to 0.003 M for the 21-suberate ester. A plot of log CMC versus chain length gave a slope of 0.24 which is close to the methylene group contribution generally found for micelle formation.[44] Below the CMC, the hydrolysis rate increase with concentration is nearly linear as expected for first order kinetics. Above the CMC reaction rates continue to increase linearly but with smaller slopes indicating that reactivity in the micelles is decreased but not totally suppressed.

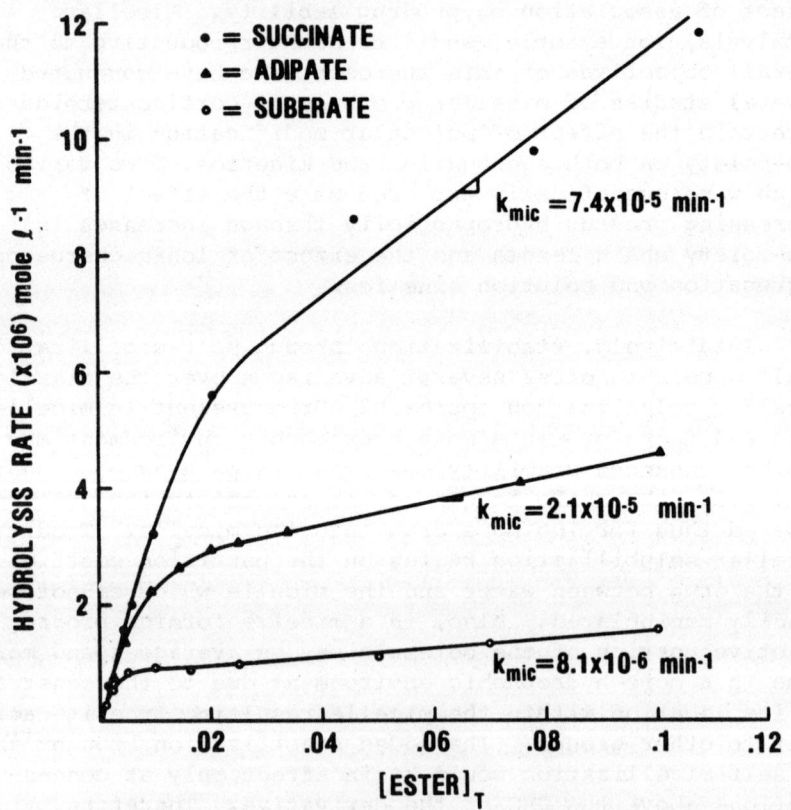

Figure 6. Absolute hydrolysis rates of dicarboxylic acid hemiesters of methylprednisolone versus ester concentration at pH 8.47 and 25°C. Key: (●) 1a; (▲) 1d; and (○) 1e.

Increasing chain length from 2 to 6 methylenes resulted in a 10-fold decrease in hydrolysis rate at high concentrations. This was due to a combination of factors: (a) a lower CMC reduced the concentration of reactive monomer by a factor of 6-7; (b) ester reactivity in the micelle was suppressed by nearly 10-fold; and (c) monomer reactivity was decreased slightly due perhaps to a steric effect. It was concluded that relatively lengthy pro-moiety chains are useful for promoting micellization and stability within the micelle.

Because of their stability in dilute solution and the chain length of their pro-moieties, 1t and 1u (see Scheme I) were expected to be ideal micellar prodrug candidates. The effects of micelle formation on the hydrolysis rates of 1t and 1u are illustrated in Figures 7 & 8.

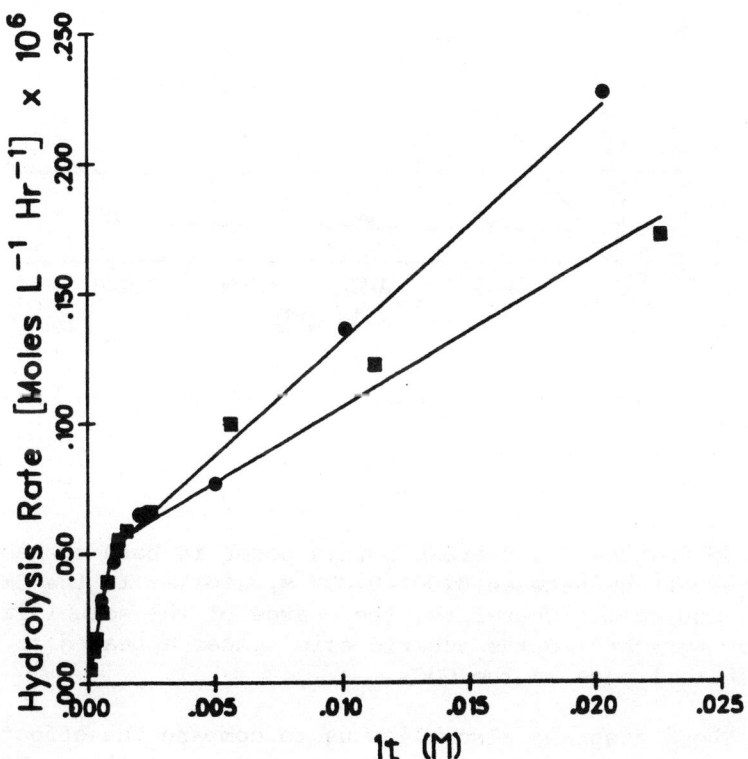

Figure 7. Absolute hydrolysis rates versus concentration of 1t at pH's of 3 (●) and 6(■).

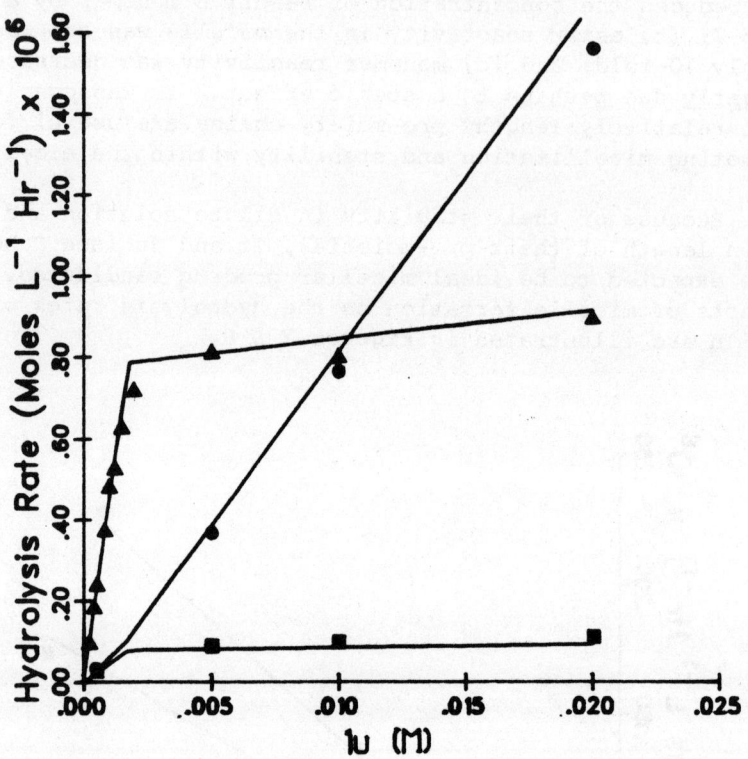

Figure 8. Absolute hydrolysis rates versus concentration of 1u at pH's of 3 (●), 6 (■), and 7 (▲).

In Figures 7 & 8 break points occur in both systems at concentrations between 0.001-0.002 M, similar to the CMC for MP 21-suberate. Therefore, the charge of the solubilizing moiety attached to the suberic acid spacer appeared to have little influence on the CMC.

These diagrams also allow us to compare the effect of prodrug charge on reactivity in associated systems. At all pH's explored, micelles of 1t are positive while 1u micelles are negatively charged. Electrostatic considerations such as those set forth by Hartley,[45] suggest that the concentration of H^+ at the aqueous solution/ micelle interface (the Stern layer) would be higher for micelles of 1u while the OH^- concentration would be lower than in the bulk solution. The converse would be true for 1t. If hydrolysis occurs in this interfacial region then we would predict acid catalyzed hydrolysis to be accelerated in micelles of 1u and retarded in micelles of 1t and vice versa for hydroxide ion catalyzed hydrolysis. While the micellar effects on acid catalyzed hydrolysis are consistent with these predictions, base catalyzed hydrolysis, contrary to the theory, is inhibited in both micellar systems. These observations are not unique and plausible theories to account for such deviations have been advanced,[46-47] but more research is needed to quantitatively explain at a molecular level the effects of self-micellization on reactivity. Nevertheless, these effects can be exploited in prodrug formulation design.

In Figure 9 are pH-hydrolysis rate profiles at 30°C for 1t and 1u in dilute and concentrated aqueous formulations.

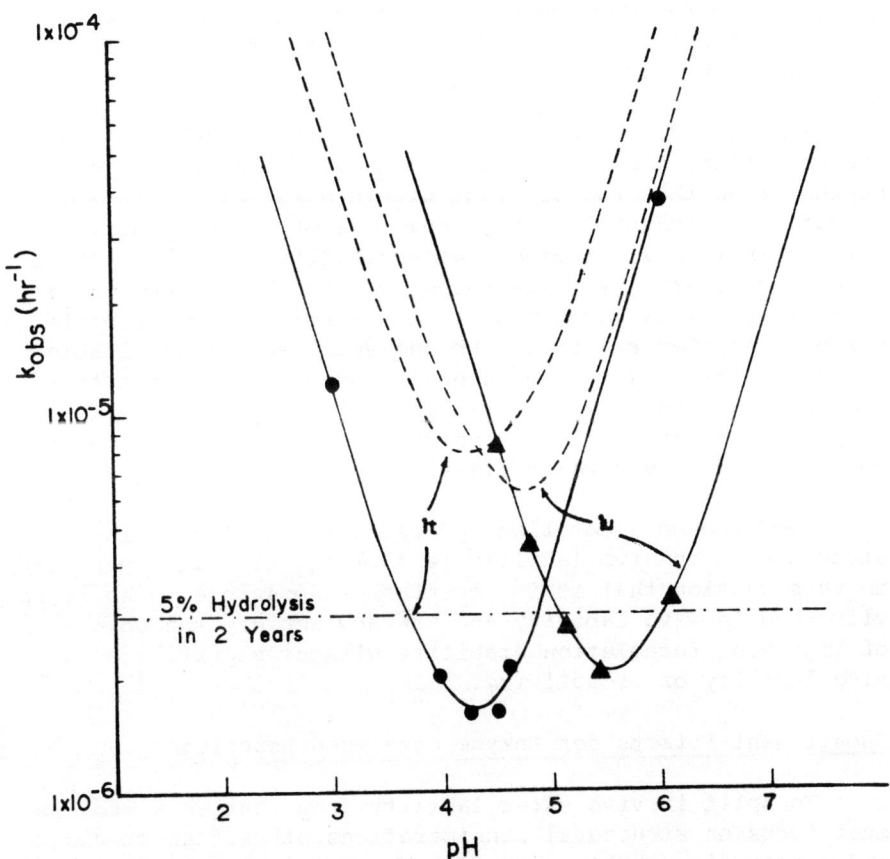

Figure 9. pH-hydrolysis rate profiles of 1t(●) and 1u(▲) in concentrated (>0.2 M, solid lines) and in dilute (5 x 10 M, dashed lines) aqueous solutions at 30°C.

Micellization lowers the pH-rate minima for both compounds
and shifts the pH-rate minimum for 1u toward a higher pH due
to an acceleration of acid catalyzed hydrolysis and an
inhibition of hydroxide ion attack. In addition to the
solubilization of any free methylprednisolone formed,
self-micellization increases the stability of concentrated
formulations by 5-fold over that expected for dilute
solutions. Due to self-micellization in concentrated
solutions these derivatives exhibit less than 5 % hydrolysis
in 2 years at $30°C$ and are therefore suitable for formulation
as ready-to-inject parenterals.

Physical Organic Considerations in In Vivo Lability Design

Though enough is known about the influence of structure
on chemical reactivity to synthesize prodrugs with improved
solution stability, the design of in vivo lability requires a
great deal more knowledge. Since there are a number of enzymes which are capable of hydrolyzing esters, one generally
will not know which enzyme is involved in the bioconversion
of a particular prodrug. Because of variation in the sensitivities of different enzymes to structure, modification of
the pro-moiety may bring about a change in the hydrolysis
mechanism so that two prodrugs within a series are hydrolyzed
by different enzymes. Also, knowledge of enzyme distributions in vivo is limited. Accessibility of the substrate
to a particular enzyme may become the rate limiting factor.
In addition, data pertaining to the influence of structure on
enzyme catalyzed reactions (Km and Vmax) are not available
for most esterases. Discussion of some of these important
factors and information currently available dealing with
enzyme-substrate specificities as related to prodrug design
may be found in several reviews.[22,26,48]

Even though a detailed understanding of the influence of
structure on in vivo lability is lacking, we will demonstrate
in this section that it is nevertheless possible to split in
vitro and in vivo lability and thereby achieve the objective
of improving formulation stability without sacrificing in
vivo lability or bioactivity.

Substituent Effects for Enzyme Catalyzed Reactions

To split in vivo ester lability from that in vitro, we
must focus on structural considerations other than steric
and electronic substituent effects. We previously discussed
the fact that enzyme catalyzed reactions are quite sensitive
to steric factors - in some cases more sensitive than solution reactions. Since steric factors influence both enzyme
and bulk solution reactions in the same direction the in

vivo/in vitro lability ratio may be difficult to modify systematically via steric effects unless more is known about the particular enzymes involved.

Enzymatic reactions involving initial rate-limiting attack by a serine hydroxyl group (probably the case for most ester containing prodrugs) exhibit similar sensitivities to electron withdrawing substituents as non-enzymatic nucleophilic reactions. Thus, studies of the acylation of chymotrypsin have given ρ values of less than 1.0 for specific substrates[49,50] and around 2.0 for nonspecific substrates such as phenyl acetates.[51-55] For comparison, ρ is 1.0-1.5[56] for direct OH attack on phenyl acetates. While some degree of selectivity between in vitro and in vivo lability may be achievable, it is again difficult to predict in advance whether or not a given electron withdrawing substituent will increase bioconversion rates more than solution reactivity. Since minimizing electronic substituent effects may be necessary to optimize solution stability, it may not be feasible to use activating substituents to build back into a molecule the desired in vivo lability. However, activation by electron withdrawing substituents has been recommended as a logical approach to improving bioactivity of a prodrug which may be inactive due to slow bioconversion.[26] Such approaches are feasible when formulation stability is not a problem.

Correlations of enzyme catalyzed reaction rates with the Taft-Ingold relationship often fit poorly suggesting that factors other than polar and steric effects are important in enzymatic reactions. For example, in studies of the specificity of α-chymotrypsin toward acyl-substituted p-nitrophenyl esters Dupaix et al defined acylation and deacylation specificity constants, S_a and S_d, to account for deviations between the correlation line using the Taft-Ingold equation and the experimental points.[57] These specificity constants were analyzed in terms of chain length and hydrophobicity. The acylation specificity constant was found to depend both on the size of the acyl chain and hydrophobicity while the deacylation step was mainly size dependent. Of particular interest in the design of esters as prodrugs are the substrate specificities of esterase enzymes. Studies of reactivity and affinity of 33 esters in the presence of horse liver carboxylesterase by Webb showed that an optimum in both affinity and reactivity occurs at acyl or alkyl chain lengths of about 4-6 carbons.[58] Further increases in chain length produced a decline in reactivity but affinity continued to increase.

Acyl or alkyl chain length and hydrophobicity, apart

148   Bioreversible Carriers in Drug Design

from their contribution to steric hindrance, do not alter
aqueous solution reactivity. It may thus be possible to
modify prodrug lability in vivo independently of that in
vitro by varying pro-moiety chain length or hydrophobicity.

Relationship between Solution Hydrolysis and Serum Hydrolysis

Recent studies in our laboratories of bioconversion
rates of various water soluble, solution stable prodrugs of
methylprednisolone illustrate the difficulty in predicting in
vivo lability from non-enzymatic data. Consider, for
example, the serum hydrolysis data shown in Figures 10 and
11. Focus for a moment on compounds 1t and 1u which were

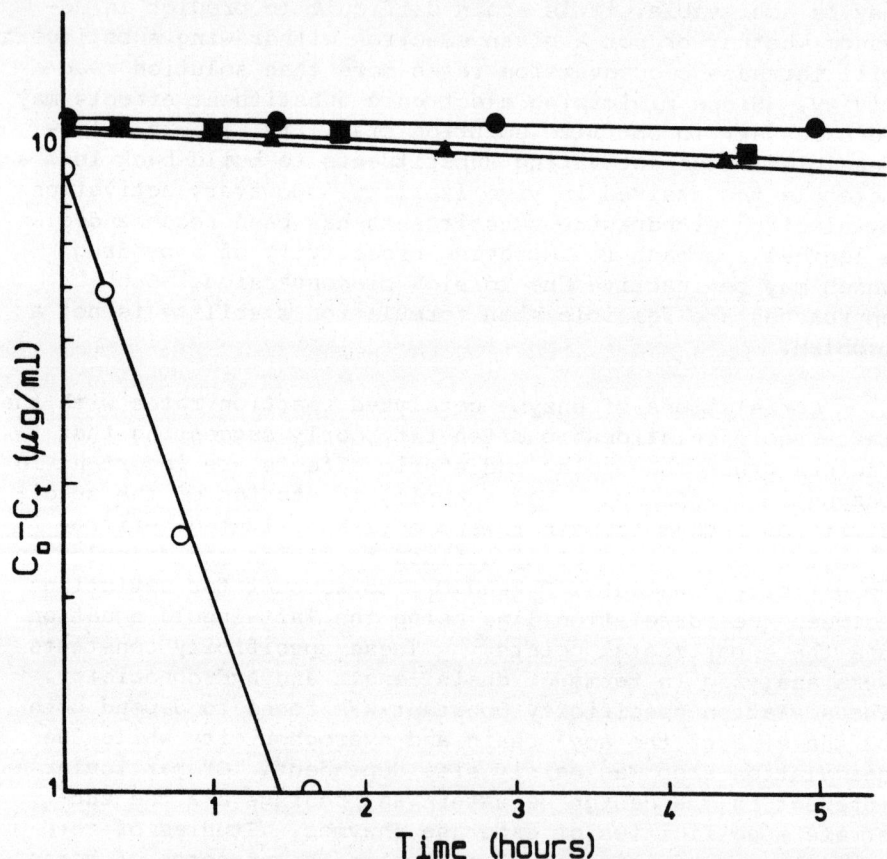

Figure 10. Semilogarithmic plots of the hydrolysis of various
esters of methylprednisolone in rhesus monkey serum at 37°C.
Key: (▲) 1a; (●) 17-succinate; (■) 1o; and (O) 1s.

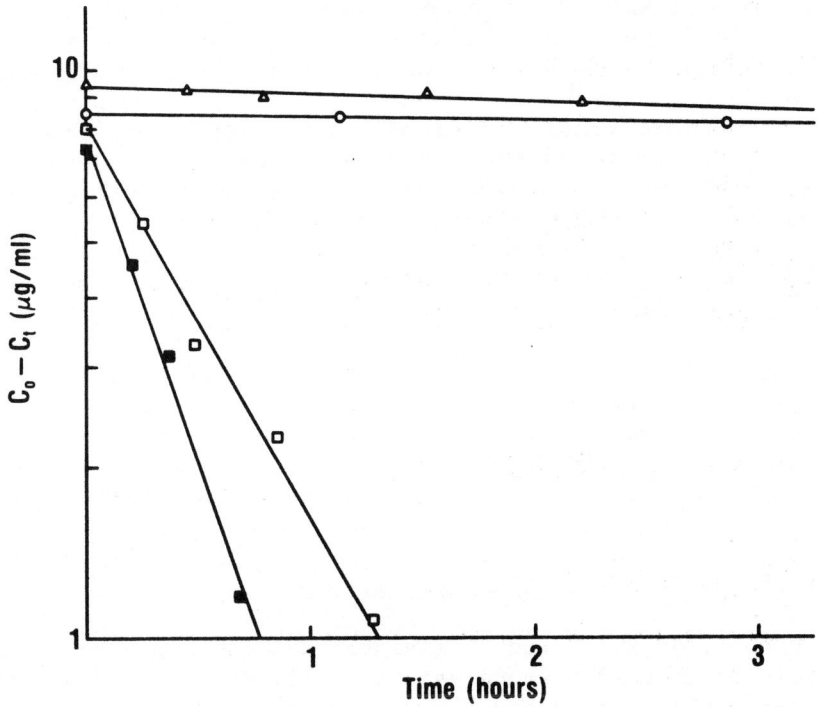

Figure 11. Semilogarithmic plots of the hydrolysis of various esters of methylprednisolone in human serum at 37°C. Key: (O) 1a; (Δ) 1u; (□) 1r; and (■) 1t.

shown previously (Figure 4) to have similar pH-hydrolysis profiles in dilute solution. Their similar reactivity in water presumably reflects minimal differences in steric bulk or electronic activation near the ester linkage due to the distances separating the solubilizing moieties from the ester bond. Semilogarithmic plots of the hydrolysis of these compounds and other derivatives of methylprednisolone in rhesus monkey serum at 37°C, shown in Figure 10, and in human serum (Figure 11) show that negatively charged compounds are not hydrolyzed by serum esterases while positively charged derivatives are cleaved relatively rapidly. In comparing compounds 1t and 1u we see that a change in one functional group a distance of 11 bonds from the ester linkage acts as an on-off switch controlling the lability of the prodrug toward serum esterases. Clearly, in vivo lability can be modified independently of in vitro reactivity.

Although the serum hydrolysis data might lead one to conclude that anionic prodrugs such as succinate esters may not be bioactive, bioavailability studies have shown that 21-succinate esters of corticosteroids are hydrolyzed in vivo to the parent drug.[8] The absence of hydrolysis of succinate esters in human serum (and blood[59]) indicates that while serum esterases may be important in cleaving some types of derivatives, other enzymes must be involved in the bioconversion of anionic esters.

Effect of Pro-Moiety Structure on Hydrolysis by Liver Carboxylesterase

Since anionic prodrugs are not hydrolyzed in the blood, and yet are active in vivo, liver esterases or esterases in other tissues may be involved. Carboxylesterases are widely distributed in vertebrate tissues with the highest activities being found in the liver, kidney, duodenum, and brain.[60] Nonspecific carboxylesterases hydrolyze a wide variety of carboxylic acid esters and may therefore play an important role in the detoxification system.

Schottler and Krisch[61] investigated the hydrolysis of a variety of steroid hormone esters catalyzed by a nonspecific carboxylesterase from pig liver microsomes and found that charged esters such as succinate esters of prednisolone and hydrocortisone were not hydrolyzed. Hattori et al,[62] however, demonstrated that methylprednisolone and hydrocortisone succinates are hydrolyzed by nonspecific liver carboxylesterase but with markedly lower Vmax's compared to the corresponding acetates. The optimum pH for hydrolysis of acetates was between 8.0 and 8.5, shifting to pH 5.5 for the hemisuccinates. The Km values for acetate and hemisuccinate esters did not vary significantly. From these results the authors concluded that the hydrolysis of charged and neutral steroid esters are catalyzed by different carboxylesterase enzymes. However, these data may also be rationalized if the reaction proceeds through an enzyme-substrate complex in which the succinate carboxyl is unionized.

To learn more about the selectivity of these enzymes, we examined the hydrolyses of 2 anionic prodrugs, MP 21-succinate (1a) and MP 21-sulfopropionate (1f) in the presence of a non-specific carboxylesterase enzyme from pig liver(EC 3.1.1.1, Sigma Chemical Co.). These compounds are nearly isosteric but differ markedly in pKa. Apart from intramolecular catalysis by the terminal carboxylic acid, the two compounds have similar reactivity in aqueous solution with the sulfopropionate being slighly more reactive in basic solution. If the enzymatic reaction depends on the fraction of ester unionized in the enzyme-substrate complex, then one would expect the sulfopropionate's hydrolysis to be much slower at a pH of 7.4, due to its lower pKa.

Solutions of the enzyme were prepared in pH 7.4 phosphate buffer at concentrations selected to provide a convenient hydrolysis rate. Reactions were conducted at $37°C$ using substrate concentrations varying from $10^{-5} - 10^{-3}$ M. Initial rates of formation of free MP were monitored by HPLC.

Shown in Figure 12 are plots of initial velocity versus ester concentration with and without carboxylesterase.

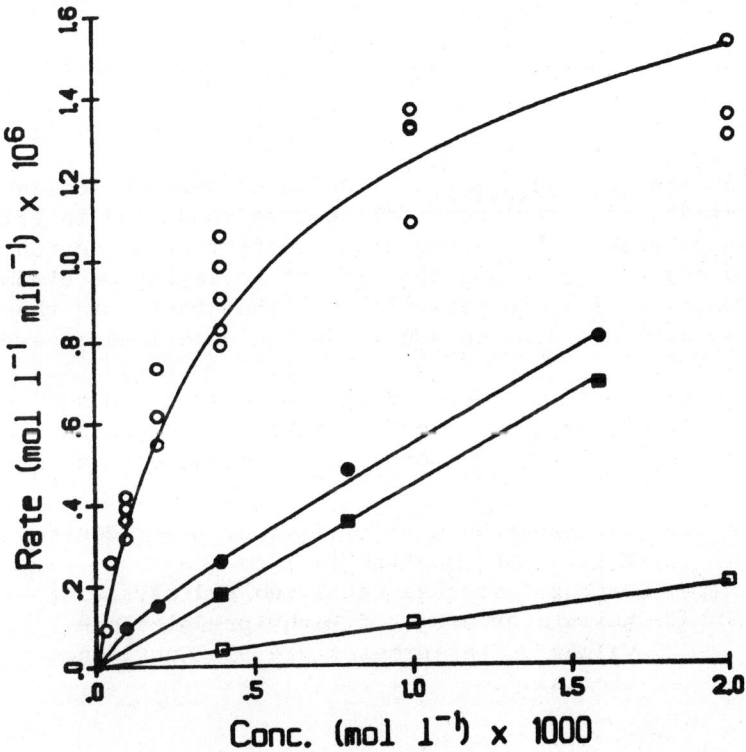

Figure 12. Initial rates of hydrolysis versus ester concentration in the presence and absence of carboxylesterase enzyme at pH 7.4 and 37°C. Key: (O) 1a with 2 µg/ml enzyme; (□) 1a without enzyme; (●) 1f with 10 µg/ml enzyme; and (■) 1f without enzyme.

Enzyme concentrations were 2 μg/ml and 10 μg/ml for the succinate and sulfopropionate studies, respectively. The curves were fitted to equation [11] by computer using a least squares optimization routine.

$$V = k_{hyd}[S] + k_{cat}[E][S]/(K_m + [S]) \qquad [11]$$

where k_{hyd} reflects the hydrolysis rate constant in the absence of enzyme and $[E]$ is the molar concentration of enzyme based on an assumed molecular weight of 166,000.[63] Values for the fitted parameters are listed in Table IV. Due to the wide confidence limits of K_m for the sulfopropionate (a higher concentration of enzyme would have improved this value) it cannot be concluded with certainty that K_m was similar for both compounds though this appears to be the case. However, it is clear that k_{cat} for the sulfopropionate is markedly lower than that of the succinate, consistent with the hypothesis that the fraction of acid unionized in the enzyme-substrate complex governs reactivity.

Effect of Pro-Moiety Structure on In Vivo Bioconversion

Several pharmacokinetic studies of various ionizable derivatives of methylprednisolone were conducted in rats or in rhesus monkeys to determine the effect of variation in pro-moiety structure and the site of acylation on bioconversion rates and bioavailability. The studies in rhesus monkeys used a 4x4 Latin square design described elsewhere.[3]

In the first of these studies we compared blood levels of methylprednisolone in rhesus monkeys after intravenous injections of 1.5 mg/kg (methylprednisolone equivalents) of

Table IV. Parameter Values Obtained by Least Squares Fitting of Equation [11] to the Carboxylesterase Catalyzed Hydrolysis of Anionic Prodrugs of Methylprednisolone. Values in Parentheses are 95% Confidence Limits.

Cmpd. No.	-R (Scheme I)	k_{hyd} (min^{-1} x 10^4)	k_{cat} (min^{-1})	K_m (M x 10^4)
1a	$-CH_2CH_2COO^-$	1.01 (0.8-1.22)	131 (100-161)	3.8 (2.3-5.3)
1f	$-CH_2CH_2SO_3^-$	4.45 (4.07-4.82)	1.9 (0.64-3.2)	1.33 (0.21 - 2.5)

each of the following compounds: methylprednisolone 21-succinate (2a), methylprednisolone 17-succinate, the sulfonate containing derivative 1o, and the amine containing compound 1s (see Scheme I). In Figure 13 are the average (n=4, error bars represent standard deviations) free corticosteroid blood concentrations resulting from each compound.

As shown in Figure 13 substantial differences in areas under the blood concentration versus time curves (AUC's) resulted depending on the pro-moiety and position of attachment of the pro-moiety. The amine containing derivative, which was previously shown to hydrolyze more readily in human serum, also exhibited significantly higher blood levels than the 21-succinate. The finding that the

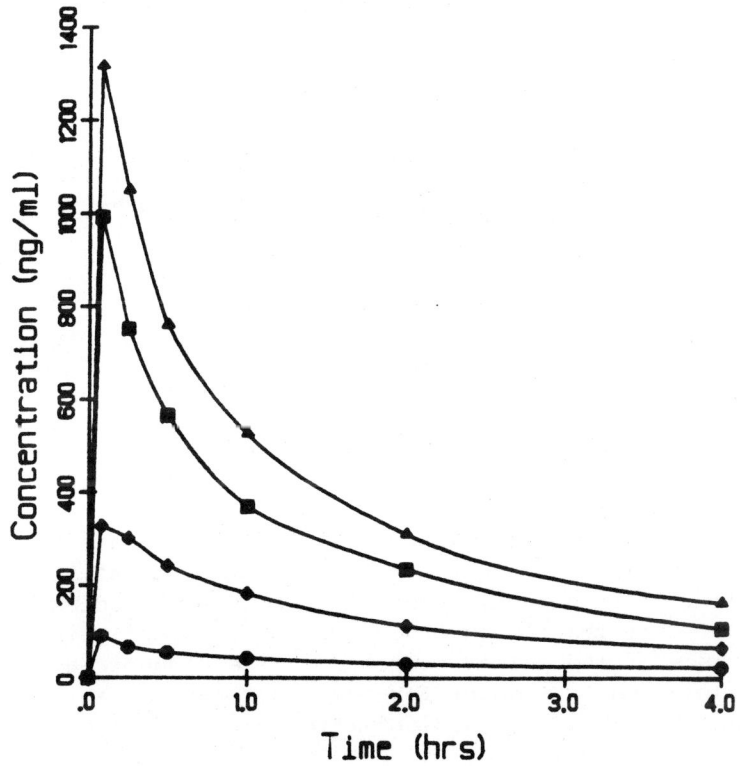

Figure 13. Average blood concentrations of methylprednisolone in rhesus monkeys (n=4) at various times after intravenous injections of 1.5 mg/kg (methylprednisolone equivalents) of prodrugs varying in pro-moiety and site of acylation. Key: (●) 17-succinate; (◆) 1o; (■) 1a; and (▲) 1s.

Table V. Relative AUC's of Methylprednisolone After Injections of Various Prodrugs in Rats or in Rhesus Monkeys.

No.	R (Scheme I)	Rat[b] 30 mg/kg	Monkey[c] 1.5 mg/kg	Monkey[c] 7.5 mg/kg
1a	$-CH_2CH_2COOH$	1.0	1.0	1.0
--	$-CH_2CH_2COOH(17\text{-ester})$	---	0.12	---
1f	$-(CH_2)_2SO_3^-$	0.26	---	---
1g	$-(CH_2)_5SO_3^-$	0.98	---	---
1o	$-CH_2CH_2CON(CH_3)CH_2CH_2SO_3^-$	---	0.52	---
1u	$-(CH_2)_6CON(CH_3)CH_2CH_2SO_3^-$	1.12	---	0.97
1t	$-(CH_2)_6CON(Et)CH_2CH_2N(Et)_2$	---	1.52	1.80
1s	$-(CH_2)_6CON(CH_3)CH_2CH_2N(CH_3)_2$	---	1.39	---

[a] Doses were calculated based on methylprednisolone equivalents.

[b] n=2; 1a and 1u were compared in a 2x2 crossover design.

[c] n=4; all results were obtained in 4x4 crossover experiments.[3]

bioavailability of methylprednisolone 21-succinate in rhesus monkeys is less than 100% correlates well with similar observations in humans.[8] Competing pathways leading to metabolism of the intact prodrug prior to hydrolysis and appearance of the parent compound in the bloodstream have been suggested to account for the lower bioavailability of succinate esters. Bioavailabilities relative to the 21-succinate are listed in Table V.

Blood levels obtained from the sulfonate containing prodrug were significantly lower than those from either the succinate or the amine. Qualitatively, the lower in vivo bioavailability of the sulfonate containing derivative correlates with the reduced ability of carboxylesterase enzyme to hydrolyze prodrugs in their anionic form. However, the conversion which did occur was relatively rapid, resulting in very early peak plasma levels of methylprednisolone (at the five minute sampling point) in rhesus monkeys. Other metabolic pathways competing with hydrolysis may have accounted for the lower bioavailability even though bioconversion was fairly rapid. The discovery that the sulfonate ester exhibited low bioavailability led us for a time to abandon the development of a solution stable sulfonate containing prodrug until it was found that in vivo lability can be built back into sulfonate containing derivatives by increasing chain length.

An additional, less surprising indication of the selectivity of the anionic prodrug hydrolyzing enzymes was found in the comparison of the AUC's resulting from the 17-succinate compared to the 21-succinate. Although the half-lives for elimination of the intact esters were comparable - about 9 min. for the 17-ester and 6 minutes for the 21-succinate - the 17-succinate was not converted to free methylprednisolone in vivo to a significant extent. Considering the steric parameters of the alkyl oxygen substituents, the base-catalyzed hydrolysis rate of 17-esters should be $<.01$ times that of 21-esters. Relative rates of conversion in vivo may also reflect this steric hindrance at the 17-position.

To further explore the variability in bioavailability of anionic prodrugs, another pharmacokinetic study was conducted in rats comparing the 21-succinate (a) with the sulfopropionate (1f) and two sulfonate containing compounds having longer alkyl chain lengths - the sulfocaproate (1d) and compound 1u. The relative AUC's resulting from each of these prodrugs are listed in Table V. Qualitatively consistent with the relative carboxylesterase activities, the sulfopropionate's bioavailability was found to be markedly lower than that of the succinate. However, increasing the distance separating the sulfonate moiety from the ester linkage reversed this effect. Thus the sulfocaproate's bioavailability was 3-4 times that of the sulfopropionate. While many factors may enter into relative bioavailabilities, these findings again support our prior conclusions that in vitro and in vivo lability can be split.

A third set of bioavailability data in rhesus monkeys further illustrates the effect of pro-moiety charge and pro-moiety chain length on relative bioavailabilities of prodrugs of methylprednisolone. In Figure 14 are plotted normalized plasma concentrations in rhesus monkeys after intravenous doses of four prodrugs as noted. Compounds 1t and 1u are structurally quite similar, differing primarily in terminal charge. Yet this charge difference accounts for a

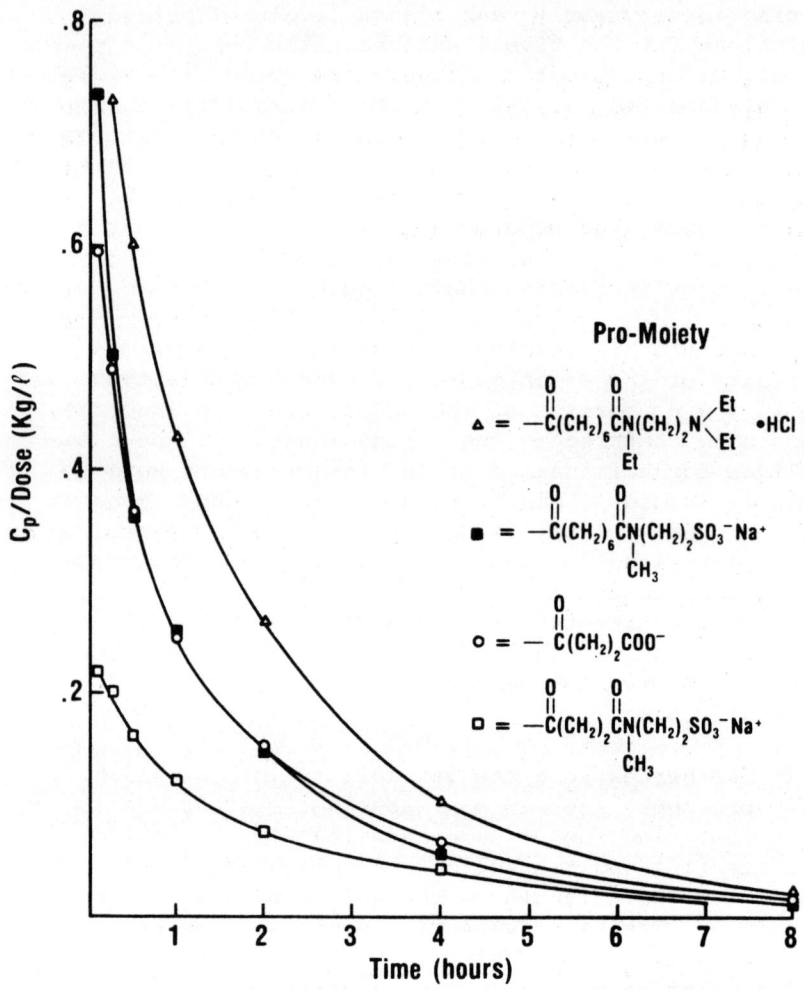

Figure 14. Normalized MP plasma concentrations (Cp/Dose) in rhesus monkeys after iv doses of various prodrugs varying in charge and chain length. Key: (Δ) 1t; (■) 1u; (O) 1a; (□) 1o.

difference in bioavailability of 1.67. Compounds 1o and 1u, both sulfonates, differ only in chain length. Consistent with the effect of sulfonate chain length seen earlier in rats, increasing chain length increased bioavailability - here by a factor of two for an increase in chain length of 4 methylene groups. Interestingly, compound 1u, shown previously to exhibit a solution stability of >2 years at 30 C is bioequivalent to the 21-succinate in rhesus monkeys. This demonstrates convincingly that one can design solution stability into a prodrug without sacrificing in vivo lability. The relative AUC's obtained from this study at two dosage levels are listed in Table V.

Influence of Pro-Moiety on Prodrug Safety

It would be dangerously shortsighted to design a prodrug having the required stability and bioavailability without considering the influence of pro-moiety on prodrug safety. In this section we will review some preliminary toxicity data generated for three compounds: MP 21-succinate, the amine containing compound, 1t, and the sulfonate, 1u.

Intuitively one might argue that the safety of a prodrug is assured if the pro-moiety is removed rapidly and the pro-moiety itself is non-toxic. Using these criteria, we would conclude that the compounds of interest would be relatively safe since each of the pro-moieties were shown to be well tolerated and the intact prodrugs are hydrolyzed quite rapidly after an intravenous injection (in rhesus monkeys). Compound 1t was cleared the fastest, its concentration in plasma being undetectable 15 minutes after injection, and yet, as shown in the following data, 1t was also the most toxic.

Table VI. Average Lesion Size and Blood Levels of Creatine Phosphokinase (CPK) After Intramuscular Injection[a] of Various Prodrugs Into Rabbits[b]

Cmpd. No.	R (Scheme I)	Avg. Lesion Size (mm^3)	Pre-Test CPK's	24 hr. CPK's
--	Control	0	462± 134	488± 161
1a	$-CH_2CH_2COOH$	5844± 2002	494± 204	4922± 1092
1t	$-(CH_2)_6CON(Et)CH_2CH_2N(Et)_2$	11361± 4453	236± 80	7442± 2397
1u	$-(CH_2)_6CON(CH_3)CH_2CH_2SO_3H$	2024± 2056	145± 38	3252± 1447

[a] Each animal received 1 ml of a solution containing 50 mg/ml of prodrug.
[b] Ref. 64.

Intravenous LD_{50} determinations in mice gave the following results:[64] 21-succinate, 953 mg/kg; compound 1u, 932 mg/kg; and compound 1t, 159 mg/kg. While the anionic prodrugs were well-tolerated, the amine containing derivative was significantly more toxic.

Compound 1t was also found to be inferior in rabbit intramuscular irritation studies and in its tendency to cause red blood cell lysis. Shown in Table VI are average lesion sizes and units of creatine phosphokinase in blood after intramuscular injections of each compound. Regardless of the criterion employed to assess muscle irritation 1t was significantly more irritating than the anionic derivatives of which 1u appeared to be slightly less irritating than the succinate. Another revealing indication of the tendency of the amine containing derivative to promote cell lysis was found in measurements of free hemoglobin in the serum of a dog given equivalent intravenous doses of the three compounds, shown in Table VII. Hemolysis was evident after administration of the amine containing derivative but minimal for the anionic compounds.

Clearly, prodrugs must be considered new drugs from the standpoint of toxicology. Even though bioconversion may be very rapid, significant toxicity may be elicited in the first minute after injection as a result of the direct action of the intact prodrug or due to the altered distribution of parent drug resulting from differences in prodrug structure.

Table VII. Free Serum Hemoglobin After Equivalent Intravenous Doses[a] of Various Prodrugs in a Single Dog.[b]

Cmpd. No.	R (Scheme I)	Free Serum hemoglobin (mg/l) Post Injection[c]		
		40 min.	1.5 hrs.	3 hrs.
1a	$-(CH_2)_2COOH$	305	300	98
1t	$-(CH_2)_6CON(Et)CH_2CH_2N(Et)_2$	2020	1760	1880
1u	$-(CH_2)_6CON(CH_3)CH_2CH_2SO_3H$	93	218	146

[a] 30 mg/kg (methylprednisolone equivalents).
[b] Ref. 65.
[c] Pre-injection value was 100 mg/l.

We conclude that the design of safety must be an integral component of a prodrug design program. Preliminary toxicity studies should be conducted in parallel with in vitro stability determinations and bioavailability studies.

Acknowledgements

The authors wish to thank C.H. Spilman, A.D. Forbes, and W.J. Bryan, The Upjohn Company, for their aid in carrying out the in vivo studies. We also thank R. Ochoa, J.T. VanderLugt and D.J. Weber of The Upjohn Company for supplying the in vivo toxicology data and for their support in the design program.

References

1. B.D. Anderson, R.A. Conradi, and K.E. Knuth, J. Pharm. Sci., 74, 365(1985).

2. B.D. Anderson, R.A. Conradi, K.E. Knuth, and S.L. Nail, J. Pharm. Sci., 74, 375(1985).

3. B.D. Anderson, R.A. Conradi, C.H. Spilman, and A.D. Forbes, J. Pharm. Sci., 74, 382(1985).

4. "Physicians' Desk Reference", 35th Ed., Medical Economics Company, Oradell, NJ, 1981.

5. E.R. Garrett, J. Med. Pharm. Chem., 5, 112(1962).

6. B.D. Anderson and V. Taphouse, J. Pharm. Sci., 70, 181(1981).

7. R.J. Townsend, A.H. Puchala, and S.L. Nail, Am. J. Hosp. Pharm., 38, 1319(1981).

8. J.C. Melby and M. St. Cyr, Metabolism, 10, 75(1961).

9. A.J. Glazko, W.A. Dill, A.W. Kinkel, J.R. Goulet, W.J. Holloway, and R.A. Buchanan, Clin. Pharmacol. Ther., 21, 104(1977).

10. L. Strebel, J. Miceli, R. Kauffman, R. Poland, A. Dajani, A. Done, Clin. Pharmacol. Ther., 27, 288(1980).

11. A.J. Kirby in "Comprehensive Chemical Kinetics: Vol 10. Ester Formation and Hydrolysis and Related Reactions", C.H. Bamford and C.F.H. Tipper, Eds., Elsevier Pub. Co., Amsterdam, 1972, p. 57.

12. B.D. Anderson, R.A. Conradi, and W.J. Lambert, J. Pharm. Sci., 73, 604(1984).

13. A. Martin, J. Swarbrick, and A. Cammarata, "Physical Pharmacy", Lea & Febiger, Philadelphia, 1983, p. 298.

14. B.D. Anderson, R.A. Conradi, and K. Johnson, J. Pharm. Sci., 72, 448(1983).

15. S.S. Davis, T. Higuchi, and J.H. Rytting in "Advances in Pharmaceutical Sciences", Vol. 4, H.S. Bean, A.H. Beckett, and J.E. Carless, Eds., Academic Press, New York, 1974, p.73.

16. A. Leo, C. Hansch, and D. Elkins, Chem. Rev., 71, 525(1971).

17. B.D. Anderson in "Physical Chemical Properties of Drugs", S.H. Yalkowsky, A.A. Sinkula, and S.C. Valvani, Eds., Marcel Dekker, Inc., New York, 1980, p. 231.

18. B.D. Anderson and R.A. Conradi, J. Pharm. Sci., 69, 4666(1980).

19. R.W. Taft in "Steric Effects in Organic Chemistry", M.S. Newman, Ed., Wiley, New York, 1956, Chpt. 13.

20. L.P. Hammett, Chem. Rev., 17, 125(1935).

21. D.D. Perrin in "Physical Chemical Properties of Drugs", S.H. Yalkowsky, A.A. Sinkula, and S.C. Valvani, Eds., Marcel Dekker, Inc., New York, 1980, p. 1.

22. M. Charton in "Design of Biopharmaceutical Properties through Prodrugs and Analogs", E.B. Roche, Ed., American Pharmaceutical Association, Washington, D.C., p. 228.

23. B. Capon and S.P. McManus, "Neighboring Group Participation", Vol. 1, Plenum Press, New York, 1976.

24. S.A. Bernard, A. Berger, J.H. Carter, E. Katchalski, M. Sela, and Y. Shalitin, J. Amer. Chem. Soc., 84, 2471(1961).

25. C.K. Ingold, J. Chem. Soc., 1032(1932).

26. W. Morozowich, M.J. Cho, and F.J. Kezdy in "Design of Biopharmaceutical Properties through Prodrugs and Analogs", E.B. Roche, Ed., American Pharmaceutical Association, Washington, D.C., p. 344.

27. M. Kawamura, R. Yamamoto, and S. Fujisawa, Yakugaku

Zasshi, 91, 863(1971).

28. E.R. Garrett, J. Pharm. Sci., 51, 445(1962).

29. E.R. Garrett and M.E. Royer, J. Pharm. Sci., 51, 451(1962).

30. C. Hansch in "Physico-Chemical Aspects of Drug Action", Vol. 7, Pergamon Press, Oxford, 1966, pp. 141-167.

31. M. Charton, J. Amer. Chem. Soc., 97, 1552(1975).

32. V. Stella, T. Higuchi, A. Hussain, and J. Truelove in "Prodrugs as Novel Drug Delivery Systems", T. Higuchi and V. Stella, Eds., American Chemical Society Symposium Series #14, 1975, pp. 154-183.

33. S.A. Varia, S. Schuller, and V.J. Stella, J. Pharm. Sci., 73, 1074(1984).

34. G.L. Flynn and D.J. Lamb, J. Pharm. Sci., 59, 1433(1970).

35. J.L. Kurz, J. Phys. Chem., 66, 2239(1962).

36. C.A. Bunton, S. Diaz, L.S. Romsted, and O. Valenzuela, J. Org. Chem., 41, 3037(1976).

37. A.T. Florence in "Techniques of Solubilization of Drugs", S.H. Yalkowsky, Ed., Marcel Dekker, New York, 1981, pp. 79-81.

38. "Guide to the Physiological Suitability of Atlas Surfactants", I.C.I. Americas Inc., 1977.

39. D. Attwood and A.T. Florence, "Biology Surfactant Systems, Their Chemistry, Pharmacy", Chapman and Hall, London, 1982.

40. K. Shinoda, "Principles of Solution and Solubility", Marcel Dekker, New York, 1978, pp. 157-199.

41. D.E. Guttman, W.E. Hamlin, J.W. Shell, and J.G. Wagner, J. Pharm. Sci., 50, 305(1961).

42. M.I. Amin and J.T. Bryan, J. Pharm. Sci., 62, 1768(1973).

43. W.K. Anderson, C.P. Chang, and H.L. McPherson, Jr., J. Med. Chem., 26, 1333(1983).

44. S.S. Davis, T. Higuchi, and J. H. Rytting, in "Advances in Pharmaceutical Sciences", Vol. 4, Academic, London, 1974, p. 232.

45. G.S. Hartley, Trans. Faraday Soc., 30, 444(1934)

46. N. Funasaki and A. Murata, Chem. Pharm. Bull., 28, 805(1980).

47. H. Al-Lohedan, C.A. Bunton, and L.S. Romsted, J. Phys. Chem., 85, 2123(1981).

48. G.L. Amidon, R.S. Pearlman, and G.D. Leesman, in "Design of Biopharmaceutical Properties through Prodrugs and Analogs", E.B. Roche, Ed., American Pharmaceutical Association, Washington, D.C., p. 281.

49. R.E. Williams and M.L. Bender, Canad. J. Biochem., 49, 210(1971).

50. A. Williams, Biochemistry, 9, 3383(1970).

51. M.L. Bender and K. Nakamura, J. Amer. Chem. Soc., 84, 2577(1962).

52. N. Shimamoto and H. Fukutome, J. Biochem. (Tokyo), 78, 663(1975).

53. C.D. Hubbard and T.S. Shoupe, J. Biol. Chem., 252, 1633(1977).

54. A.R. Butler, I.H. Robertson, and L.A. Rudkin, J. Chem. Soc. Perkin Trans. II, 351(1977).

55. K. Ikeda, S. Kunugi, and N. Ise, Archives of Biochemistry and Biophysics, 217, 37(1982).

56. E. Tommila and C.N. Hinshelwood, J. Chem. Soc., 1801(1938).

57. A. Dupaix, J.J. Bechet, and C. Roucous, Biochemistry, 12, 2559(1973).

58. M. Dixon and E.C. Webb, "Enzymes", 3rd ed., Academic Press, New York, 1979, p. 252.

59. D.J. Weber, unpublished data.

60. K. Krisch in "The Enzymes", 3rd ed., Vol. V, Academic Press, New York, 1971, p. 43.

61. C. Schottler and K. Krisch, Biochem. Pharmac., 23, 2867(1974).

62. K. Hattori, M. Kamio, E. Nakajima, T. Oshima, T. Satoh, and H. Kitagawa, Biochem. Pharmac., 30, 2051(1981).

63. A.J. Adler and G.B. Kistiakowsky, J. Biol. Chem., 351, 81(1970).

64. R. Ochoa, unpublished data.

65. D.J. Weber and J.T. Vanderlugt, unpublished data.

Chapter 5
Physical Model Based Optimization of Local and Systemic Delivery of Prodrugs

Jeffrey L. Fox

Department of Pharmaceutics
University of Utah
College of Pharmacy
Salt Lake City, UT 84112

Introduction

The application of the physical model approach to therapeutics is discussed in general, and the approach is illustrated with a detailed description of its application to a research problem that has been studied in our laboratories for nearly a decade. The problem is the optimization of the topical delivery of vidarabine to its presumed site of action in the vaginal membrane. For reasons to be discussed below, the application of prodrug esters has been shown to be more effective in the topical delivery of vidarabine than is the application of vidarabine itself. The goal of this research has thus been the rational determination of that prodrug structure that will be most optimal as judged by its ability to deliver vidarabine to its presumed site of action.

The physical model approach to this problem will be discussed in some detail, with the intent of providing the reader with an idea as to what is involved in such an approach. The organization of this chapter will therefore center on the physical model approach and the general steps involved with applying it to therapeutics. Thus the content of this chapter is intended to be applicable to a broad range of problems in drug delivery. The use of a specific example research problem throughout should help the reader develop a fairly complete picture of how the method is used in practice, from the initial statement of the problem to the use of the model in interpreting clinical observations.

The Physical Model Approach as a Research Strategy

The role of the physical model approach in the larger context of research problem solving is frequently misunderstood and will therefore be briefly commented upon. The terms "approach" and "strategy" are suggestive of the niche that the use of physical models occupies in the arsenal of laboratory techniques, data analysis techniques, thought processes, etc. that a scientist can bring to bear on a research problem. We would like the reader to regard the notion of a research strategy as occupying a level above that occupied by techniques and below that of the overall research philosophy employed.

Consider the overall goal of gaining a conceptual and mechanistic understanding of the behavior of the system being studied. In many cases, qualitative approaches are appropriate and entirely adequate. The determination of the mechanism of action of drugs is a prominent example of such a qualitative problem. Other problems may be dealt with effectively only by quantifying the concepts involved. The physical model strategy is a means of accomplishing this concept quantification. The physical model approach should therefore not be seen as synonymous with the overall goal of understanding a system, but should be seen only as a strategy to be employed when concept quantification is useful to achieving this overall goal.

On the other hand, the physical model approach is much more than just a technique for data analysis. There is a tendency (often justified, unfortunately) to perceive the use of physical models as limited in scope to "exercises in data fitting, in an attempt to 'explain' results". Such data fitting can, indeed, be extremely useful, a case in point being the use of simple compartmental models in pharmacokinetics. Uses such as this amount to what might be called a "physical model technique" for data analysis as opposed to the broader idea of the physical model approach as a research strategy.

As will become readily apparent, the physical model approach is much more than a data analysis technique. It will be seen to be an integrated approach that encompasses both experimental design and model based data interpretation into the overall research strategy.

The Mechanics of the Physical Model Approach

A simplistic view of the physical model approach might characterize the approach as a sequence of steps to be carried out in a prescribed fashion with the goal of fitting some physical model to a given experimental system. The steps in accomplishing this might be something like the following:

(1) Write down a physically realistic model for the system.

(2) Solve the mathematical equations that describe the system.

(3) Design a set of experimental studies that will enable the model to be tested.

(4) Determine the values for any unknown parameters that appear in the model.

(5) Try to think of something useful to do with the results of steps 1 - 4.

This naive view is deficient at best. While these steps may represent an effective means of fitting experimental data to a physical model, they do not necessarily bear an obvious relationship to any question that needs answered. In other words, these steps alone do not represent anything useful when not in the context of a research problem. At most these steps comprise a recipe or technique for data fitting that is not complete enough even for this limited use.

Our view is that the use of the physical model approach should be integrated in a natural fashion into the overall research strategy as opposed to being used only as an isolated technique for data analysis. Since we are presenting the approach as a research strategy, we will describe it in terms of a series of questions to be addressed. The answering of these questions comprises a physical model based strategy for studying a research problem.

As is the case with other research strategies, it is not generally most productive to answer these questions in an obvious predetermined sequence, with each question being considered in isolation from the others. Instead, all these should be kept in mind while any one of them is being actively pursued, since there are many interrelationships among them. In particular, we must constantly be aware of developments that might suggest abandoning or changing the direction of our studies.

The questions we will consider are the following:

o   what physical model is appropriate for the system being studied?

o   can values be assigned to the parameters appearing in the model?

o which of these parameters are important in determining the behavior of the system?

o can these parameters be manipulated to control the behavior of the system?

o can the model be used to make useful correlations with experimental data or predictions as to how new systems will behave?

o if so, what are the optimum values for the parameters that can be manipulated?

o is the physical model approach a cost effective one for the system being studied?

The remainder of this chapter will take each of these questions in turn and show how it has been addressed in the research problem of optimizing the topical delivery of vidarabine to its presumed site of action.

The Problem: Topical Delivery of Vidarabine

The topical delivery of vidarabine was chosen for investigation by the physical model strategy for the following reasons:

The Problem is Clinically Important

Vidarabine (9-beta-arabinofuranosyladenine, ara-A) has been reported to be intrinsically active against herpes viruses replicating in cell culture (1-4), in laboratory animals (3, 5-12) and in human patients (13-23). In spite of its intrinsic activity, vidarabine has been found to be ineffective in some important therapeutically situations, most notably in the treatment of genital herpes infections.

In mice inoculated either intranasally or intravaginally with herpes simplex virus type II and treated either systemically (24-26) or topically (24) with vidarabine, the drug was ineffective. No difference could be seen between control and treatment groups in a double-blind evaluation of topical vidarabine treatment of herpes progenitalis in humans (27). The investigators in this latter study noted the low solubility of the drug and its inability to penetrate lesions and suggested that the therapeutic ineffectiveness might be attributable to poor delivery of the agent to its site of action.

The Prodrug Approach Appeared Promising

The ineffectiveness of vidarabine itself could be linked to several physical factors that could be subject to manipulation by chemical structural modifications. Low solubility, poor permeability through biological tissues, and susceptibility to inactivation by adenosine deaminase had all been noted as factors limiting the effectiveness of vidarabine. In addition, a number of monoesters, diesters and triesters of vidarabine had been synthesized (28-29) having a wide range of solubilities and lipophilicities. Furthermore, a potent inhibitor of adenosine deaminase had been developed (30), opening the possibility to a combination therapy consisting of the inhibitor along with either vidarabine or a selected vidarabine prodrug.

The Behavior of the System was Dependent on a Large number of Physical Chemical and Biological Factors

The presumed site of action of vidarabine is between the site of application and the systemic circulation, and the drug is partially metabolized in its transit between these two sites. The situation with prodrugs is even more complex, as prodrug conversion to active drug also occurs in this region. Thus a quantitative understanding of the system can only be obtained via a detailed analysis. Such a quantitative understanding in many cases would be of academic interest, but not necessary to the development of effective therapy, since serious candidate compounds are usually those that perform well in screening tests, and therefore have high enough potency to be effective even in the non-optimal delivery systems employed in such tests. Vidarabine, unfortunately, is not so potent as to afford the luxury of non-optimal delivery and a quantitative understanding of its behavior is therefore required for success in delivery system design.

What Experimental Model(s) are Appropriate?

There are two therapeutic situations for which the topical delivery of vidarabine might be useful: the treatment of cold sores and the treatment of vaginal herpes infections. In the former, the relevant experimental system would be an infected skin lesion and the in the latter situation the target tissue would be the vaginal membrane. Since these systems are similar in their morphology and in the enzyme profiles relevant to vidarabine delivery (at least qualitatively), there is the possibility for considerable application of facts learned in the study of one system to the understanding of the other. A similar argument suggests that experiments conducted on the same tissues from different species might be qualitatively similar, even though species might differ considerably in values for tissue permeabilities, enzyme levels and other quantifiable factors. So long as we remain aware of these likely quantitative differences, we are free to choose our experimental systems on the basis of considerations such as convenience, reproducibility and cost.

In the early stages of working with a given physical model, much of the effort is focused on establishing the model and verifying that it is useful in explaining a variety of experimental observations. In this stage, it is appropriate to choose model experimental systems on the basis of their likelihood of providing quantitatively reproducible data. Once the model is firmly established, it can then be productive to switch the emphasis to systems that more closely mimic the real therapeutic situation. That is, animal models may be more productive in the early phase when models are being established and verified, while less reproducible experiments using human tissue (or better yet, infected human tissue) may be more useful later on in testing the usefulness of the model under more clinically relevant conditions.

What Physical Model is Appropriate?

Two sets of considerations must be satisfied for the realization of a useful physical model. The model must include those physical chemical factors most important in determining the behavior of the system and the model must be representable in terms of mathematical expressions that show the relationship of these factors to both variables that are experimentally measurable and those that are important, but for which direct measurement is difficult or impossible. A corollary to this second consideration is that the equations chosen must be solvable. Each of these considerations will now be discussed in turn for the topical delivery of vidarabine via the prodrug approach.

Physical Chemical Considerations

The chemical structures and solubilities of vidarabine and several of its prodrugs are shown in Figure 1. Vidarabine is an adenine nucleoside, structurally very similar to adenosine. Table 1 shows solubility and partition coefficients for vidarabine and a number of its ester prodrugs, including those formed by the acylation of the 2' and 3' hydroxyls, as well as the 5' hydroxyl. Even a cursory consideration of this table suggests that a prodrug might be found that will be much more effective than vidarabine in the delivery of this species.

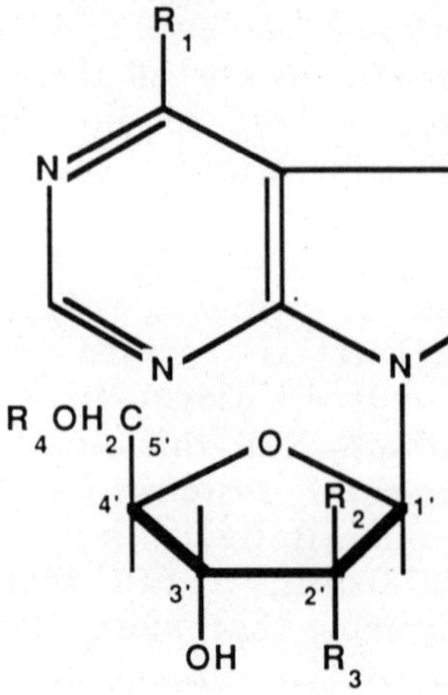

COMPOUND	R_1	R_2	R_3	R_4
Adenosine	NH_2	H	OH	H
Vidarabine	NH_2	OH	H	H
-5' Acetate	NH_2	OH	H	CH_3CO
-5' Valerate	NH_2	OH	H	$CH_3(CH_2)_3CO$
-5' Octanoate	NH_2	OH	H	$CH_3(CH_2)_6CO$
Ara-Hx	OH	OH	H	H

Figure 1. The structures of vidarabine and related compounds.

Vidarabine possesses the unfortunate combination of both low solubility (in water) and low lipophilicity relative to the other compounds. Therefore if the drug delivery goal were simply to effect the delivery of either vidarabine or one of its esters through a lipoidal membrane, almost any of the esters listed in Table 1 would be superior to vidarabine. It was this line of thinking that motivated the synthesis of many of the compounds shown.

In addition to solubility and lipophilicity, two other major concerns in the choice of a prodrug from this table are readily apparent. First, the prodrug must itself possess intrinsic antiviral activity or else be readily hydrolyzed to release vidarabine. Secondly, adenosine deaminase may inactivate vidarabine as rapidly as it is formed or, even worse, may deaminate the prodrug before its hydrolysis to liberate vidarabine. An awareness of this latter concern was the driving force behind the development of coformycin (30), an inhibitor of adenosine deaminase, as a possible adjuvant to enhance the effectiveness of vidarabine.

Table 1. Physical properties of vidarabine and some ester prodrugs of vidarabine

Type	Ester Moiety	Aqueous Solubility (mg/ml)	Log K_p (pentanol/H_2O)
Vidarabine	--	-0.4	-0.48
2'-mono	acetate	very soluble	-1.8
	propionate	---	0.19
3'-mono	acetate	---	0.15
	propionate	---	0.60
5'-mono	acetate	6.6 - 9.9	0.12
	propionate	9.2	0.58
	n-butyrate	16.1	0.90
	n-valerate	8.4	1.33
	isovalerate	19.8	1.39
	trimethylacetate	7.0	1.63
	n-hexanoate	2.5	1.78
	n-octanoate	0.23	approx. 2
	benzoyl	0.08	1.35
	hydroxycinnamoate	1.5	1.73
2',3'-di	acetate	33.0	0.20
	propionate	4.5	1.10
	isobutyrate	0.42	1.74
	benzoyl	very low	---
3',5'-di	acetate	4.7	0.71
	propionate	2.28	1.55
	isobutyrate	0.02	1.66
2',3',5'-tri	acetate	3.5	0.66
	propionate	0.23	2.15
	butyrate	---	---

For simplicity we will focus most of the detailed discussion of the physical models and their application on one series of monoesters chosen from those listed in Figure 1, namely the 5' esters of vidarabine. If we consider only the n-alkanoic acid esters, we see that lipophilicity increases monotonically with increasing alkanoate chain length. Aqueous solubility is highest for the butyrate and decreases with increasing chain length as would be expected. Not expected *a priori* is the decrease in solubility as chain length is shortened from C_4 to C_2 with the vidarabine solubility being lower than that of any of these short chain length alkanoate esters.

In addition to the information in Figure 1, it is apparent that the kinetics of vidarabine liberation by each of these esters must be determined. An unexpected property of these prodrugs that also must be considered is that they competitively inhibit the deamination of vidarabine by adenosine deaminase (31).

Mathematical Representation of the Physical Model

The model used to represent the vaginal membrane is shown schematically in Figure 2. Each of the three regions is assumed to be a continuous homogeneous phase. The physical

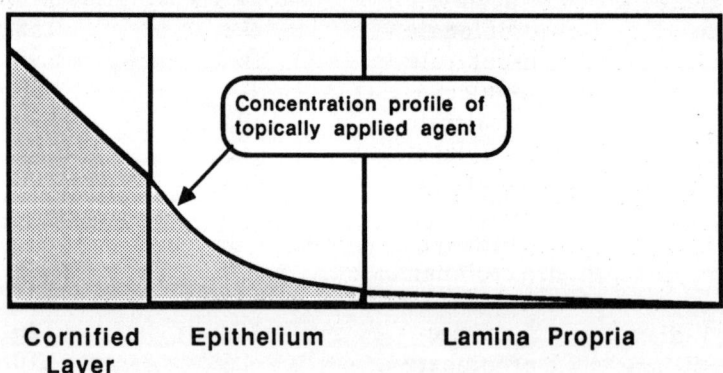

Figure 2. Schematic of the physical model for the vaginal membrane.

chemical properties of each layer that determine the attainable levels of the active drug are diffusivity of prodrug and drug, the partition coefficients of each and the levels of esterase and deaminase present. For studies with skin, the model used is essentially the same, with the stratum corneum, epidermis and dermis in the skin corresponding to the cornified layer, epithelium and lamina propria in the vaginal membrane, respectively.

A more physically realistic model would attempt to portray each layer in more detail. For example, the epithelium might consist of a packed bed of spherical cells and in this case transport into and out of the cells, diffusion between and through the cells and levels of enzymes both inside and outside the cells would need to be considered to calculate the concentration of the active drug attainable at the presumed site of action inside the cells. The mathematics of such a complex model are not conceptually different from those of the homogeneous phase model and could be solved using similar mathematical approaches. However, the experimental effort required to characterize this more complex model would be considerable. We will therefore employ the simpler homogeneous phase model so long as it is useful in interpreting the available data.

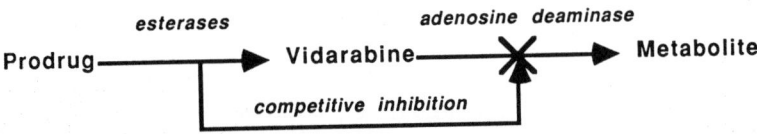

Figure 3. Metabolic scheme for the monoester prodrugs of vidarabine.

The general metabolic scheme is shown in Figure 3. Both the esterase and deaminase enzymes are presumed to be saturable. In addition, the deaminase enzyme has been found to be competitively inhibited by the prodrug. The non-steady state partial differential equations for the concurrent diffusion and metabolism of the prodrug, the active drug and the inactive metabolite are:

$$\frac{\partial P}{\partial t} = D_P \frac{\partial^2 P}{\partial x^2} - \frac{Vmax_P [P]}{Km_P + [P]}$$

$$\frac{\partial V}{\partial t} = D_V \frac{\partial^2 V}{\partial x^2} + \frac{Vmax_P [P]}{Km_P + [P]} - \frac{Vmax_V [V]}{(1 + \frac{[P]}{k_1}) * Km_V + [V]}$$

$$\frac{\partial M}{\partial t} = D_M \frac{\partial^2 M}{\partial x^2} + \frac{Vmax_V [V]}{(1 + \frac{[P]}{k_1}) * Km_V + [V]}$$

These equations are used for each lamina of the model. At the interfaces between laminae, continuity of concentrations and fluxes are assumed. If this multilaminar membrane is mounted in a diffusion cell, the boundary condition at each extreme of the membrane is that the rate of change in the amount of each species in each diffusion cell compartment is equal to the flux of that species from the membrane into the compartment. The initial conditions generally used are that the concentrations of all species are initially zero throughout the membrane and the initial concentrations of each species (most of which are zero) are specified in each diffusion cell compartment.

Solution of the Model Equations

Up to this time, factors such as computer speed, expense and convenience have provided an incentive to simplify the differential equations and then design experimental procedures that legitimize the use of these mathematically simpler models. As computing power becomes even cheaper and the appropriate software more widely available, the mathematical difficulty of solving models will be less and less a problem, even when carrying out lengthy sequences of calculations in which models may have to be solved tens or hundreds of times with different values of some of the physical parameters.

Even if complexity of computation were not an issue, however, there would still be incentive to simplify the model. Simpler models tend to have fewer unknown parameters associated with them; indeed simpler models often lead to data collection in such a way that less information is available from which to determine parameter values. For example, in studying the transport of a solute through a simple membrane it is common to measure the limiting steady state flux of solute through the membrane. That is, the transport is characterized by a single quantity, the permeability, which is readily calculated from the steady state flux. A more complex model that also accounts for the pre steady-state data, on the other hand, can enable one to deduce both diffusivity and partition coefficient, the physical quantities that together determine the permeability. Thus the price paid for simplicity in mathematics and data treatment is often a sacrifice in the information that can be deduced from the data. This is a price that is often worth paying, however, as there is usually greater certainty in the values of quantities that are determined in clean simple experiments that are not confounded by multiple unknown quantities to be deduced.

There are three independent simplifying assumptions that can be made for this system: infinite volumes of donor and receiver compartments, linear enzyme kinetics and attainment of the steady state. The most general approach to solving this system would be to develop a model with none of these assumptions built in. Each special case resulting from various combinations of the assumptions could then be computed by the appropriate choice of model parameters. If calculations entailed no expense in terms of either time or money, this would be a most attractive approach. However, the use of computing resources entails costs in terms of both time and money. Furthermore, experiments based on this most general case would be the most difficult to quantitatively interpret. Therefore, we seek computational and experimental approaches that take advantage of these simplifying assumptions.

The eight possible combinations of assumptions can be divided into two groups with respect to the approaches to solution of the model, based on whether the enzyme kinetics are assumed to be linear. The discussion of approaches to the solution of the model will therefore be divided accordingly.

In the simplest of the linear models, the steady state is also assumed and an explicit analytic solution is available in principle. Even for the simple case of a single enzymatic reaction and a two layer membrane, however, this analytical solution becomes extremely unwieldy (32), with some 70 numbered equations being involved in its development. A simpler approach is clearly desirable to attack problems involving either more complex chemistry or multiple lamina membranes.

Carslaw and Jaegar (33) described a matrix Laplace transform approach to the problem of non-steady state heat conduction in a multilaminar system. We have adapted this approach to the problem at hand. Briefly, each lamina is considered as a separate problem for which the Laplace transform of the solute concentration and flux profiles can be readily written in matrix form. The Laplace transform for the entire membrane involves the matrix product of these individual matrices for each lamina.

These Laplace transform matrices readily lead to matrices for the actual steady state concentrations and fluxes. When expressed in this matrix notation, the solution can be developed in about a dozen equations, no matter how complex the chemistry or how many layers comprise the membrane (34). By shifting to this matrix notation we have sacrificed the availability of an explicit solution in exchange for the ability of expressing the problem concisely. This is not a great loss as the explicit solution is so cumbersome as to be of little or no value in terms of lending insight into the behavior of the model.

As to the non-steady state case, Carslaw and Jaegar note that while the Laplace transform is readily written in the matrix notation as a product of matrices, its inversion involves "extremely heavy algebra" and, although possible in principle, is impractical in practice. Very recently, however, a computer routine has been published (35) capable of reliably inverting Laplace transforms by a numerical technique. The inversion of Laplace transforms is an extremely ill-conditioned numerical problem, when the value of the Laplace variable is restricted to lie on the real axis (36) and previous algorithms using only real numbers (reference 37, for example) were of very limited use. The new inversion routine requires that the user supply a routine to evaluate the Laplace transform for complex as well as real values of the Laplace variable. We have recently begun using this technique for the solution of non-steady state transport problems in multilaminar systems and have found it to be quite promising. For the problem at hand, this approach could be used without the assumption of infinite volumes of donor and receiver compartments, and these assumptions brought in if need be by simply choosing appropriate values for parameters in the model.

The final case involving linear kinetics is the so-called quasi-steady state case, in which the transport processes in the membrane are assumed to be at steady state but the donor and receiver compartments, having finite volumes, experience changes in the concentrations of the diffusants. This problem is essentially a system of ordinary differential equations for the concentrations of species in the donor and receiver compartments as functions of time. The most straightforward method of solution is therefore by means of numerical integration. For any given set of values of donor and receiver compartment concentrations, the steady state problem is solved by the matrix technique described above (34) and rates of change of these concentrations calculated from the fluxes into and from the donor and receiver. This technique for calculating time derivatives can be used along with a capable differential equation solver (38) and the quasi-steady state problem solved.

The cases involving nonlinear kinetics are much more complicated since there are no analytical solutions available for the unilaminar problem that can be simply combined to yield multilaminar solutions as in the linear case. Even if such unilaminar solutions were to be calculated numerically (they readily can be), the manipulations done in the linear case would not be valid because they implicitly depend on the principle of superposition of solutions, which is valid only when working with linear systems. Thus the nonlinear problem cannot be divided into a series smaller problems, one for each lamina, but must be solved for the entire membrane at once. In the steady state case, with infinite reservoir volumes (i.e., unchanging concentrations in each reservoir), we have used a shooting method (39) to solve the nonlinear boundary value problem (40). For the quasi-steady state case, a method analogous to that used for the linear quasi-steady state problem would be appropriate.

For the nonlinear non-steady state case, a general numerical technique suitable for parabolic partial differential equations is required. We have found the method of lines to be a suitable technique and have used the software designed by Sincovec and Madsen (41) for such problems. The case where the donor and receiver compartments have finite volumes is not handled by the above software without modification, but the required changes are minor and can be done fairly simply.

Determination of Parameter Values

Once the mathematical techniques are in hand for calculating the behavior of the model we must develop methods for determining the values of the various parameters that appear in the model. In so far as is possible, we endeavor to directly measure these parameter values. When this can not be done, we must resort to indirect methods such as parameter fitting. This latter method should be a last resort and its use must be scrutinized critically to ensure its validity. For the model system considered here, the experimentally measured parameters are as follows.

Directly Measured Parameters

In this system the relevant parameters are those affecting the transport and metabolism of each species in each lamina of the membrane. The total activities of the relevant enzymes (esterases and adenosine deaminases) in each tissue lamina can be measured by conducting experiments with homogenates of each lamina. By varying the concentrations of substrates, the parameters that characterize the saturability of the enzymes and the competitive nature of the deaminase inhibition by the prodrugs can be determined.

It is not experimentally feasible, however, to isolate each lamina of membrane while maintaining physical integrity so that solute permeation can be readily measured. However, there are available enough subsets of the full skin so that permeabilities of solutes through each layer can be estimated. With skin, for example, the stratum corneum can be removed by "stripping" with cellophane tape (42), leaving an epidermis / dermis composite membrane through which permeation can be measured. The dermis can be removed with trypsin, leaving a stratum corneum / epidermis composite through which transport can be measured. Combining the results obtained from these two preparations with measurements made on the full membrane allows the permeability of each individual lamina to be calculated. More recently Raykar et al. (43) have succeeded in removing the stratum corneum from human skin samples in such a way that the integrity of the stratum corneum is maintained. Incorporation of this preparation into experimental protocols affords a direct check on the inferences made from the other preparations. To eliminate the confounding of permeation measurements by the production of metabolites, enzyme inhibitors can be used as appropriate (44).

Indirectly Measured Parameters

Models as complex as the ones described here often include parameters for which values can be indirectly estimated by use of the physical model along with an appropriate data fitting procedure. In some cases this is the only means available for estimating these parameter values. In other cases, indirect estimation may involve simpler or less costly experimental procedures than direct means. In any case, parameter values obtained by indirect means should be independently checked for reasonableness if at all possible.

In the model systems being studied, the activities of enzymes in the various layers of membrane can be determined by such indirect means. *In vitro* permeation experiments are conducted in which a membrane is mounted in a diffusion cell, one chamber charged with either vidarabine or one of its prodrugs, and fluxes of all relevant species into both donor and receiver chambers measured. For simplicity in fitting the model, these experiments are usually conducted under sink conditions and with the donor chamber charged with only a tracer level of the compound being studied. In the receiver chamber, the fluxes of this compound and its metabolites are measured. As a result of the metabolism occurring in the membrane, there are fluxes of metabolites back into the donor chamber, which are also measured.

A typical application of this technique is with vaginal membrane or skin stripped of the less permeable outer layer of cornified tissue. The membrane being studied then consists of two layers, both of which have appreciable esterase and deaminase activity. Generally, three experimental runs are performed, with the roles of donor and receiver chambers alternating with each run. With the skin for example, the donor chamber might be on the epidermis side of the membrane during the first and third runs and on the dermis side during the second run. The first and third runs can be compared as a check on the invariance of the behavior of the membrane. The second run provides somewhat different information than the others, since the back flux of metabolites is most sensitive to the enzyme activity in that part of the membrane nearest the donor chamber. Fluxes through the membrane into the receiver chamber, on the other hand, are independent of the orientation of the membrane (so long as the permeabilities of the various chemical species are assumed to be equal).

If permeabilities of each species are assumed to be known from direct measurement as described above, then enzyme activities in each of the lamina of the membrane can be estimated from the fluxes measured in these permeation experiments. For any assumed set of values for enzyme activities, the model can be used to calculate the fluxes expected experimentally. A procedure for calculating these fluxes as a function of enzyme activities is embedded into a nonlinear least squares minimization program (45, 46) and the enzyme activities adjusted until those values are found which give the best agreement between calculated and experimentally observed fluxes.

For the model system described here, these enzyme activities are also estimable from experiments with homogenates of the various membrane lamina. This latter technique would appear to be more direct and thus obviate the need for the indirect estimation from the flux measurements. This would be true if there were no assumptions in the model subject to doubt (i.e., if the model were unquestionably valid). This model, however, contains the assumption of homogeneity within each lamina of the membrane. Even the most cursory morphological examination would clearly reveal that such an assumption is not strictly true. Nonetheless, the enzyme activities calculated from the permeation experiments and those measured with homogenate experiments are in good agreement (44). Insofar as transport and metabolism are concerned, then, the assumption of homogeneous laminae is consistent with experimental observation. This suggests that as the compounds diffuse across the membrane, there is free access to the enzymes; otherwise, the enzyme activities calculated from the permeation experiments would be smaller than those measured with the more direct homogenate technique. Thus the use of the physical model to indirectly infer a redundant piece of information serves as a check on the validity of the model.

Sensitivity Analysis

The physical model approach thus far has enabled us to calculate or simulate experimental results for assumed values of the parameters of the model; and, furthermore, to couple these calculations with the appropriate experiments in such a way that values for unmeasured parameters can be deduced. Were this all that could be accomplished, the approach would be little more than an academic exercise, for these parameter values are of interest only insofar as they lead to an understanding of the therapeutic performance of the system being studied. The power of the physical model approach, then, lies in its ability to relate probable therapeutic efficacy to the values of measurable (by direct or indirect means) parameters, thereby leading to effective strategies for optimizing the system by the manipulation of these parameters.

The process of optimization with respect to the parameters of a physical model consists of finding the set of values of these parameters for which some object function takes on its maximum value. The choice of an object function is not as simple as one might imagine. In general, such a function could include measures of therapeutic efficacy, costs of production of the final dosage form, estimates of the likely market and so forth, all expressed in some common unit of measure, such as dollars. Even if the scope of the optimization is restricted to maximizing therapeutic efficacy, the choice of object function is not always obvious. For the system being studied, possible choices might involve either steady-state concentrations of vidarabine or peak levels attained at some presumed site of action. We will later briefly discuss a proposed technique for determining the appropriate object function for this system. For now, we will use the simple assumption that therapeutic efficacy can be related to the total amount of vidarabine in the viable portion of the membrane (i.e.: the integral of the concentration vs. position profile, disregarding the dead cornified region of the skin or vaginal membrane).

In choosing the prodrug most effective at delivering vidarabine, the several physical chemical parameters that change with prodrug structure must be considered. These parameters are:

(1) solubility of the prodrug;

(2) permeability of the prodrug (especially to the stratum corneum or cornified layer);

(3) esterase mediated conversion of the prodrug to vidarabine; and

(4) the ability of the prodrug to competitively inhibit the conversion of vidarabine to the inactive metabolite.

The effects of changing the values of each of these parameters has been discussed in detail elsewhere (40) and will be summarized briefly here.

The baseline for these calculations was taken to be the calculated performance of the 5'-valerate monoester of vidarabine. Each of the parameters above was then varied in turn to assess its effect on the object function described above. Two membrane systems were simulated in the calculations, both based on experiments conducted with hairless mouse skin. The first system assumed the skin to be intact, with the full stratum corneum barrier present, while in the second system no stratum corneum barrier was assumed. These two simulated systems were intended to mimic the extremes in permeability characteristics of the vaginal membrane during the estrous cycle. More importantly, from a practical point of view, the comparison of the two systems would indicate whether the degree of cornification would have any effect on the choice of optimal prodrug.

For the intact skin with stratum corneum present, calculations showed that any increase or decrease in prodrug solubility or stratum corneum permeability would lead to a proportional change in the amount of vidarabine delivered. While such a result could easily be regarded as intuitively obvious, further calculations suggest that this apparently simple result is an accident of the parameter values that apply in this case. In particular, this apparently simple dependence of vidarabine availability on solubility or stratum corneum permeability is the result of stratum corneum penetration being the factor that limits vidarabine in this case. Even for this case, however, this simple dependence may not always hold. Calculations showed that if the solubility or permeability were increased by two orders of magnitude (conceivable with the use of penetration enhancers), the cleavage of prodrug by esterase would be the rate limiting factor and no additional gain would be available from further solubility or permeability enhancement. Nonetheless, the calculation clearly indicates that prodrug modifications designed to increase solubility or permeability would be effective in improving vidarabine delivery in this case.

A possible alternative strategy for increasing the availability of vidarabine is to inhibit its deamination to the inactive metabolite, vidarabine hypoxanthine. Preliminary studies conducted in our laboratories had shown that the use of covidarabine, an adenosine deaminase inhibitor, could increase intracellular vidarabine levels by several orders of magnitude in cell suspension experiments. In addition, Lipper (31) had shown that the vidarabine prodrugs were inhibitors of the deamination of vidarabine. This led to the idea of designing a prodrug that would not only release vidarabine, but prevent its subsequent inactivation by adenosine deaminase. Physical model calculations, however, quickly dashed the hopes for this strategy. The difference between no inhibition of deaminase and its complete inhibition was only a factor of two to three in the steady-state availability of vidarabine. Thus the use of model calculations clearly showed that an intuitively attractive strategy would yield no improvement in vidarabine delivery and a potentially expensive and unproductive development pathway was avoided.

The final parameter considered for manipulation is the lability of the prodrug to esterases. Calculations showed that esterase lability of the 5'-valerate prodrug was nearly optimal. Any significant decrease in this quantity would shift the availability-limiting factors from solubility and permeability to esterase lability, after which further decreases would result in proportional decreases in vidarabine availability. Increases in lability would be ineffective, since solubility and permeability were the performance limiting factors. In fact, increases in esterase lability were calculated to lead to a decrease in vidarabine availability as a result of depletion of the prodrug and consequent loss of its deaminase inhibition activity. The magnitude of this decrease was minor and of no practical significance, consistent with the previous result that inactivation of vidarabine by deaminase was shown to be unimportant.

Calculations of the sensitivity of the model to prodrug physical properties gave much different results when the stratum corneum was assumed to not be present. For this system, permeability through the stratum corneum obviously could not be a factor, although solubility of the prodrug conceivably might. The physical model calculations showed, however, that levels of vidarabine attainable would be sufficiently high that the esterases would become saturated and vidarabine availability would be limited by the lability of the prodrug to esterase cleavage. In spite of the limiting rate of conversion to vidarabine, the calculated concentrations of vidarabine were high enough to result in saturation of the adenosine deaminase in these simulations. This apparent lower deaminase activity caused the calculated effect of deaminase inhibition to be even less significant than with the intact stratum corneum model. Finally, the effect of increasing the solubility was shown to be minimal, as a result of esterase lability being the availability-limiting factor. Significant decreases in solubility, however, would result in the esterases no longer being saturated and the solubility would become the availability-limiting factor. Any further solubility decreases would then result in proportional decreases in vidarabine availability.

The foregoing exploration of the sensitivity of the model calculations to the various physical parameters dramatically illustrates the potential value of the physical model approach to the rational design of prodrugs. Several factors, all dependent on the structure of the prodrug, were considered and their relative importances shown to depend on the system being studied. In the intact skin model, vidarabine availability could be substantially increased only by increasing the solubility of the prodrug or its ability to penetrate the stratum corneum. With no stratum corneum present, however, vidarabine availability could only be improved by increasing the susceptibility of the prodrug to the esterases. In neither case was the deamination of vidarabine an important factor, in spite of its overwhelming importance in cell suspension systems.

Thus these systems possess not only quantitative differences in vidarabine availability, but more importantly, the choice of an effective prodrug design strategy depends on which system is being used. This result is non-intuitive and can only be obtained by a quantitative physical model analysis of the systems. It should be emphasized that this shift in most appropriate strategy is not a rare happening that occurs only because there are qualitative geometric differences in the intact stratum corneum and no stratum corneum systems. The shift is a result of a shift in the quantitative relationships among the physical parameters of the system when the stratum corneum is removed.

We should interpret this as a warning that the results obtained in this system, besides not being quantitatively reproduced in another system, may even show significant qualitative differences as well. If we take these models to be valid indicators of the behavior of real systems, we should expect that quantitative differences between various animal tissues might lead to qualitative differences in the behavior of these prodrug systems with respect to vidarabine delivery. For example, the choice of most effective prodrug for vidarabine delivery might depend on the species being studied. It should be no great surprise, then, that various animal models are frequently inconsistent with each other, and may conceivably all be inconsistent with human results for a given drug delivery problem.

Can the Key Parameters be Manipulated to Control the System?

Once the sensitivity analysis has identified the variables that would be most useful to manipulate, the means for doing so must be explored. For the example system, there are several avenues that might be pursued to accomplish this.

Most obvious are changes to the structure of the prodrug. For the 5'-monoesters of vidarabine, it has been shown that changing the length of the ester side chain affects solubility, stratum corneum permeability, lability to esterase and potency as an inhibitor of adenosine deaminase. These changes are obviously not independent of each other, a constraint that will be briefly discussed later.

A second approach to parameter manipulation is to enhance solubility by manipulation of the formulation. This approach must be applied with care if it is to be effective, however, since vehicle changes that increase the absolute solubility of the prodrug (by lowering the free energy of prodrug in the vehicle relative to its free energy in its crystalline state) will decrease (by the same degree, to a first approximation) the tendency of the prodrug to partition into the stratum corneum. The key to increasing availability by solubility enhancement then is to increase the free energy of the prodrug in its solid state. Approaches for doing so include the formation of coprecipitates and polymorphs.

More recently, permeability of compounds through the stratum corneum has been enhanced by the use of various adjuvants such as dimethylsulfoxide (DMSO) and 1-dodecylaza-cycloheptan-2-one (Azone^{TM}). The mechanism(s) of action of these extremely potent penetration enhancers is not yet well understood although it is being actively investigated in a number of laboratories.

For the model system, then, there appear to be adequate means available to manipulate the various parameters that appear in the model and that affect the topical delivery of vidarabine.

Can the Model Make Useful Correlations and Predictions?

Up to this point we have shown the use of the physical model approach to provide quantitative corroboration for a number of *in vitro* experimental results. We have also shown that the model can be used to predict how the availability of vidarabine at its presumed site of action depends on the parameters of the model. Furthermore, the values of these parameters have been shown to be controllable. It would appear, then, that these parameters could be chosen in such a way that the therapeutic efficacy of the system is maximized. Before doing so, however, we should ask if any evidence exists to demonstrate that the physical model developed for this system can, indeed, be used to predict the results of *in vivo* experimental studies from model parameters determined from *in vitro* experiments. In this section we will discuss the use of the model to quantitatively predict the results of *in vivo* transport studies and to corroborate the findings of efficacy studies in infected animals. Then we will briefly describe a technique currently being developed for the prediction of efficacy of a treatment applied to a population of animals.

Transport Studies Using Vascularly Isolated Skin Grafts

Krueger (47) has recently described a technique whereby grafts of human or other foreign animal skin can be made onto hypothalamic rats and maintained for several months. These grafts appear to behave biochemically in a fashion similar to their behavior in the donor animal, rather than taking on characteristics of the host animal. Furthermore, microsurgical techniques allow these grafts to be made in such a way that their blood supply can be cleanly isolated from that to other tissues. It is possible, then, to devise transport experiments that are similar to traditional diffusion cell experiments, except that the function of the receiver cell is assumed by the venous blood flow from the skin graft. Thus transport and metabolism studies that have previously been done *in vitro* can now be done with living skin.

It is especially noteworthy that this system can be used for human skin as well as animal skin. This leads to the very exciting possibility of conducting an entire series of quantitative transport studies with the same piece of skin, perhaps over a period of weeks or months, with the viability of the skin being maintained throughout.

We have used this skin flap system to test the hypothesis that our *in vitro* studies are quantitatively consistent with studies done with viable grafted hairless mouse skin (48). These studies have been conducted by applying a transdermal patch with a known zero-order release rate of compound to the skin graft. Concentrations of prodrug and drug have been measured in the venous blood coming from the graft and systemically as well. The rate of blood flow through the isolated graft is determined independently. These measurements can be used to calculate permeability of the grafted skin and the extent of metabolism in the grafted skin. Both are consistent with values measured in *in vitro* diffusion cell experiments. Additionally, the systemic pharmacokinetics following intravenous administration of drug or prodrug have been measured. This data can be combined with the known input from the skin graft to predict the systemic pharmacokinetics resulting from the application of the transdermal patch. Again, the prediction is consistent with experiment.

This grafted skin system has thus far been quantitatively consistent with *in vitro* diffusion cell experiments as well as with systemic pharmacokinetics. This technique, in concert with the physical model approach, promises to become an extremely valuable tool in the study of transdermal drug delivery.

Efficacy Studies With Infected Animals

Several studies with infected animals have been done that enable the model to be tested for its ability to predict therapeutic efficacy. As already noted, vidarabine itself has been shown to be an ineffective agent for the topical treatment of herpes virus infections. Calculations with the physical model described above (40) indicate that such topical treatments will lead to local vidarabine concentrations some two orders of magnitude lower than the minimum inhibitory concentration measured for this compound.

Efficacy prediction calculations (49) for a series of vidarabine 5'-monoesters applied topically to hairless mouse skin indicated that the valerate ester would be the most effective of the series, but that it would lead to local vidarabine concentrations only about equal to the minimum inhibitory concentration. Subsequent topical *in vivo* studies using this compound showed it to only be marginally effective in reducing lesion scores and mortality rates of hairless mice infected topically with herpes simplex virus type I. Model calculations for the topical application of the valerate ester in the presence of the potent permeation enhancer, Azone^{TM}, predicted local tissue vidarabine concentrations some 50 to 200 times higher than those obtained by application of the valerate ester alone. Accordingly, topical application of the valerate ester in the presence of Azone^{TM} was found to be quite effective, with significantly reduced lesion scores and a mortality rate of zero, as compared to 100% mortality in the untreated infected control animals.

The effect of Azone^{TM} is essentially the same as removal of the relatively impermeable cornified layer of the membrane. We would therefore expect that the vaginal membrane would be similar in behavior to the Azone^{TM} treated skin. This expectation was realized in studies using guinea pigs given intravaginal inoculations of herpes simplex type II virus. Vidarabine 5'-valerate was found to completely abort the primary infection when twice daily treatments were given within 6 hours of inoculation (50). When the initiation of treatment was delayed until 24 hours post-infection, the 5'-valerate ester was no longer effective. The 2'-3'-diacetate ester of vidarabine, however, was found to be effective even with this delay. This compound is now being studied in our laboratories using the same physical model approach described here.

The above studies, while certainly not providing an exhaustive test of the ability of the model to corroborate theory with efficacy, are encouraging. The hypothesis that the model can predict efficacy needs further testing with physical model studies and infected animal studies using several more combinations of animal models and prodrugs.

Physical Model Based Prediction of Efficacy

Recent studies in our laboratories have shown that the permeability of the vaginal membrane to vidarabine prodrugs varies tremendously as a function of the stage of the estrous cycle in animal models. In both the mouse (51) and the guinea pig (52) the vaginal membrane permeability is from 1 to 2 orders of magnitude greater in the diestrus phase of the estrous cycle than during the estrus phase.

Accordingly, physical model calculations have been done to calculate the expected efficacy of various 5'-monoesters of vidarabine during the various stages of the estrous cycle of the mouse (53). Some of these predictions are as follows.

Vidarabine itself or its octanoate ester would be expected to be ineffective during the estrus and late diestrus phases and marginally effective during early diestrus. Topical application of the valerate is expected to be effective during early diestrus, marginally effective during late diestrus and ineffective during estrus.

The acetate is expected to perform more evenly as a function of stage of the estrous cycle than is the valerate. During diestrus, the acetate is expected to lead to lower vidarabine concentrations than does the valerate, although the acetate would still produce vidarabine concentrations well above the minimum inhibitory concentration. During late diestrus and estrus, the acetate is expected to perform better than the valerate. The primary reason for these differences is the much smaller lability to esterase exhibited by the acetate; consequently there is slow release of vidarabine as the acetate diffuses across the epithelium. The valerate is acylated much more rapidly, releasing vidarabine before penetrating deeply into the epithelium. These differences in effective site of vidarabine release would be of little significance were it not for the high levels of adenosine deaminase activity in the vaginal membrane. The enzyme activity is high enough so that vidarabine is deactivated before it can diffuse an appreciable fraction of the way through the epithelium. The acetate therefore leads to higher vidarabine concentrations of vidarabine deeper into the epithelium as a result of its delayed vidarabine release.

The complexity of the above predictions is as noteworthy as the predictions themselves. These predictions do not lead in a simple way to a statement of which prodrug is "best", for the choice depends on the situation as the relative performances of the prodrugs are functions of the stage of the estrous cycle being considered. Similarly, we might expect even larger differences in relative performances when different animal models are used for studies. It is no small wonder then that studies employing different animal models often do not agree with each other and, even worse, may fail to be even qualitative indicators of the outcome of similar studies in humans.

The physical model approach can potentially be used to elicit useful information regarding drug or therapy design from situations such as this that are too complex to otherwise be profitably analyzed. If the results in the above situation were observed experimentally in the absence of a physical model analysis, there would be little to be gained from them in terms of devising strategies for designing prodrugs. The availability of the model analysis, however, suggests two strategies for overcoming the rapid deamination that limits vidarabine availability in this case:

(1) inhibit the adenosine deaminase; or

(2) optimize the rate of prodrug deacylation.

The qualitative complexity of the results discussed above arises partially because of the borderline effectiveness of the compounds studied. If these compounds were more potent, much of this complexity with respect to the question of effectiveness would disappear. In such a case the model would still be a valuable tool for the optimization of dosing. This problem becomes quite complex if we consider the performance of a delivery system on an entire population as opposed to an individual subject with some assumed well defined mean response.

We have recently observed (54) that activities of esterase and deaminase vary as a function of stage of the estrous cycle as does the permeability of the guinea pig vaginal membrane. In addition, the distributions of these quantities for each stage of the estrous cycle over the limited population sample studied have been determined. In a study now in progress, the physical model is being used to calculate the population distribution of epithelial concentrations of vidarabine to be expected from treatment with the various prodrugs studied. Such calculations will lead to a prediction of the probability of effective treatment in an individual subject as a function of dose or for populations, a prediction of the likely fraction of subjects in which the treatment will be effective for any given dose. In other cases where threshold concentrations for both effectiveness and toxicity are known, probabilities of both as a function of dose could be calculated.

Determination of Optimum Parameter Values

In the sensitivity analysis above, we varied model parameters one by one to show the effect of each on the performance of the system. In actuality, parameters that depend on molecular structure are not independent and therefore cannot be manipulated one at a time. Ideally, the dependence of each of these parameters on changes in molecular structure should be determined, and the sensitivity analysis conducted with respect to molecular structure. That is, molecular structure should be the independent variable.

As already alluded to above, the choice of dependent variable (or object function to be maximized) for the optimization is not necessarily an obvious one. For this system we have arbitrarily chosen the area under the steady-state vidarabine concentration versus distance profile as a measure of activity. An equally defensible choice would be the vidarabine concentration at some presumed site of action, either in the membrane or systemically. The locus of this site of action and dependence of therapeutic response on vidarabine concentration at this site can, in principle, be simultaneously determined by the physical model approach. We have recently worked out a procedure for doing so, assuming the availability of dose-response data from series of both topical and systemic administrations of an active agent. As of this writing, the precision with which the site of action and local dose-response dependency can be determined is uncertain. Nonetheless, this information is not directly accessible experimentally and the physical model approach may be the only currently available technique by which it can be deduced.

Cost Effectiveness of the Physical Model Approach

Our own experience with the physical model approach suggests that its cost effectiveness is related to the importance of obtaining quantitative information that is not measurable by more direct techniques. When such information is required, the physical model approach may be the only means available to obtain it.

Based on our own experiences up to the present time, the effort required to develop the numerical techniques to carry out model calculations has often been a significant fraction of the total effort required in a given study. The widespread availability of software tools for machines ranging from personal microcomputers to large mainframes has greatly reduced the effort that must be expended in writing computer problems to perform model calculations. The costs of actual computation, of course, continually decline and place more and more sophisticated models within practical reach. On the other hand, there is still an unavoidable amount of pencil and paper mathematical activity required to translate the concepts underlying a model to the equations to be solved, and this effort increases with increasing complexity of the model being considered. Even so, the effect of the continuing expansion of computer related resources is to decrease the effort required to implement a given physical model.

The biggest expense in implementing the physical model approach is usually the cost of conducting the experiments necessary to quantitatively determine the parameters of the model. Not surprisingly, these costs are directly related to the complexity of the model and the certainty with which parameters need to be determined. In the model described in this report, the assumption of homogeneous lamina as opposed to the more physically appealing picture of packed layers of discrete cells not only simplified the calculations, but also the experiments required to determine the model parameters. There are generally choices such as this available as to how complex the model should be, with the answer determined by balancing costs of the more complex model against the importance of the additional information likely to be deduced from it.

The above comments apply to situations such as the prodrug optimization problem, where the physical model analysis is a complex undertaking requiring a serious commitment of effort to implement. In cases such as this, the development of the model and the techniques for using it must be considered as a research problem. We should therefore be prepared for unforeseen difficulties requiring the expenditure of more effort than anticipated in the development and validation of any aspect of such a model.

After the model has been developed and validated, however, it may find uses in many studies beyond the initial one for which it was developed. The cost effectiveness, therefore, depends on both initial development costs and anticipated future uses over which these costs can be effectively amortized.

The great majority of situations, however, involve much simpler models and much more limited experimental studies. Most such models are simple and require little enough effort to work out that their development can be justified even if there are no further anticipated uses for them. The implementation of even such simple models is, of course, dependent on the availability of the appropriate computing resources and knowledge of their use. Such resources and knowledge are becoming so common that their availability will cease to be an issue in considering the use of simple physical models.

It should be noted that the advantages of using more complex models (i.e., ability to make predictions, ability to optimize systems, ability to deduce quantities difficult or impossible to measure directly) are shared by even the simplest physical models. Given these advantages and the increasing ease with which models can be implemented, the use of such approaches will likely continue to increase.

Summary

Many aspects of the use of physical models have been touched on in the preceding pages. We have tried to present an overview of the considerations attending the use of the physical model approach and show examples of the kinds of information that can be inferred with this approach. We will close this discourse by briefly discussing the factors that motivate us to adopt this approach to scientific problem solving.

The Approach is Useful in Identifying Critical Variables

In many situations, the quantities of most interest are not directly measurable, but may be calculable from the appropriate physical model. Additionally, the model may contain variables that are manipulable, but only with a significant investment of effort. An empirical experimental study of the effects of such variables would not only be costly, but frequently unproductive. The use of a physical model based sensitivity analysis can identify variables that are expected to have no influence on the outcome of experiments as well as those that may be most important. The model thus serves as a vital guide in the informed planning of experimental studies.

Complex Biological Systems can be Studied Quantitatively

Physical models of biological systems necessarily contain many assumptions and approximations. Even so, models that capture the essence of the behavior of the system can be extremely useful as they enable the system to be manipulated in ways not readily accessible experimentally. So long as we are cognizant of the implications of these assumptions and approximations, the models can provide useful valuable information not obtainable otherwise.

Relatively Cheap Calculations Can Often be Used in Place of More Expensive Animal Experiments

Physical models can not now eliminate the need for animal models and human clinical studies, nor will they in the foreseeable future. The validity of models will continue to be dependent on their verification by experiment. When models are used in situations in which there is confidence in their validity, however, calculations can be used to predict outcomes of more expensive *in vivo* experiments. This is not particularly useful if only a few experiments are involved, since they will likely be done even if model calculations are available. When optimization of some experimental system is the goal, however, the situation changes dramatically. In this case, literally hundreds or thousands of simulations can be rapidly done and a selected few of the most interesting of these situations chosen to be verified experimentally. The physical model approach thereby provides access to information that is simply not available by any other practical means. This is the primary motivation for its use.

Literature Cited

1. M. Privat de Garilhe and J. De Rudder, C. R. Acad. Sci. D (Paris), 259:2725 (1964).
2. F. A. Miller, G. J. Dixon, J. Ehrlich, B. J. Sloan, and I. W. McLean, Jr., Antimicrob. Agents Chemother.--1968, p. 136 (1969).
3. F. M. Schabel, Jr., Chemotherapy, 13:321 (1968).
4. W. M. Shannon, in Adenine Arabinoside: An Antiviral Agent (D. Pavan-Langston, R. A. Buchanan, and C. A. Alford, Jr., eds.) Raven Press, New York, 1975, p. 1.
5. R. W. Sidwell, G. J. Dixon, F. M. Schabel, Jr., and D.H. Kaump, Antimicrob. Agents Chemother.--1968, p. 148 (1969).
6. B. J. Sloan, F. A. Miller, J. Ehrlich, I. W. McLean, Jr., and H. E. Machamer, Antimicrob. Agents Chemother.--1968, p. 161 (1969).

7. H. E. Kaufman, E. D. Ellison, and W. M. Townsend, Arch. Ophthalmol., 84:783 (1970).
8. L. B. Allen and R. W. Sidwell, Antimicrob. Agents Chemother., 2:229 (1972).
9. B. J. Sloan, F. A. Miller, and I. W. McLean, Jr., Antimicrob. Agents Chemother., 3:74 (1973).
10. B. J. Sloan, in Adenine Arabinoside: An Antiviral Agent (D. Pavan-Langston, R. A. Buchanan, and C. A. Alford, Jr., eds.), Raven Press, New York, 1975, p. 45.
11. J. F. Griffith, J. F. Fitzwilliam, S. Casagrande, and S. R. Butler, J. Infect. Dis., 132:506 (1975).
12. E. Lefkowitz, M. Worthington, M. A. Conliffe, and S. Baron, Proc. Soc. Exp. Biol. Med., 152:337 (1976).
13. L. T. Ch'ien, F. M. Schabel, Jr., and C. A. Alford, Jr., in Selective Inhibitors of Viral Function (W. A. Carter, ed.), CRC Press, Cleveland, Ohio, 1973, p. 227.
14. L. T. Ch'ien, N. J. Cannon, L. J. Charamella, W. E. Dismukes, R. J. Whitley, R. A. Buchanan, and C. A. Alford, Jr., J. Infect. Dis., 128:658 (1973).
15. L. T. Ch'ien, R. J. Whitley, L. J. Charamella, R. A. Buchanan, N. J. Cannon, W. E. Dismukes, and C. A. Alford, Jr., in Adenine Arabinoside: An Antiviral Agent (D. Pavan-Langston, R. A. Buchanan, and C. A. Alford, Jr., eds.), Raven Press, New York, 1975, p. 205.
16. R. J. Whitley, L. T. Ch'ien, A. J. Nahmias, R. A. Buchanan, and C. A. Alford, Jr., in Adenine Arabinoside: An Antiviral Agent (D. Pavan-Langston, R. A. Buchanan, and C. A. Alford, Jr., eds.), Raven Press, New York, 1975, p. 225.
17. D. Pavan-Langston and C. H. Dohlman, Am. J. Ophthalmol., 74:81 (1972).
18. R. A. Hyndiuk, R. O. Schultz, and D. S. Hull, in Adenine Arabinoside: An Antiviral Agent (D. Pavan-Langston, R. A. Buchanan, and C. A. Alford, Jr., eds.), Raven Press, New York, 1975, p. 331.
19. D. Pavan-Langston, in Adenine Arabinoside: An Antiviral Agent (D. Pavan-Langston, R. A. Buchanan, and C. A. Alford, Jr., eds.), Raven Press, New York, 1975, p. 345.
20. R. Abel, Jr., H. E. Kaufman, and J. Sugar, in Adenine Arabinoside: An Antiviral Agent (D. Pavan-Langston, R. A. Buchanan, and C. A. Alford, Jr., eds.), Raven Press, New York, 1975, p. 393.
21. J. R. McKinnon, J. I. McGill, and B. R. Jones, in Adenine Arabinoside: An Antiviral Agent (D. Pavan-Langston, R. A. Buchanan, and C. A. Alford, Jr., eds), Raven Press, New York, 1975, p. 401.
22. C. A. Alford, Jr. and R. J. Whitley, J. Infect. Dis., 133(Suppl.):A101 (1976).
23. M. D. Aronson, C. F. Philips, D. W. Gump, R. J. Albertini, and C. A. Phillips, JAMA 235:1339 (1976).

24. E. R. Kern, J. C. Overall, and L. A. Glasgow, Abstr. Ann. Mtg. Am. Soc. Microbiol., 1975, Abstr. No. A26, p.5.
25. J. C. Overall, E. R. Kern, and L. A. Glasgow, in Adenine Arabinoside: An Antiviral Agent (D. Pavan-Langston, R. A. Buchanan, and C. A. Alford, Jr., eds.), Raven Press, New York, 1975, p. 95.
26. E. R. Kern, J. C. Overall, Jr., and L. A. Glasgow, Antimicrob. Agents Chemother., 7:587 (1975).
27. E. L. Goodman, J. P. Luby, and M. T. Johnson, Antimicrob. Agents Chemother., 8:693 (1975).
28. D. C. Baker, T. H. Haskell, and S. R. Putt, J. Med. Chem., 21:1218 (1978).
29. D. C. Baker, T. H. Haskell, S. R. Putt, and B. J. Sloan, J. Med. Chem., 22:273 (1979).
30. E. Chan, S.R. Putt, H.D.H. Showalter and D.C. Baker, J. Org. Chem., 47:3457 (1982).
31. R. A. Lipper, S. M. Machkovech, J. C. Drach, and W. I. Higuchi, Mol. Pharmacol., 14:366 (1978).
32. C. D. Yu, J. L. Fox, N. F. H. Ho, and W. I. Higuchi, J. Pharm. Sci., 68:1341 (1979).
33. H. S. Carslow and J. C. Jaeger, Conduction of Heat in Solids, 2nd ed., p. 326, Oxford University Press (1959).
34. C. D. Yu, N. A. Gordon, J. L. Fox, W. I. Higuchi, and N. F. H. Ho, J. Pharm. Sci., 69:775 (1980).
35. R. Piessens and R. Huysmans, ACM Trans. on Math. Software, 10(3):348 (1984).
36. R.E. Bellman, R.E. Kalaba and J.A. Lockett, Numerical Inversion of the Laplace Transform, American Elsevier, New York (1966).
37. F. Veillon, Commun. ACM, 17(10):587 (1974).
38. A. C. Hindmarsh and H. Byrne, ACM Trans. on Math. Software, 1:75 (1975).
39. J. S. Shipman and S. M. Roberts, Two Point Boundary-Value Problems: Shooting Methods, American Elsevier, New York (1972).
40. J. L. Fox, C. D. Yu, W. I. Higuchi, and N. F. H. Ho, Int. J. Pharmaceutics, 2:41 (1979).
41. R. F. Sincovee and N. K. Madsen, ACM Trans. Math. Software, 1(3):232 (1975).
42. H. Schaefer, G. Stuttgen, A. Zesch, W. Schalla and J. Gazith, Curr. Probl. Dermatol., 7:80 (1978).
43. P. Rayker, J. Mizutani, W.I. Higuchi and B.D. Anderson, in preparation.
44. N. A. Gordon, Ph.D. Thesis, The University of Michigan, 1981.
45. C.H. Metzler, G.L. Elfring and A.J. McEwan, A User's Manual for NONLIN and Associated Programs, The Upjohn Co., Kalamazoo, Mich. (1978).
46. J.L. Fox, MINSQ: An Interactive Nonlinear Least Squares Program for Microcomputers, in preparation.

47. G.G. Krueger, Z.J. Wojciechowski, S.A. Burton, A. Gelhar, S.E. Huether, L.G. Leonard, U.D. Rohr, T.J. Petelenz, W.I. Higuchi and L.K. Pershing, completed manuscript.
48. U.D. Rohr, Z.J. Wojciechowski, S.A. Burton, G.G. Krueger, J.L. Fox and W.I. Higuchi, in preparation.
49. W. I. Higuchi, W. M. Shannon, J. L. Fox, G. L. Flynn, N. F. H. Ho, R. Vaidyanathan, and D. C. Baker, in Recent Advances in Drug Delivery Systems (J. Anderson, ed.), Plenum Press, New York, 1984.
50. W. M. Shannon, G. Arnett, D. C. Baker, S. D. Kumar, and W. I. Higuchi, Antimicrob. Agents Chemother., 24:706 (1983).
51. C. C. Hsu, J. Y. Park, N. F. H. Ho, W. I. Higuchi, and J. L. Fox, J. Pharm. Sci., 72:674 (1983).
52. M. J. Durrani, A. Kusai, N. F. H. Ho, J. L. Fox, and W. I. Higuchi, Int. J. Pharmaceutics, 24:209 (1985).
53. W. I. Higuchi, A. Kusai, J. L. Fox, N. A. Gordon, and N. F. H. Ho, Controlled Release Delivery Systems (T. J. Roseman and S. Z. Mansdorf, eds.), Marcel Dekker, Inc., New York, 1983, p. 43.
54. M. J. Durrani, J. L. Fox, and W. I. Higuchi, in preparation.

Chapter 6
Biological Evaluation of Soluble Macromolecules as Bioreversible Drug Carriers

R. Duncan, J. Kopecek*, and J. B. Lloyd

Department of Biological Sciences
University of Keele
Keele, Staffordshire ST5 5BG U.K.
and
Institute of Macromolecular Chemistry
Czechoslovak Academy of Sciences
162 06 Prague 6, Czechoslovakia*

Introduction

Binding drugs to macromolecules will, in most cases, alter their pharmacokinetics and this can be used to advantage in at least three different therapeutic contexts (1). These are illustrated in Fig. 1. Drugs that exert their effect via cell surface receptors may have their action prolonged if conjugation to a macromolecule serves to protect the drug from rapid metabolism or excretion. Drugs that act by interaction with intracellular receptors normally reach these by passing across cell membranes, therefore conjugation inevitably prevents their normal penetration into cells. As macromolecular drug-carriers can only be captured by cells by pinocytosis, they have obvious potential for use in limiting the body distribution of drugs, i.e. drug targeting. In recent years there has been growing interest in the use of natural macromolecules (2,3) and synthetic polymers (4-6) as targetable drug-carriers. We and our colleagues have devoted considerable effort to the development of N-(2-hydroxypropyl)methacrylamide (HPMA) copolymers as drug carriers (reviewed in (7)) and this work will be used in the present article to illustrate some of the basic concepts relating to the design of, and biological testing of, macromolecular drug-carriers. Thirdly, soluble polymeric drug conjugates can also be used as a sustained release formulation. If administered directly into a body compartment e.g. intramuscularly, drug will be progressively released, providing that the polymer-drug linkage is degradable. However, at present there are probably better systems available for controlled release, such as polymeric matrices and liposomes.

In this Chapter we limit ourselves to discussion of the development of bioreversible drug-carriers designed for intacellular drug delivery. In vitro and in vivo techniques used

i. at the cell surface

ii. intracellularly

iii. an extracellular depot

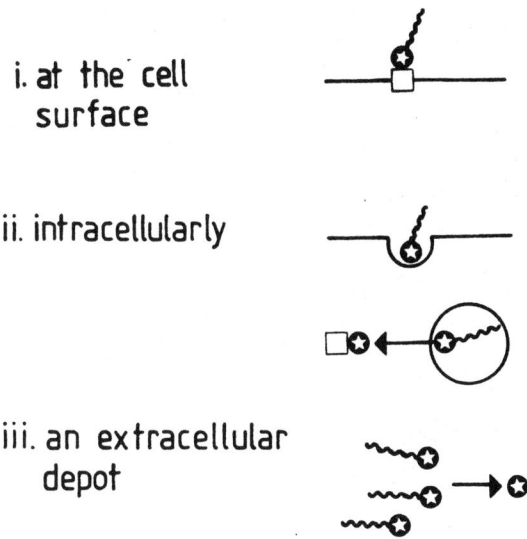

Fig.1. Mechanisms of action of macromolecular drug conjugates.

for their evaluation will be described. As stated above these conjugates connot pass across membranes, but gain access to the cells' interior by the mechanism of pinocytosis. This process has been described at length elsewhere (7,8) but, briefly, the cell membrane infolds and then pinches off to form intracellular vesicles (Fig. 2). Macromolecules present in the extracellular fluid are captured by either fluid-phase pinocytosis (if taken up as solutes) or adsorptive pinocytosis (if they bind to the infolding plasma membrane). It is the known cell specificity of adsorptive pinocytosis that provides the possibility to achieve cell-specific targeting of macromolecular drug conjugates.

Newly formed pinocytic vesicles move into the cell and eventually fuse with lysosomes. These are vesicles of intracellular origin containing many different hydrolytic enzymes capable of degrading all naturally occurring materials. Enzymes present include; proteinases, glycosidases, esterases, phosphatases and sulphatases. The known specificities of these enzymes enables the design of bioreversible drug-carriers that are stable during transport to the cell, but that can be cleaved intracellularly by lysosomal enzymes following pinocytic internatlization.

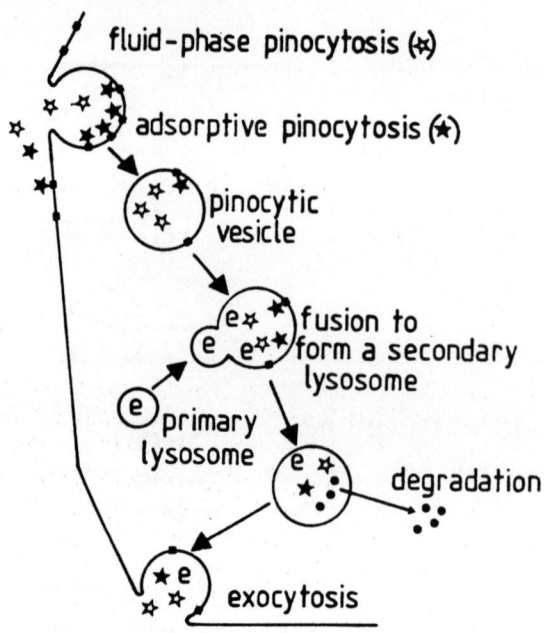

Fig.2. Adsorptive and fluid-phase pinocytosis. Intracellular fate of materials ingested by pinocytosis. Lysosomes containing lysosomal enzymes (e) are shown.

Bioreversible Polymer-Drug Linkages

Oligopeptide drug-carrier linkages should be ideal as they are relatively stable in the biological environment and amino acid sequences susceptible to cleavage by specific proteinases have been described. HPMA copolymers have been synthesized that contain either drugs or drug analogues bound to the polymer via oligopeptide side-chains (Fig. 3). Firstly, a polymeric precursor is prepared by radical polymerization of HPMA with p-nitrophenyl esters of N-methacryloylated oligopeptides and this is then reacted with compounds containing an aliphatic amino group (9). In order to study the suitability of oligopeptide side-chains as bioreversible linkages, a large number of different sequences were synthesized, each terminating in p-nitroaniline (NAp). Cleavage of NAp from the side-chain can be monitored with ease spectrophotmetrically, so this terminal group proved a useful drug analogue. Kopecek has recently discussed the biodegradation of this type of HPMA copolymer in some depth (10).

For sucessful targeted drug delivery it is essential

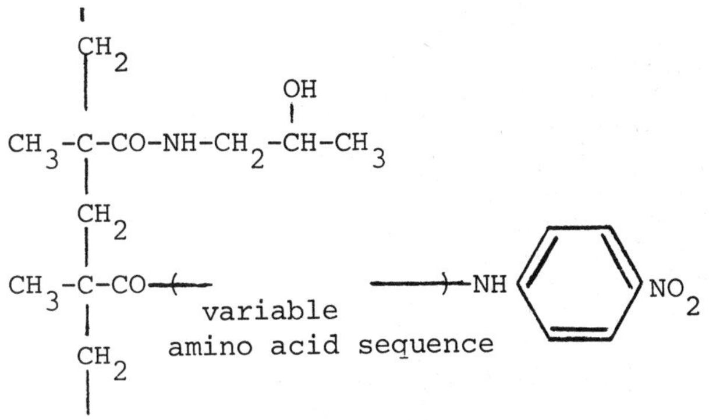

```
         |
         CH₂
         |                  OH
                            |
    CH₃-C-CO-NH-CH₂-CH-CH₃
         |
         CH₂
         |
    CH₃-C-CO-(―      ―)-NH―⟨  ⟩-NO₂
         |        variable
         CH₂   amino acid sequence
         |
```

Fig. 3. Structure of HPMA copolymers whose oligopeptide side-chains terminate in p-nitroaniline

that the polymer-drug linkage is stable during transport to the target cell, but effectively degraded intralysosomally. Incubation of HPMA copolymers with either rat liver lysosomal enzymes (11-13) or rat plasma or serum (14) has shown that these requirements can be achieved in vitro. For example a HPMA copolymer containing the side-chain sequence P-Gly-Phe-Leu- Gly-Phe-NAp releases more than 52% of the bound NAp during an incubation (5h) with lysosomal enzymes (13), whereas only 3-4% of the bound NAp is released from this side-chain during the same incubation period with rat plasma or serum (14).

Using enzyme inhibitors (12) and purified lysosomal enzymes (15,16), it has been shown that the lysosomal thiol-proteinases are the enzymes most important in cleavage of oligopeptide drug-polymer linkages. In fact, it would appear that one particular enzyme, cathepsin B, is most active against these polymeric substrates (10,16). Identification of the enzyme(s) responsible for the hydrolysis of drug-carrier linkages is very important as it permits:

(i) design of linkages that will be cleavaged intralysosomally rather than in the extracellular milieu.
(ii) design of linkages that are hydrolysed to give optimum rate of drug liberation intracellularly.
(iii) in certain cases it may be useful in preventing drug liberation in cells other than a target cell rich in the necessary enzyme.

Incubation of radiolabelled HPMA copolymer with rat visceral yolk sacs cultured in vitro confirmed that lysosomal enzymes can selectively degrade the oligopeptide copolymer side-chains and in this case resulted in the release of low molecular weight radiolabelled degradation products which escape from the cell (17). Likewise experiments performed <u>in vivo</u> have shown that a radiolabelled drug analogue can be released from a polymeric carrier and excreted in the urine within 5h of intravenous administration of ^{125}I-labelled HPMA copolymer to rats (18).

Endocytic Capture of Polymeric Drug-Carriers Measured In Vitro

Membrane invagination leading to the capture of extra-cellular material (endocytosis) can be divided into two distinct processes: phagocytosis, the uptake of particulate matter (usually > 1_μ in diameter) and pinocytosis, uptake of soluble macromolecules by the small vesicles continually forming at the surface of all cells. Phagocytosis, in contrast with pinocytosis, is initiated by particle attachment to the surface of the cell and is limited to specialized cells in the body (so-called phagocytes). Phagocytic uptake of particles by these cells is extremely efficient and it is this phenomenon that has severely limited the usefulness of particles/liposomes in targeted drug delivery (19). As soluble macromolecules are internalized by pinocytosis, a mechanism common to most, if not all, cell types (2), they can potentially act as carriers of any pharmaceutical agent.

Quantitation of Rates of Pinocytosis

It is important to discover the rate at which a drug-carrier is internalized by cells, as this relates directly to the rate of intracellular drug delivery. Comparison of rates of pinocytic capture by different cell types is also important for discovering whether a particular conjugate may be useful for cell-specific delivery.

Measurement of rates of pinocytosis has been achieved using a number of techniques including morphometric analyses, biochemical measurements e.g. using a pinocytic substrate that has enzymatic activity, or radiolabelled or fluorescent-labelled substrates. In our studies we have used ^{125}I-labelling of tyrosine residues in HPMA copolymers as a method of monitoring polymer fate <u>in vitro</u> and <u>in vivo</u>. The schematic diagram shown in Fig. 4 indicates the patterns of tissue accumulation of radioactivity measured with time, showing pinocytic uptake of macromolecular substrate that is not degraded intracellularly (Fig. 4a) and uptakes one that is (Fig. 4b). Providing the rate of regurgitation of the macromolecule (exocytosis) is negligible, the accumulation of radioactivity relating to a non-degradable substrate (Fig. 4a) represents the rate of pinocytic

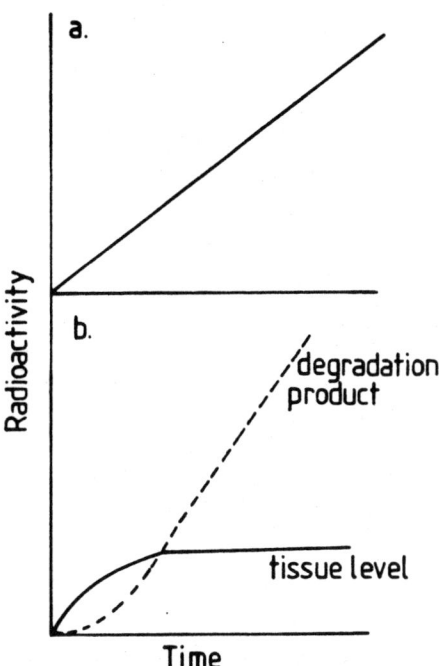

Fig.4. Tissue accumulation of radiolabelled pinocytic substrates, (a) a non-degradable substrate (b) a degradable sustrate. Release of low molecular weight degradation products back into the incubation medium is also shown in (b).

capture. However, it can be seen from Fig. 4b that tissue radioactivity soon begins to plateau if degradation of substrate is occurring within the cell which is followed by loss of low molecular weight degradation products from the cell. In this case the extent of degradation at any time must be assessed and added to tissue accumulation to give a value representing total capture.

HPMA copolymers whose side-chains contained tyrosine residues were radiolabelled with ^{125}I iodide and incubated with rat visceral yolk sacs cultured in vitro (17). A copolymer containing the side chain Gly-Ala-Tyr-NAp was captured linearly with time by the tissue, whereas one containing Gly-Gly-Tyr-NAp side-chains showed a pattern of tissue accumulation of radioactivity suggestive of intracellular degradation. Examination, using Sephadex G-15 chromatography, of the incubation medium after yolk sacs had been exposed to radiolabelled copolymer for 5h showed that low molecular weight degradation products had indeed been generated and released by the cells. Uptake of four different HPMA copolymers was measured (each bearing a different oligopeptide side-chain) and, although their side-chains were degraded to different extents, the measured rates of pinocytic uptake of these polymers were very similar. In fact the rate of pinocytic uptake of HPMA copolymers was the same as that previously reported for uptake of ^{125}I-labelled poly-(vinylpyrrolidone) (PVP) which is a marker of fluid-phase pinocytosis in the yolk sac (21). This observation indicates that HPMA copolymers containing small amounts of side-chain (approximately 2 mol%) do not have natural affinity for the infolding cell surface, and thus, providing an efficient address system can be incorporated, have maximum potential for cell-specific targeting.

Factors Governing Non-Specific Capture

Although attachment of macromolecules to the cell surface does not seem necessary to trigger pinocytic internalization, substrate size and chemical characteristics do greatly affect the rate of capture of a macromolecule. For example in the case of a polymer captured by fluid-phase pinocytosis (^{125}I-labelled PVP in the yolk sac), the rate of capture has been shown to be greatly affected by molecular weight (22). Polydisperse ^{125}I-labelled PVP fractions of M_w 84000 and 700 000 were captured half as fast as a similar fraction M_w 50 000. Likewise ^{125}I-labelled HPMA copolymer fractions M_w 34 000 - 400 000 showed increasing rates of pinocytic uptake of yolk sacs cultured in vitro with decreasing size (23).

The relationship between the size of a macromolecule and its rate of pinocytosis is not, however, the same in all cell types. Phagocytic cells capture high molecular weight polymers more avidly (22) and it has been shown that rat jejunal sacs cultured in vitro capture higher molecular weight ^{125}I-labelled HPMA copolymers more rapidly than lower molecular weight species (24). If the material is unable to stimulate pinocytosis, the higher rate of capture must reflect an increased affinity for the cell surface and hence capture by adsorptive pinocytosis.

Size, charge, and hydrophobicity have been shown to influence the rates of adsorptive pinocytosis of natural macromolecules (25-27) and synthetic polymers (22,23,28-30). Incorporation of side-chains bearing a terminal tyrosinamide residue into HPMA copolymers caused an increase in their rate of pinocytic capture by rat yolk sacs cultured in vitro which was related to the degree of substitution of the polymer (30). Increased uptake was attributed to the substituted molecules becoming more hydrophobic and this having an increased affinity for the yolk sac surface. If macromolecular drug-carriers are heavily loaded with pharmacological agents that are hydrophobic or cationic in nature, it is likely that they will acquire significant affinity for cell surfaces in general. This would obviously be disadvantageous if they were intended to reach a particular cell type.

Cell-Specific Targeting

To increase the therapeutic index of drugs that display non-specific side-effects, such as cytotoxic anticancer agents, it is important to concentrate them within the cells or tissues where action is required. A macromolecular drug-carrier will be taken up slowly by fluid-phase pinocytosis by all cells encountered unless it has non-specific affinity for cell surfaces or contains some feature that promotes binding to a particular cell type. During investigation of endocytic phenomenon a number of receptor-mediated pinocytic processes have been discovered in which cell-specific membrane receptors recognise and bind moieties on passing macromolecules (31,32). Many of these are dependent on carbohydrate recognition systems are shown in Table 1.

Table 1. Carbohydrate-Related Cell-Specific Recognition Systems.

Carbohydrate Residue on the Macromolecule	Cell Possessing Receptor	Reference
Galactose	Liver hepatocytes Liver macrophages Hepatoma	33 34 35
Mannose N-Acetylglucosamine/ Fucose	Macrophages	36, 37, 38
Mannose-6-Phosphate	Fibroblasts Liver cells	39 40
Fucose	Mouse leukaemia (L1210)	41
Glucose	Lewis lung carcinoma	42

Although the absolute cell-specificity of most of these carbohydrated-dependent recognition systems has yet to be verified, and many would seem to be detectable on more than one cell type, they appear to be useful for efficient concentration of macromolecules within particular cell types in vivo. As a result they may hold considerable potential for use in targeting drug conjugates. Already it has been shown that receptor-mediated pinocytosis can be used to target natural macromolecules carrying drugs (e.g. asialofetuin carrying drugs (43)) and to alter the body distribution of synthetic polymers (18,44,45).

^{125}I-labelled HPMA copolymers administered intravenously to rats were found to be removed from the bloodstream at a rate proportional to their molecular weight (46). Rapid removal from the circulation was accompanied by appearance of low molecular weight polymer chains in the kidney and urine, indicating that glomerular filtration was the cause of polymer disappearance. Tissue levels of radiolabelled polymer were found to be low, and therefore compatible with cellular capture by fluid-phase pinocytosis. Even 1h after administration only 5 - 12% of the radioactivity recovered was associated with the liver (18,46). Modification of the HPMA copolymers by incorporation of galactosamine (approximately 2mol%) radically altered their fate in vivo. Following intravenous administration radioactivity rapidly disappeared from the bloodstream, subsequently appearing in the liver (60-70% after 1h (18,46)). Separation of liver into its two major cell types, hepatocytes and Kupffer cells (liver macrophages), showed that the majority of radiolabelled material is associated with hepatocytes (R. Duncan, L. Scarlett, J.B. Lloyd, P. Rejmanová and J. Kopeček, unpublished data) and this confirmed that it is the galactose receptor on the hepatocyte membrane that mediates this efficient and rapid uptake.

Subsequent experiments using ^{125}I-labelled HPMA copolymers containing a range of galactosamine substitutions (1 - 11 mol%) have shown that a substitution of 4mol% is sufficient to promote efficient targeting to the liver (44) and experiments using rat hepatocytes cultured in vitro have confirmed that polymers with higher galactosamine contents interact more strongly with the hepatocyte membrane (44).

Although low molecular weight carbohydrate moieties would appear promising as an address system for macromolecular drug-carriers, there is still insufficient knowledge of their receptor cell-specificity and indeed whether, important target cells, such as tumour cells, can be reached/addressed in this way. An alternative approach would be to utilize antibodies directed against a specific cell surface determinant for drug targeting. Already antitumour antibodies have found uses as diagnostics.

Direct conjugation of drugs to antibodies has certain problems (47), but conjugation via an intermediate can lead to preservation of both antibody and pharmacological activity. It is envisaged that antibodies will provide a useful address system for polymeric drug-carriers. It has already been shown that antibodies can be bound to HPMA copolymers (48) and that following binding, they still display antigen-binding activity (44, 49).

Rat IgG is efficiently captured by adsorptive pinocytosis by the rat visceral yolk sac, protected from lysosomal degradation and passed across the tissue and on to the developing embryo (50). This is the normal route for transfer of passive immunity from mother to fetus. Heterologous rat IgG was bound to HPMA copolymers and the pinocytic properties of the resultant conjugate investigated (44). It was shown that conjugation of copolymer with antibody slightly raised the polymer's rate of uptake by the yolk sac cultured in vitro, but markedly increased its rate of transport across. These observations indicate preservation of antibody function when attached to a polymer.

Fate of Polymer-Drug Conjugates In Vivo

Demonstration of macromolecule handling in vitro is valuable in defining precise cellular interactions, since the number of experimental variables can be limited to some extent. However, there is always concern about the validity of extrapolation to the whole animal and, of course, the latter is the only matter of importance in the therapeutic context. Parallel experiments in vitro and in vivo allow both definition of cellular mechanisms and indicate the fate of materials in the body.

In the context of a targeted drug delivery system, there are many potential complications arising from the movement of a drug-carrier from the site of administration to the target tissue. Many of these relate equally to drug delivery, e.g. premature excretion, metabolism, inactivation due to protein binding etc., but others affect the drug-carrier specifically, such as limitation of movement from one body compartment to another owing to molecular size, poor vascularisation of the target tissue etc. Movement of HPMA copolymers from one body compartment to another was studied in rats, using I-labelled soluble crosslinked copolymers (M_w 64 000 - 74 000) without or with galactosamine residues (2.1 mol%) (45). As reported earlier for the single chain HPMA copolymer bearing galactosamine (18), the soluble crosslinked polymer bearing this moiety was efficiently captured by the liver after intravenous administration (Table 2). Following intraperitoneal administration radioactivity associated with both copolymers gradually left the peritoneal cavity, but only in the case of the galactosamine-HPMA copolymer did radioactivity appear in the liver. The unsubstituted polymer was excreted in the urine. Likewise subcutaneous administration was followed by liver targeting of the galactosamine-HPMA copolymer, but not of the unmodified polymer.

Table 2. Targeting of Soluble Crosslinked HPMA copolymers Following Different Routes of Administration In Vivo[a].

HPMA Copolymer	Route of Administration[b]						
	Intravenous	Intraperitoneal			Subcutaneous		
	1h	1h	2.5h	24h	1h	5h	24h
P$<$ TyrNH$_2$ / GlyGlyGal	60.4	13.4	29.1	51.9	18.6	20.4	23.6
P$<$ TyrNH$_2$ / GlyGlyaminopropanol	7.5	2.8	4.0	4.0	6.0	1.8	1.2

[a] S.A.Cartlidge, P.Rejmanová, R.Duncan, J.B.Lloyd and J.Kopeček unpublished data.

[b] Results are expressed as a percentage of the total radioactivity recovered in the organs studied at each time point.

After subcutaneous administration the radiolabelled polymer was slow to leave the site of injection. Radioactivity recovered, expressed as a percentage of the injected dose, was only 14% after 1h, but rose to approximately 60% after 24h. These experiments demnstrate organ targeting from a sustained release formulation.

There is obvious need for basic scientific evaluation of polymers designed as drug-carriers in in vivo experiments,as well as their pharmacological evaluation. Manipulation of macromolecular drug-carrier characteristics to ensure drug delivery in the right place at the right time will help to ensure optimum pharmacological activity.

Biocompatibility of Macromolecular Drug-Carriers

The term biocompatibility is used in a general sense to describe the interaction of synthetic materials with the biological environment. Movement of soluble macromolecules within the body suggests that interactions with tissues are likely to occur at sites remote from the place of administration, and therefore of particular interest is the systemic biocompatibility of these soluble materials. It is essential that any macromolecular drug-carrier is well tolerated by the organism. Ideally it should be non-toxic, non-immunogenic, degradable and the degradation products either innocuous or efficiently excreted. These requirements must be considered at an early stage in the development of any drug-carrier system, as, if any one is not fulfilled, the system may be worthless.

Natural macromolecular drug-carriers are attractive in that they can usually be degraded enzymically. However, they are likely to be immunogenic. Soluble polymers can be synthesized so that they too are biodegradable, eg. polyamino acids, or alternatively they may hydrolyse spontaneously, eg. polyesters. The HPMA copolymers described here are not biodegradable, but it has been shown that limited degradability can be introduced into their structure by synthesis of soluble crosslinked HPMA copolymers whose polymer chains are connected by oligopeptide crosslinks (51). Experiments performed in vivo have shown that such crosslinked HPMA copolymers are cleaved in the animal, resulting in the excretion of lower molecular weight polymer chains in the urine (52).

Development and use of synthetic polymers eg. PVP as plasma expanders has lead to considerable investigation in the organism. Although PVP is not biodegradable, and accumulates in the body for some time after administration, it was given to over 500 000 patients during the second world war without adverse reactions (53). Studies on the immunogenicity of HPMA (54) and HPMA copolymers (55,56) showed that no antibodies were produced against the homopolymer and only a weak reaction occurred against copolymers bearing peptide side-chains. However, if the ends of these side-chains were modified to include hapten groups, such as 4-azophenyl-arsonate, the immune response was significant. This is an important consideration when the terminal groups are drugs.

Concluding Remarks

Since the mid-seventies, when macromolecules were first proposed as potential drug-carriers (4,57) there has been growing interest in their development in clinical situations. This interest has been heightened with the realization that liposomes have limited potential in therapeutic applications, particularly drug targeting. In this Chapter our own progress with HPMA copolymers has been discussed, but thers have reported drug delivery systems based on protein carriers (58), polyglutamic acid (59), dextran and inulin (60,61) and antibodies (62), to give just a few examples. Elsewhere in this volume the potential targets for site-directed drug delivery are reviewed in depth.

As yet there are no sucesses to report from the clinic, but with careful tailor-made design of a macromolecular drug-carrier, it is surely only a matter of time.

Acknowledgements

The authors would like to thank sincerely their coworkers who are mentioned by name throughout the publications list. R.D. and J.B.L. thank the (British)Cancer Research Campaign, Medical Research Council and the Science and Engineering Research Council for supporting their work. The Royal Society and British Council are thanked for supporting the collaboration between the University of Keele and Institute of Macromolecular Chemistry, Prague.

References

1. R.Duncan, Biological effects of soluble synthetic polymers as drug carriers, CRC Critical Reviews in Therapeutic Drug Carrier Systems, 1, (1985) in press.
2. G.Gregoriadis, J.Senior and A.Trouet (Eds.) Targeting of Drugs, Plenum Press, New York, 1982, pp.1-430.
3. G.Möller, (Ed.) Antibody carriers of drugs and toxins in tumor therapy, Immunological Rev., 62,1 (1982).
4. H.Ringsdorf, Structure and properties of pharmacologically active polymers, J. Polymer Sci.Polymer Symp.,51, 135 (1975)
5. J.B.Lloyd, R.Duncan and M.K.Pratten, Soluble synthetic polymers and targetable agents for intracellular drug release, Brit. Polymer J., 15, 158 (1983).
6. J.Kopeček and K.Ulbrich, Biodegradation of biomedical polymers, Prog. Polymer Sci., 9, 1 (1983).
7. R.Duncan and J.Kopeček, Soluble synthetic polymers as potential drug carriers, Adv. Polymer Sci., 57, 51 (1984).
8. R.Duncan, Selective endocytosis. In: " Sustained and Controlled Release Drug Delivery Systems", 2nd Edition, J.R. Robinson and V.H.L.Lee (Eds.), Marcel Dekker, New York, 1985, in press.
9. J.Kopeček, P.Rejmanová and V.Chytry, Polymers containing enzymatically degradable bonds. 1. Chymotrypsin catalysed hydrolysis of p-nitroanilides of phenylaniline and tyrosine attached to side-chains of copolymers of N-(2-hydroxyprop-

yl)methacrylamide, Makromol.Chem., 182, 799 (1981)
10. J.Kopeček, Controlled biodegradability of polymers- a key to drug delivery systems, Biomaterials, 5, 19 (1984).
11. R.Duncan, J.B.Lloyd and J.Kopeček, Degradation of side-chains of N-(2-hydroxypropyl)methacrylamide copolymers by lysosomal enzymes, Biochem. Biophys. Res.Commun., 94, 284 (1980).
12. R.Duncan, H.C.Cable, J.B.Lloyd, P.Rejmanová and J.Kopeček, Degradation of side-chains of N-(2-hydroxypropyl)methacrylamide copolymers by lysosomal thiol-proteinases, Bioscience Reps., 2, 1041 (1982).
13. R.Duncan,H.C.Cable,J.B.Lloyd, P.Rejmanová and J.Kopeček, Polymers containing enzymatically degradable bonds,7. Design of oligopeptide side-chains in poly[N-(2-hydroxypropyl)methacrylamide] copolymers to promote efficient degradation by lysosomal enzymes, Makromol. Chem., 184, 1977 (1983).
14. P.Rejmanová, J.Kopeček, R.Duncan, and J.B.Lloyd, Stability in rat plasma and serum of lysosomally degradable oligopeptide sequences in N-(2-hydroxypropyl)methacrylamide copolymers, Biomaterials, 6, 45 (1985).
15. P.Rejmanová, J.Pohl, M.Baudyš, V.Kostka and J.Kopeček, Degradadtion of oligopeptide sequences in N-(2-hydroxypropyl)methacrylamide copolymers by bovine spleen cathepsin B,Makromol. Chem.,184, 2009 (1983).
16. P.Rejmanová, J.Pohl, V.Šubr,M.Baudyš, V.Kostka and J. Kopeček, in preparation.
17. R.Duncan, P.Rejmanová, J.Kopeček, and J.B.Lloyd, Pinocytic uptake and intracellular degradation of N-(2-hydroxypropyl)methacrylamide copolymers . A potential drug delivery system. Biochim. Biophys. Acta,678, 143 (1981).
18. R.Duncan, J.Kopeček, P.Rejmanová and J.B.Loyd, Targeting of N-(2-hydroxypropyl)methacrylamide copolymers to liver by incorporation of galactose residues, Biochim. Biophys. Acta, 755, 518 (1983).
19. G.Poste, Liposomes targeting in vivo : problems and opportunities, Biol. Cell., 47, 19 (1983).
20. M.K.Pratten, R.Duncan and J.B.Lloyd, Adsorptive and passive pinocytic uptake, In : "Coated Vesicles", C.J. Okleford and A.Whyte (Eds.), Cambridge University Press, Cambridge, 1980, pp. 179-218.
21. K.E.Williams, E.M. Kidston, F.Beck and J.B.Lloyd, Quantitative studies of pinocytosis. 1. Kinetics of uptake of [^{125}I]polyvinylpyrrolidone by rat yolk sac cultured in vitro, J.Cell Biol., 64, 113 (1975).
22. R.Duncan, M.K.Pratten, H.C.Cable, H.Ringsdorf and J.B. Lloyd, Effect of molecular size of ^{125}I-labelled poly(vinylpyrrolidone) on its pinocytosis by rat visceral yolk sacs and rat peritoneal macrophages, Biochem.J., 196, 49 (1981).

23. S.A.Cartlidge, R.Duncan, J.B.Lloyd, P.Rejmanová and J. Kopeček, Pinocytic capture of poly N-(2-hydroxypropyl)-methacrylamide chains connected by oligopeptide sequences Abstract from the International Conference on Biomedical Polymers, Durham, U.K., 1982.
24. R.Duncan and J.B.Lloyd, Biological evaluation of soluble synthetic polymers as drug carriers, In:"Recent Advances in Drug Delivery Systems", J.M.Anderson and S.-W. Kim, (Eds.), Plenum Press, New York, 1984, pp. 9-22.
25. T.Kooistra, A.Duursma, J.M.W.Bouma and M.Gruber, Endocytosis and breakdown of proteins by sinusoidal liver cells, Acta biol. med. germ., 36, 1763 (1977).
26. T.Kooistra, M.K.Pratten and K.E.Williams, Endocytosis of simple proteins by rat yolk sacs and by rat peritoneal macrophages incubated in vitro, Acta biol. med. germ., 40 1637, (1981).
27. G.Livesey, and K.E.Williams, Heterogeneity of binding sites for adsorptive pinocytosis of simple proteins by rat yolk sacs, Eur.J.Biochem., 122, 147 (1982).
28. M.K.Pratten, H.C.Cable, H.Ringsdorf and J.B.Lloyd, Adsorptive pinocytosis of polycationic copolymers of vinylpyrrolidone with vinylamine by rat yolk sac and peritoneal macrophage, Biochim. Biophys. Acta, 719, 424 (1982).
29. R.Duncan, D.Starling, F.Rypaček, J.Drobnik and J.B.Lloyd, Pinocytosis of poly(α,β-(2-hydroxyethyl)-DL-aspartamide and a tyramine derivative by rat visceral yolk sacs cultured in vitro. Ability of phenolic residues to enhance the rate of pinocytic capture of a macromolecule, Biochim. Biophys. Acta, 717, 248 (1982).
30. R.Duncan, H.C.Cable P.Rejmanová, J.Kopeček and J.B.Lloyd, Tyrosinamide residues enhance pinocytic capture of N-(hydroxypropyl)methacrylamide copolymers, Biochim. Biophys. Acta, 799, 1 (1984).
31. P.Cutrecasas and T.Roth (Eds.), Receptor-Mediated Endocytosis, Receptors and Recognition, Series B, Vol. 15, Chapman and Hall, London, 1983.
32. M.Monsigny, C. Kieda, and A.-C.Roche, Membrane glycoproteins, glycolipids and membrane lectins as recognition signals in normal and malignant cells, Biol. Cell., 47, 95 (1983).
33. G.Ashwell and A.G.Morrell, The role of surface carbohydrates in hepatic recognition and transport of circulating glycoproteins, Adv. Enzymol., 41, 99 (1974).
34. V. Kolb-Bachofen, J.Schrepper-Schafer and H.Kolb, Receptor-mediated particle uptake by liver macrophages. Galactose-particle receptor-mediated uptake via coated and also non-coated structures, Exp.Cell Res., 148, 173 (1983).
35. A.L.Schwartz, S.E. Fridovich and H.F. Lodish, Kinetics of internalization and recycling of the asialoglycoprotein receptor in a hepatoma cell line, J.Biol.Chem., 257, 4230

(1982).
36. V.L.Sheperd, Y.C.Lee, P.H.Schlesinger and P.D. Stahl, L-Fucose terminated glycoconjugates are recognised by pinocytosis receptors on macrophages, Proc. Natl. Acad. Sci. U.S.A, 78, 1019 (1981).
37. P.Stahl and S.Gordon, Expression of a mannosyl-fucosyl receptor for endocytosis on primary macrophages and their hybrids, J.Cell Biol., 93, 49 (1982).
38. P.Stahl, H.Six, J.S.Rodman, P.Schlesinger, D.R.P. Tulsani and O.Touster, Evidence for specific recognition sites mediating clearances of lysosomal enzymes in vivo, Proc. Natl. Acad. Sci. USA, 73, 4045 (1976).
39. E.F.Neufeld and G.Ashwell, Carbohydrate recognition systems, In:"The Biochemistry of Glycoproteins and Proteoglycans", W.J.Lennarz (Ed.), Plenum Press, New York, 1980, pp. 241-266.
40. K.Ullrich, G.Mersmann, M.Fleischer and K.Von Figura, Epithelial rat liver cells have cell surface receptors recognising a phosphorylated carbohydrate on lysosomal enzymes, Hoppe-Seyler's Z. Physiol.Chem.,359, 1591 (1978).
41. M.Monsigny, A.-C.Roche and P.Midoux, Uptake of neoglycoproteins via membrane lectin(s) of L1210 cells evidenced by quantitative flow cytofluorometry and drug targeting, Biol. Cell., 51, 187 (1984).
42. A.C.Roche, M.Barzilay, P.Midoux, S.Junqua, N.Sharon and M.Monsigny, Sugar-specific endocytosis of glycoproteins by Lewis lung carcinoma cells, J.Cell Biochem., 22, 131(1983).
43. L.Fiume, C.Busi and A.Mattioli, Targeting of antiviral drugs by coupling with protein carriers, FEBS LETTS., 153, 6 (1983).
44. R.Duncan, J.B.Lloyd, P.Rejmanová and J.Kopeček, Methods of targeting N-(2-hydroxypropyl)methacrylamide copolymers to particular cell types, Makromol. Chem., in press.
45. S.A.Cartlidge, P.Rejmanová, R.Duncan, J.Kopeček and J.B. Lloyd, Evaluation of soluble N-(2-hydroxypropyl)methacrylamide copolymers as drug carriers. In vivo distribution of copolymers in the rat following different routes of administration, Abstract from the Microsymposium on Polymers in Medicine, Prague, Czechoslovakia, 1984.
46. S.A.Cartlidge, P.Rejmanová, R.Duncan, J.Kopeček and J.B. Lloyd, Targeting of soluble crosslinked N-(2-hydroxypropyl)methacrylamide copolymers in vivo. A potential drug delivery system, Biochem. Soc. Trans., 12, 1064 (1984).
47. E.Hurwitz, R.Levy, R.Maron, M.Wilchek, R,Arnon and M.Sela, The covalent binding of daunomycin and adriamycin to antibodies with retention of both drug and antibody activities, Cancer Res., 35, 1175 (1975).
48. J.Kopeček, Synthesis of tailor-made soluble polymeric drug carriers, In:"Recent Advances in Drug Delivery Systems", J.M.Anderson and S.-W.Kim (Eds.), Plenum Press, New York,

1984, pp. 41-62.
49. B.Říhová and J.Kopeček, Immunological activity of antibodies bound to N-(2-hydroxypropyl)methacrylamide copolymers, Makromol. Chem., in press.
50. U.Weisbecker, G.E.Ibbotson, G.Livesey and K.E.Williams, The fate of homologous ^{125}I-labelled immunoglobulin G within rat visceral yolk sacs incubated in vitro, Biochem.J., 214, 815 (1983).
51. P.Rejmanová, B.Obereigner and J.Kopeček, Polymers containing enzymatically degradable bonds. 2. Poly [N-(2-hydroxypropyl)methacrylamide] chains connected by oligopeptide sequences cleavable by chymotrypsin, Makromol. Chem., 182, 1899 (1981).
52. J.Kopeček, I.Cifkova, P.Rejmanová, J.Strohalm, B.Obereigner and K.Ulbrich, Polymers containing enzymatically degradable bonds, 4. Preliminary experiments in vivo, Makromol. Chem., 182, 2941 (1981).
53. B.Hulme, P.W.Dykes, I.Appleyard and D.W.Arkall, Retention and storage sites of radioactive polyvinylpyrrolidone, J.Nucl.Med., 9, 389 (1968).
54. J.Kopeček, L.Šprincl and D.Lim, New types of synthetic infusion solutions. 1. Investigation of the effect of solutions of some hydrophilic polymers on blood, J.Biomed. Mater. Res., 7, 179 (1973).
55. B.Říhová, K.Ulbrich, J.Kopeček and P.Mančal, Immunogenicity of N-(2-hydroxypropyl)methacrylamide copolymers - potential hapten or drug carriers, Folia Microbiol., 28, 217 (1983).
56. B.Říhová, J.Kopeček, K.Ulbrich, M.Popisil and P.Mančal, Effect of chemical structure of N-(2-hydroxypropyl)methacrylamide copolymers on the immune response of inbred strains of mice, Biomaterials, 5, 143 (1984).
57. C.De Duve, T.De Barsey, B.Poole, A.Trouet, P.Tulkens and F.Van Hoof, Lysosomotropic agents, Biochem. Pharmacol. 23, 2495 (1974).
58. A.Trouet, R.Baurain, D.Deprez-de-Campeneere, M.Masquelier and P.Pirson, Targeting of antitumour and antiprotozoal drugs by covalent linkage to protein carriers, In:"Targeting of Drugs",G. Gregoriadis, J.Senior and A.Trouet (Eds.), Plenum Press, New York, 1982, pp. 19-30.
59. W.A.R. Van Heeswijk, T.Stoffer, M.J.D. Eenik, W.Potman, W.J.F. van der Vijgh, J.Vander Poort, H.M. Pinedo, P. Lelieveld and J.Feijen, Synthesis, characterisation and antitumour activity of macromolecular prodrugs of adriamycin, In:"Recent Advances in Drug Delivery Systems", J.M.Anderson and S.W.Kim (Eds.), Plenum Press, New York, 1984, pp. 77-100.
60. E.Schacht, L.Ruys, J.Vermeersch and J.P.Remon, Polymer-drug combinations, Synthesis and characterisation of modified polysaccharides containing procainamide moieties, J.Controlled Release, 1, 33 (1984).

61. J.P.Remon, R.Duncan and E.Schacht, Polymer-drug combinations: Pinocytic uptake of modified polysaccharides containing procainamide moieties by rat visceral yolk sacs cultured in vitro, J.Controlled Release, 1, 47(1984).
62. P.E.Thorpe, and W.C.J.Ross, The preparation and cytotoxic properties of antibody-toxin conjugates, Immun. Rev., 62, 119 (1982).

Chapter 7
Preferential Membrane Permeation and Receptor Recognition in Drug Targeting

T. Y. Shen

Merck Sharp and Dohme Research Laboratories
Rahway, New Jersey 07065

The selective delivery of therapeutic agents or their bioconvertible derivatives to target cells or tissues can be facilitated by optimization of a membrane permeation process favoring lipophilic molecules or by a specific mechanism involving the recognition and uptake by cell surface receptors.

The first case may be illustrated by the pharmacodynamics of a nonsteroidal antiinflammatory/analgesic drug, sulindac[1]. In the current development of antiarthritic agents with improved safety and efficacy, a general approach is to develop agents with well-defined biochemical mechanism of action and trying to achieve preferential tissue distribution, either through manipulation of the pharmacodynamics of the drug molecule or, in special instances, by means of targeted drug delivery.

The antiinflammatory drug sulindac is an indene analog of indomethacin[1]. The introduction of a methylsulfinyl (sulfoxide) group not only increases the aqueous solubility of this aromatic molecule but also provides a center for metabolism in vivo. Sulindac per se is biochemically inactive as an antiinflammatory agent. It is reversibly reduced to the sulfide metabolite which is as potent as indomethacin (Fig. 1). Thus, sulindac is an interesting example of a reversible prodrug[2]. The tissue distribution of the active sulfide is dependent upon the local capacity of the oxidizing[3] and reducing[4] enzymes and the partition characteristics of the more hydrophilic sulindac vs. the more hydrophobic sulfide. Using liposomes as vesicle models the penetration and perturbation of the bilayer membrane by sulindac sulfide, but not by sulindac itself, can readily be demonstrated by NMR[5] and differential scanning calorimetry techniques[6].

SULFIDE   **SULINDAC**

Active Metabolite
Potency ~ Indomethacin

Favorable pharmacodynamics

                                                                               Inactive Prodrug

At the cellular level, a double labeling experiment showed that the interconversion of ^{3}H-sulindac and the ^{14}C-sulfide takes place readily in leukocytes[7]. Furthermore, a marked difference in the partition and membrane permeation of the two compounds is noted. The more hydrophilic sulindac tends to remain extracellular whereas the more lipophilic sulfide accumulates inside the cell with a cell/medium ratio of 50:1. The highly increased intracellular concentration of sulindac sulfide presumably would allow an expression of its secondary biochemical actions, in addition to its inhibition of the cyclooxygenase enzyme, such as the inhibition of LTB$_4$ synthesis[8] and the neutralization of oxygen radicals[9].

In vivo, the differential distribution of sulindac and its sulfide metabolite fortuitiously contribute to its patient tolerance as well. As cyclooxygenase inhibitors, most NSAIDS produce systemic side-effects which are related to the local depletion of prostaglandins and possibly some increase of leukotrienes. Gastrointestinal irritations and renal function disturbances are two notable ones. In the case of sulindac, the exposure of gastrointestinal tract to drug action is reduced both by the oral administration of its inactive prodrug and by the lack of enterohepatic recirculation of the active sulfide metabolite. As a consequence, one would expect less inhibition of the production of gastric prostaglandins. Sulindac also appears to exert much less effect on prostaglandin-mediated renal functions than other NSAIDS[10]. These observations are supported by a recent clinical pharmacology experiment, which showed that at its therapeutic dosage of 400 mg/day, sulindac inhibits the cyclooxygenase pathway in circulating platelets and synovial tissue but, unlike several other NSAIDS, does not reduce prostaglandin synthesis in the gastric and renal tissues[11]. These data are attributable to a reversible prodrug activation process which converts a hydrophilic prodrug to a lipophilic active metabolite with differential membrane permeation characteristics.

In our laboratory, the phenomenon of preferential membrane permeation is also used to design lysosomotropic agents. Lysosomes are highly acidic intracellular vesicles which contain a variety of hydrolytic enzymes and which are involved in cellular metabolism and the phagocytosis process. The delivery of lysosomotropic agents through a piggyback endocytosis process is well known. Another class of lysosomotropic agents enters into cells through passive membrane diffusion. A group of weakly basic hydrophobic amines with pK values between 5-9 can freely penetrate the bilayer cell membrane and the lysosome membrane. Once inside the acidic medium of a lysosome, the amine molecule is protonated and becomes nondiffusible through the membrane. The trapped amine can exert its pharmacological action directly inside the lysosome, either as an enzyme inhibitor or as a membrane stabilizer like chloroquine (Fig. 2).

LYSOSOMOTROPIC AGENTS

Membrane Permeation

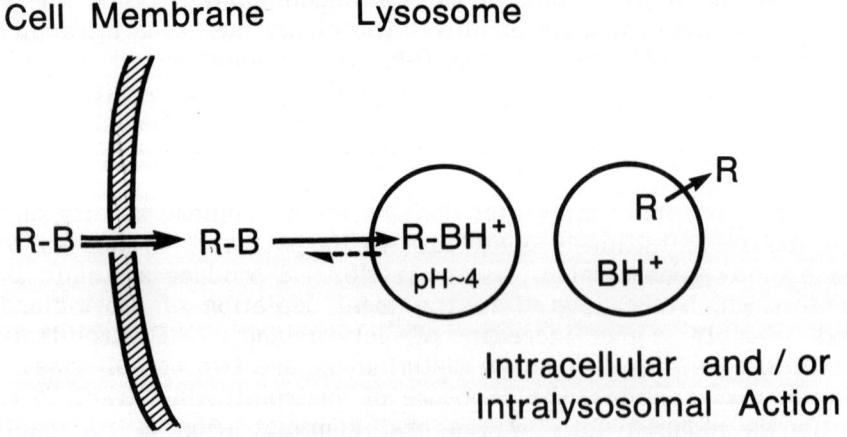

A group of lysosomotropic detergents was shown recently as membrane destabilizers as well[12]. These lysosomotropic detergents are long chain aliphatic derivatives of weak organic bases such as imidazole or morpholine. These detergents will accumulate in BHK cells, causing leakage and rupture of the lysosome membrane followed by cell rounding and cell death. Some selective toxicity of these detergents was demonstrated in cells with high pinocytic activity. They may have potential utility in the extracorporeal treatment of leukomic bone marrow cells for autologous transplantation. The cellular specificity can be improved further by the attachment of a small peptide, Z-gly-L-phe. Conjugates of Z-gly-L-phe with lysosomotropic detergent or a nitrogen mustard were shown to have a much faster rate of entry, up to 10 times, into pinocytic cells such as macrophage, P-815 mastocytoma, SV-40 3T3, and leukemia 1210 cells[13]. An active transport mechanism in cell membrane has been postulated for this accelerated entry.

Monclonal antibodies which recognize cell surface antigens have been used as carriers for drug targeting with some success. Conversely, one can use cell surface receptors as a target-specific entrance (Fig. 3). Receptors on cell-surface are noted for their high degree of specificity in their interactions with appropriate ligands. In receptor mediated drug delivery the drug is chemically attached to or physically associated with a ligand which is recognized by a specific receptor on the surface of a target cell. The ligand can be peptide or oligosaccharide. It can also be a component of a drug carrier such as a phospholipid vesical, i.e. liposome or a lipoprotein particle. After ingestion of the ligand-carrier complex, the active free drug is dissociated from the carrier or liberated from the chemical conjugate by intracellular enzymes to exert its pharmacological effect.

Cell Targeting

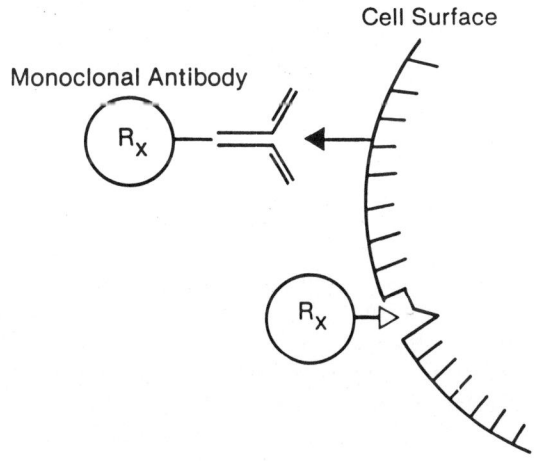

Receptor Ligand: –▷

R_x : Liposome . LDL
Enzyme . Drug

For example, the well-defined low density lipoprotein (LDL) receptors[14,15] have been investigated as a potential target for drug delivery. On the surface of many cell types there are approximately 50-100,000 LDL receptors per cell. The interaction of low density lipoprotein, or LDL, with its membrane receptor is followed by internalization and metabolism by lysosomal hydrolases. LDL is composed of an inner lipid core which contains cholesterol and esters, triglycerides and phospholipids. It is recognized by the receptor through Apoprotein B in the outer layer. The cholesterol esters in the lipid core can readily be removed by solvent extraction and replaced by lipophilic drug derivatives to form a reconstituted LDL (r-LDL), which can still be recognized by the LDL receptor and internalized into lysosomes[16].

In preliminary experiments the selective cytotoxicity of such a Trojan horse approach was demonstrated by r-LDL containing a cholesterol synthesis inhibitor, 25-hydroxy cholesterol[17], or a photosensitizer pyrene[18]. Nitrogen mustard has also been anchored by 3-oleoyl cholesterol inside reconstituted LDL with minimal leakage into the serum. After cellular uptake, free nitrogen mustard is efficiently released by lysosomal enzymes to exert cytotoxicity against SV-589 cells which have more LDL-receptor than normal human fibroblasts[19].

Clearly, the therapeutic advantage of this approach depends upon a quantitatve difference in the density of LDL receptor in different tissues. Some leukemic cells possess a higher number of LDL receptors. However, among normal tissues the adrenal gland is also noted for its high density of LDL receptor. The margin of safety of drug-LDL complex *in vivo* remains to be demonstrated[20]. It should be noted that the intracellular pathway of LDL is, with minor variations, a mechanism for the receptor mediated endocytosis of many polypeptide factors and plasma proteins[15]. The peptide region involved in their receptor interactions might also be considered as potential receptor-specific ligands.

In addition, cell-surface saccharide receptors have also been investigated as a means of selective drug delivery. Membrane polysaccharides or glycoproteins on the surface of many cells play important roles in cellular functions. Some are surface determinants involved in cellular interactions. In the coated-pit region of exterior cell surface membranes, there are saccharide receptors which recognize and internalize glycoproteins with specific carbohydrate determinants[21]. A familiar example is the D-galactose binding site on the surface of hepatocytes[22]. There are receptors on Kupffer cells and macrophages which recognize D-mannose[23] or L-fucose and, to a lesser extent, N-acetyl-D-glucosamine. Many saccharide receptors are multivalent. An oligosaccharide unit was defined as the minimal structure required for receptor binding and endocytosis by a mannose receptor of macrophages and Kupffer cells. The hepatic lectin also has higher affinity for a cluster of galactose terminals[24]. Recent study showed that optimal binding is obtained with a cluster of three galactose terminals attached to flexible backbones with triangular interdistances of 15, 22 and 25 Å[25].

These saccharide determinants have been incorporated into liposomes or chemical conjugates in several drug delivery experiments. We have synthesized a group of glycolipids by attaching a saccharide moiety through a hexamethylene spacer arm to the 3-hydroxy group in cholesterol[26] (Fig. 4). Incorporation of these glycolipids into the bilayer of liposomes introduces specific mono- and disaccharide determinants on the liposome surface. Instead of cholesterol, other lipophilic groups, e.g. diglycerides or ceramide, have also been used as anchors in the liposome bilayer. But liposomes prepared from cholesterol glycoconjugates appear to be more stable than ceramide liposomes in vivo[27].

Saccharide-Cholesterol Conjugates

Saccharide: D-Gal, Man, NAcGlu
L-Fuc, Lac, etc.

The ability of surface saccharides to enhance the uptake of liposomes by target cells in the liver was clearly demonstrated in a recent gene transfer experiment[28,29]. Hepatocytes are secretory cells capable of expressing liposome-transported insulin genes. With ordinary liposomes, after i.v. injection, the incorporated plasmid DNA was mainly taken up by the phagocytic Kupffer cells in the liver. With addition of lactosylceramide to the liposome membrane to provide surface galactose terminals, significant increases of plasmid DNA were delivered to hepatocytes and endothelial cells, both of which possess galactose receptors. On a weight basis, considering the abundance of hepatocytes in the liver, nearly 20%

of total plasmid DNA administered i.v. were delivered to hepatocytes. Parameters affecting liposome-mediated delivery of nucleic acids into eucaryotic cells have been investigated previously[30]. Further optimization of the membrane composition and physical properties of these galactose liposomes would undoubtedly improve their selectivity and efficiency in delivering genetic materials.

The cellular interactions and in vivo distribution of liposomes containing other saccharides, e.g. D-mannose, L-fucose, etc. and modified saccharides, e.g. 6-amino-6-deoxy-D-mannose, have also been studied[31,32]. The potential application of these derivatized liposomes in the delivery of drugs, biologically active substances or diagnostic agents is under active investigation.

We have also explored the feasibility of using chemical conjugates of carbohydrate ligands for drug targeting[33]. A group of synthetic saccharide ligands were prepared by attaching mannose through a mercapto propionyl group to the ε-amino group(s) in lysine, lysyl-lysine and (lys)$_3$. These model glycopeptides competitively block the binding of labeled mannosyl-BSA with the mannose receptor on macrophages. The trivalent ligand, Man$_3$Lys$_2$, with K_i = 4 µM, is approximately 200 times more potent than simple mannosides. The carbohydrate specificity of the macrophage receptor is again corroborated by the ineffectiveness of the corresponding D-galactose analog, Gal$_3$Lys$_2$. The L-fucose analog, Fuc$_3$Lys$_2$, is only moderately active.

The affinity of these mannose ligands for the macrophage receptor is not much reduced by the attachment of other chemical groups at the peptide end. Using an iodine^{125} labeled Bolton-Hunter reagent attached to the Man$_3$Lys$_2$ ligand (Fig. 5), a dissociation constant K_D of 2.7 µM and estimated maximal binding of 5.2×10^5 molecules per cell at 0°C were obtained. This number of receptors per cell is very similar to that for LDL receptors. The labeled ligand is readily endocytozed by macrophage at 21°. The Michaelis-Menten constant K_m of uptake is 5.6 µM with a maximum velocity (V_{max}) of 1.7×10^5 molecules per minute per cell. In other words, the labeled ligand conjugate enters into macrophage at a rate roughly one molecule every three minutes. This rate of entry is again comparable to the estimated rate for the uptake of LDL by its receptor.

Man₃Lys₂BH Conjugate

For possible targeted delivery, the Man₃Lys₂ ligand was coupled to corticosteroids and other drugs. Furthermore, the possible application of Man₃Lys₂ in enzyme replacement therapy was also explored. Gaucher's disease is a genetic disorder caused by a deficiency of β-glucocerebrosidase in Kupffer cells of the patient. The polysaccharide portion of this enzyme has several galactose terminals. As a consequence, intravenously administered exogenous enzyme is mainly taken up by hepatocytes of the patient and less by Kupffer cells. It would seem that attachment of mannose ligands to the enzyme should in theory increase the distribution to Kupffer cells via their mannose receptors. For this purpose as partially purified human placental enzyme supplied by Dr. Brady's group at NIH was chemically coupled with Man₃Lys₂[34]. A modified enzyme preparation contains approximately 8 to 9 molecules of the ligand per each subunit and retains its enzymatic activity in full. In the macrophage culture the cellular uptake of this modified enzyme is indeed faster and to a greater extent than the native enzyme. At an enzyme concentration of 0.7 μM, alveolar macrophages endocytose an amount of (Man₃Lys₂)ₙ-β-glucocerebrosidase equal to more than 11 times their endogenous β-glucosidase level after one hour. The modified enzyme also appears to be reasonably stable inside the macrophage, its activity is maintained for several hours *in vitro*. In the rat it is cleared from the circulation more rapidly than the native enzyme. The clearance of the modified enzyme, but not the native enzyme, can be inhibited significantly by coinfusion with mannan. An analysis of enzyme activity in isolated liver cells indicates that there is an 18-fold increase in enzyme specific activity in non-parenchymal cells and only 1.5 fold in hepatocytes as compared with uninjected control animals[35] (Table 1). These data clearly indicate that mannan receptors are largely responsible for the enzyme uptake. In this experiment the increase in enzyme activity in non-parenchymal cells is more than 1/3 of the increase obtainable after injection of partially deglycosylated glucocerebrosidase. Further optimization of enzyme-modification may yield a higher uptake preparation suitable for therapeutic trials.

Glucocerebrosidase Distribution in Liver Cell Populations

	Hepatocytes		Non-Parenchymal Cells	
	Total Activity (u/mg Protein)	Total Activity in Hepatocyte Fraction U/Liver	Total Activity (u/mg protein)	Total Activity in Non-Parenchymal Cell Fraction (U/Liver)
Control	67 ± 11		44 ± 17	
G (400,000 U)	87 ± 7	47,000	251 ± 116	7,000
MAN$_3$LYS$_2$-G (400,000 U)	102 ± 5	82,000	766 ± 346	24,000
AHEXO-G (300,000 U)	122	129,000	2,200	73,000

In conclusion, selective drug delivery is receiving increasing attention as an important aspect in new drug development. The reversible activation of sulindac in different tissue compartments provides a complex but fortuitously favorable pharmacodynamic pattern, supported by extensive clinical pharmacological experiments. Several experimental approaches based on lysosomotropism, and ligand-receptor recognition have also demonstrated the methodology and feasibility of drug targeting via molecular mechanisms. Certainly the selective delivery of plasmid-DNA and genetically-deficient enzymes to their target cells in vivo with the help of specific carbohydrate ligands are encouraging examples for further development in this exciting area.

References

1. T. Y. Shen and C. A. Winter, Chemical and Biological Studies on Indomethacin, Sulindac and Their Analogs, Advances in Drug Research, 12, 89-245 (1977).
2. D. E. Duggan, K. F. Hooke, E. A. Risley, T. Y. Shen and C. G. Van Arman, Identification of the Biologically Active Form of Sulindac, J. Pharmacol. Expt. Therap., 201, 9-13 (1977).
3. D. R. Light, D. J. Waxman and C. Walsh, Studies on the Chirality of Sulfoxidation Catalyzed by Bacterial Flavoenzyme Cyclohexanone Monooxygenase and Hog Liver Flavin Adenine Dinucleotide Containing Monooxygenase, Biochemistry, 21, 2490-2498 (1982).

4. J. H. Ratnayake, P. E. Hanna, M. W. Anders and D. E. Duggan, Sulfoxide Reduction - In Vitro Reduction of Sulindac by Rat Hepatic Cytosolic Enzymes, Drug Metabolism and Disposition, 9, 85-87 (1981).
5. S. S. Fan and T. Y. Shen, Membrane Effects of Anti-Inflammatory Agents. 1. Interaction of Sulindac and its Metabolites with Phospholipid Membrane, A Magnetic-Resonance Study, J. Med. Chem., 24, 1197-1202 (1981).
6. S. B. Hwang and T. Y. Shen, Membrane Effects of Anti-Inflammatory Agents. 2. Interaction of Non-Steroidal Anti-Inflammatory Drugs with Liposome and Purple Membranes, J. Med. Chem., 24, 1202-1211 (1981).
7. D. E. Duggan, Sulindac: Therapeutic Implications of the Prodrug/Pharmacophore Equilibrium, Drug Metabolism Reviews, 12, 325 (1981).
8. J. L. Humes, S. Sadowski, M. Galavage, M. Goldenberg, E. Subers, F. A. Kuehl, Jr., and R. J. Bonney, Pharmacological Effects of Non-Steroidal Antiinflammatory Agents on Prostaglandin and Leukotriene Synthesis in Mouse Peritoneal Macrophages, Biochem. Pharmacol., 32, 2319 (1983).
9. R. W. Egan, P. H. Gale and F. A. Kuehl, Jr., Reduction of Hydroperoxides in the Prostaglandin Biosynthetic Pathway by a Microsomal Peroxidase, J. Biol. Chem., 254, 3295-3302 (1979).
10. G. Ciabattoni, G. A. Cinotti, A. Pierucci, B. M. Simonetti, M. Manzi, F. Pugliese, P. Barositti, G. Pecci, F. Taggi and C. Patrono, Effects of Sulindac and Ibuprofen in Patients with Chronic Glomerular Disease, New Eng. J. Med., 310, 279-283 (1984).
11. G. Ciabattoni, G. Bianchi Porro, I. Caruso, M. Fumagalli, F. Publiese and C. Patrono, Differential Inhibition of Prostaglandin (PG) and Thromboxane (TX) Synthesis in Human Tissues by Non-Steroidal Antiinflammatory Drugs (NSADs), Clin. Res., 32, PA462 (1984).
12. D. K. Miller, E. Griffiths, J. Lenard and R. A. Firestone, Cell Killing by Lysosomotropic Detergents, J. Cell Biol., 97, 1841-1851 (1983).
13. R. A. Firestone, J. M. Pisano, P. J. Bailey, A. Sturm, R. J. Bonney, P. Wightman, R. Devlin, C. S. Lin, D. L. Keller and P. C. Tway, Lysosomotropic Agents. 4. Carbobenzoxyglycylphenylalanyl, A New Protease-Sensititve Masking Group for Introduction Into Cells, J. Med. Chem., 25, 539-544 (1982).
14. J. L. Goldstein and M. S. Brown, The Low Density Lipoprotein Pathway and Its Relation to Atherosclerosis, An. Rev. Biochem., 46, 897-930 (1977).
15. R. W. Mahley and T. L. Innerarity, Lipoprotein Receptors and Cholesterol Homeostasis, Biochem. Biophys. Acta, 737, 197-222 (1983).
16. M. Krieger, M. S. Brown, J. R. Faust and J. L. Goldstein, Replacement of Endogenous Cholesteryl Esters of Low Density

- Reconstitution of a Biologically Active Lipoprotein Particle, J. Biol. Chem., 253, 4093-4101 (1978).
17. M. Krieger, J. L. Goldstein and M. S. Brown, Receptor-Mediated Uptake of Low-Density Lipoprotein Reconstituted with 25-Hydroxycholesteryl Oleate Suppresses 3-Hydroxy-3-methylglutaryl-coenzyme-a Reductase and Inhibits Growth of Human Fibroblasts, Proc. Natl. Acad. Sci. USA, 75, 5052-5056 (1978).
18. S. T. Mosley, J. L. Goldstein, M. S. Brown, J. R. Falck and R. G. Anderson, Targeted Killing of Cultured Cells by Receptor Dependent Photosensitization, Proc. Natl. Acad. Sci. USA, 78, 5717-5721 (1981).
19. R. A. Firestone, J. M. Pisano, J. R. Falck, M. M. McPhaul and M. Krieger, Delivery of Cyto-Toxic Compounds to Cells by the LDL Pathway, J. Med. Chem., 27, 1037-1043 (1984).
20. R. E. Counsell and R. C. Pohland, Lipoproteins as Potential Site-Specific Delivery Systems for Diagnostic and Therapeutic Agents, J. Med. Chem., 25, 1115-1120 (1982).
21. M. C. Willingham, Microscopic Aspects of Receptor-Mediated Endocytosis, J. Amer. Med. Assoc., 244, 2092 (1980).
22. G. Ashwell and A. G. Morell, Membrane Glycoproteins and Recognition Phenoma, Trends Biochem. Sci., 2, 76-78 (1977).
23. V. L. Shepherdt, M. G. Konish and P. Stahl, Dexamethasone Increases Expression of Mannose Receptors and Decreases Extracellular Lysosomal Enzyme Accumulation in Macrophages, J. Biol. Chem., 260, 160-164 (1985).
24. J. U. Baenziger and Y. Maynard, Human Hepatic Lectin. Physiochemical Properties and Specificity, J. Biol. Chem., 255, 4607-4613 (1980).
25. R. T. Lee, P. Lin and Y. C. Lee, New Synthetic Cluster Ligands for Galactose/N-Acetylgalactosamine Specific Lectin of Mammalian Liver, Biochem., 23, 4255-4261 (1984).
26. M. M. Ponpipom, R. L. Bugianesi, and T. Y. Shen, Cell Surface Carbohydrates for Targeting Studies, Canadian J. of Chem., 58, 214-220 (1980).
27. P. S. Wu, H. M. Wu, G. W. Tin, J. R. Schuh, W. R. Croasmun, J. D. Baldeschwieler, T. Y. Shen and M. M. Ponpipom, Stability of Carbohydrate Modified Vesicles In Vivo: Comparative Effects of Ceramide and Cholesterol Glycoconjugates, Proc. Natl. Acad. Sci. USA, 79, 5490-5493 (1982).
28. P. Soriano, J. Dijkstra, A. Legrand, H. Spanjer, D. Londos-Gagliardi, F. Roerdink, G. Scherphos and C. Nicolau, Targeted and Nontargeted Liposomes for In Vivo Transfer to Rat Liver Cells of Plasmid Containing the Preproinsulin I Gene, Proc. Natl. Acad. Sci. USA, 80, 7128-7131 (1983).
29. C. Nicolau, A. Legrand and P. Soriano, Liposomes for Gene Transfer and Expression In Vivo, Ctr. Biophys. Molec., CNRS, Ciba Foundation Symposia, No. 103, 254-264 (1984).

30. M. J. Ostro, D. Lavelle, W. Paxton, B. Matthews and D. Giacomoni, Parameters Affecting the Liposome-Mediated Insertion of RNA Into Eucaryoticc Cells In Vitro, Archives of Biochem. and Biophys., 201, 392-402 (1980).
31. P. S. Wu, G. W. Tin, J. D. Baldeschwieler, T. Y. Shen and M. M. Ponpipom, Effect of Surface Modification on Aggregation of Phospholipid-Vesicles, Proc. Natl. Acad. Sci. USA, 78, 6211-6215 (1981).
32. M. M. Mauk, R. C. Gamble and J. D. Baldeschwieler, Targeting of Lipid Vesicles: Specificity of Carbohydrate Receptor Analogues for Leukocytes in Mice, Proc. Natl. Acad. Sci. USA, 77, 4430-4434 (1980).
33. J. C. Robbins, M. H. Lam, C. S. Tripp, R. L. Bugianesi, M. M. Ponpipom and T. Y. Shen, Synthetic Glycopeptide Substrates for Receptor Mediated Endocytosis by Macrophages, Proc. Natl. Acad. Sci. USA, 78, 7294-7298 (1981).
34. T. W. Doebber, M. S. Wu, R. L. Bugianesi, M. M. Ponpipom, F. S. Furbish, J. A. Barranger, R. O. Brady and T. Y. Shen, Enhanced Macrophage Uptake of Synthetically Glycosylated Human Placental β-Glucocerebrosidase, J. Biol. Chem., 257, 2193-2199 (1982).
35. G. J. Murray, T. W. Doebber, M. S. Wu, R. L. Bugianesi, M. M. Ponpipom, T. Y. Shen, R. O. Brady and J. A. Barranger, Targeting of Synthetically Glycosylated Human Placental Glucocerebrosidase, in press.

Chapter 8
Carrier Mediated and Receptor Mediated Transport Across the Endothelelial Cells of the Vasculature

Kenneth L. Audus and Ronald T. Borchardt

Department of Pharmaceutical Chemistry
School of Pharmacy
The University of Kansas
Lawrence, Kansas

Introduction

Microvascular endothelium is composed of a single layer of simple squamous epithelial cells that varies in thickness from 0.1 to 1.0 micrometers. Three types of endothelium are found in the microvasculature: continuous, fenestrated, and discontinuous (1,2). Continuous endothelium, comprised of closely apposed endothelial cells, is the most predominant type of endothelium and typical of the microvasculature of the heart, lungs, skeletal muscle, and the central nervous system. The endothelium of the renal glomerulus and the intestinal mucosa has relatively large transcellular openings called fenestrae and is referred to as fenestrated endothelium. Discontinuous endothelium possesses much larger transcellular openings or gaps between cells and is found in the spleen and hepatic sinusoids (1,3).

A critical physiological function of microvascular endothelium is to form a physical partition and semipermeable porous membrane between the blood and extravascular tissue. The permeability properties and transport processes of the endothelial barrier participate in the regulation and specificity of the exchange of fluid, water-soluble solutes (including drugs), macromolecules, and cells between the blood and the extravascular tissue (1,3). Accordingly, anatomical and functional differences among the three types of endothelium account for the variability in microvascular permeability among different tissues. For example, the permability of the continuous type of endothelium is limited to molecules that pass through intercellular junctions or utilize transendothelial carrier systems. Conversely, the discontinuous endothelium is permeable to molecules of all sizes including proteins (2).

Discussion here will be limited to the continuous endothelium of the brain microvasculature known as the blood-brain barrier. Specifically, unique cellular and cytochemical characteristics, examples of carrier and receptor mediated transport systems, and recently developed in vitro models of brain endothelium will be briefly reviewed. Additionally, the potential of blood-brain barrier transport systems and their study in the in vitro model systems as related to delivery of drugs to the brain will be addressed.

Brain Endothelium

The continuous microvascular endothelium of the brain represents the most restrictive type of endothelium and is of particular importance as the blood-brain barrier (4,5). Endothelium of the blood-brain barrier, as illustrated in Figure 1A, is distinguishable from peripheral endothelium, Figure 1B, by the presence of highly resistant epithelial tight junctions, few pinocytotic vesicles, and the virtual absence of fenestrations (6). Permeability and transport properties of the blood-brain barrier, then, are those associated with the plasma membranes of the endothelium. Consequently, the blood-brain barrier has a low filtration coefficient and is impermeable to most polar solutes (7).

Unlike peripheral endothelium, cerebral endothelium also possesses a high activity of enzymes normally identified with active epithelial transport systems such as those found in the small intestine or the proximal renal tubule (7). For instance, the blood-brain barrier is enriched in gamma-glutamyl transpeptidase an enzyme thought to be directly involved in the gamma-glutamyl cycle, a mechanism postulated to be a component of the transmembrane transport of amino acids (8). Although its relationship to blood-brain barrier transport is not understood, gamma-glutamyl transpeptidase is currently considered to be a specific marker for brain endothelium (7,9). Other enzymes often associated with actively transporting epithelium and of high activity in brain endothelium include alkaline phosphatase, butyrylcholinesterase, aromatic amino acid decarboxylase, monoamine oxidase, and sodium, potassium-ATPase (7,9,10). Consistent with the idea of the blood-brain barrier as an active interface is the observation that there is five to six times more mitochondria per cross-section of brain endothelial cells than in skeletal muscle endothelial cells (11).

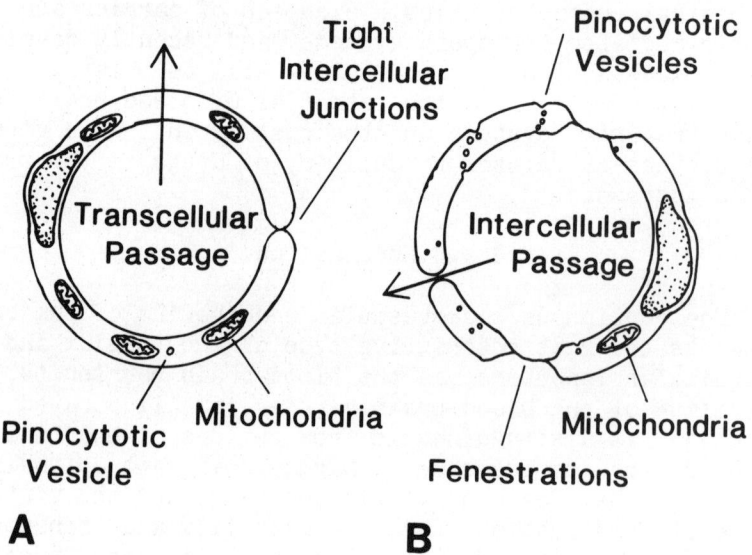

Figure 1. Fundamental Morphological Differences between Endothelium of the Brain and Peripheral Microvessels. A) Endothelial cells of brain microvessels possess tight intercellular junctions, few pinocytotic vesicles, and numerous mitochondria. B) Endothelial cells typical of the peripheral microvessel often contain fenestrations, intercellular clefts, and few mitochondria. Permeability of brain capillaries is restricted to molecules that undergo transcellular passage as opposed to peripheral capillaries where molecules cross the cell layers intercellularly and transcellularly.

Carrier Mediated Transendothelial Transport

Carrier-mediated transport is a major mechanism by which water soluble nutrients and certain drugs cross the blood-brain barrier (12,13). At present seven different bidirectional carrier systems in brain endothelium are known. In general, these carrier systems are concentration-dependent, saturable, stereospecific, and can be competed for by related substrates (12). Table I lists the individual transport systems and representative substrates. Certain drugs and other non-nutrients may also gain access to the brain environment by utilizing these carriers. Of the seven transport systems, the neutral amino acid carrier is particularly relevant as a mechanism for delivery of drugs to the brain (13).

Table I. Carrier Systems of the Blood-Brain and Representative Subtrates (12).

Carrier	Representative Substrate
Hexose	Glucose
Monocarboxylic Acid	Lactate
Neutral Amino Acid (L-System)	Phenylalanine
Basic Amino Acid	Lysine
Amine	Choline
Purine	Adenine
Nucleoside	Adenosine

The neutral amino acid carrier, like the other blood-brain barrier transport systems, is bidirectional and equilibrative in nature. The role of this amino acid transport system as a transporter of neutral amino acids is also similar to the amino acid carrier of other tissues. The carrier of brain endothelium is different from the carrier in other tissues in two respects. First, it is a sodium-independent carrier. Second, and perhaps most important in terms of selective delivery of neutral amino acids to the brain, there is a great difference in the affinity of the blood-brain amino acid carrier as compared to the affinity of the carrier in other tissues. The affinity constant, K_m, of the blood-brain barrier amino acid transport system is 0.10 to 0.60 mM, or approximately equivalent to plasma amino acid levels. In peripheral tissues the K_m of the neutral amino acid carrier is tenfold greater. As a consequence of this large difference in K_m's, especially under conditions where plasma levels of amino acids are low, competition among amino acids for tissue uptake only occurs at the blood-brain barrier (12,13).

Certain neutral amino acids that are centrally acting drugs (e.g. L-DOPA, alpha-methyltyrosine, alpha-methyldopa, and phenylalanine nitrogen mustard (melphalan)) are transported across the blood-brain barrier by the neutral amino acid carrier (13, 14-16). In addition, recent <u>in vivo</u> studies demonstrate that perhaps because of the sensitivity of neutral amino acid carrier to competition among amino acids for uptake into the brain, the pharmacological action of certain drugs may be altered. For example, the therapeutic effects of both L-DOPA and alpha-methyldopa are attenuated in the presence of postprandial hyperaminoacidemia (17,18). Moreover, the "on-off" phenomenon in L-DOPA treatment of Parkinson's disease may be related to fluctuating plasma amino acid levels resulting from the chronological distribution of daily protein intake (18). While elevated plasma amino acids may reduce the effectiveness of certain centrally-acting neutral amino acid drugs, the depletion of plasma amino acids might enhance central drug delivery. Pardridge (1985) has suggested that in the presence of insulin-induced hypoaminoacidemia, enhanced delivery of high concentration of melphalan might be accomplished (13). Though not conclusive, there is evidence to suggest that insulin slightly enhances neutral amino acid delivery to the brain (19,20).

It is unfortunate that at present, the precise mechanism by which neutral amino acids are transported across the blood-brain barrier is not understood. Neutral amino acid transport across endothelial cell membranes could involve the gamma-glutamyl cycle shown in Figure 2A. As proposed by Orlowski et al. (1974), either glutathione or gamma-glutamyl-glutamine may serve as glutamyl donors (21). Inhibitors of the gamma-glutamyl cycle have been shown to decrease the transport of neutral amino acids from the blood to the brain (22). Alternatively, a simple protein mediated exchange system, shown in Figure 2B, might exist where one amino acid from the blood is exchanged for an amino acid in the brain extracellular fluid. Glutamine has been proposed as an amino acid in the brain extracellular fluid that may be exchanged for plasma amino acids (23). Despite the association of glutamine with both proposed carrier mechanisms, recent findings leave unresolved a definitive role for glutamine in neutral amino acid transport at the blood-brain barrier (24). Further study of the neutral amino acid carrier and the processes involved in regulating the carrier is required before the potential of selective delivery of drugs by this pathway might be realized.

Receptor Mediated Transendothelial Transport

The presence of few pinocytotic vesicles in brain endothelium under normal conditions (4) suggests that transendothelial vesicular transport is not a major blood-brain barrier transport system. However, Pardridge et al. (1985) have recently demonstrated receptor-mediated endo- and exo-cytosis, and therefore perhaps transcytosis, of insulin in isolated human cerebral microvessels (25). In

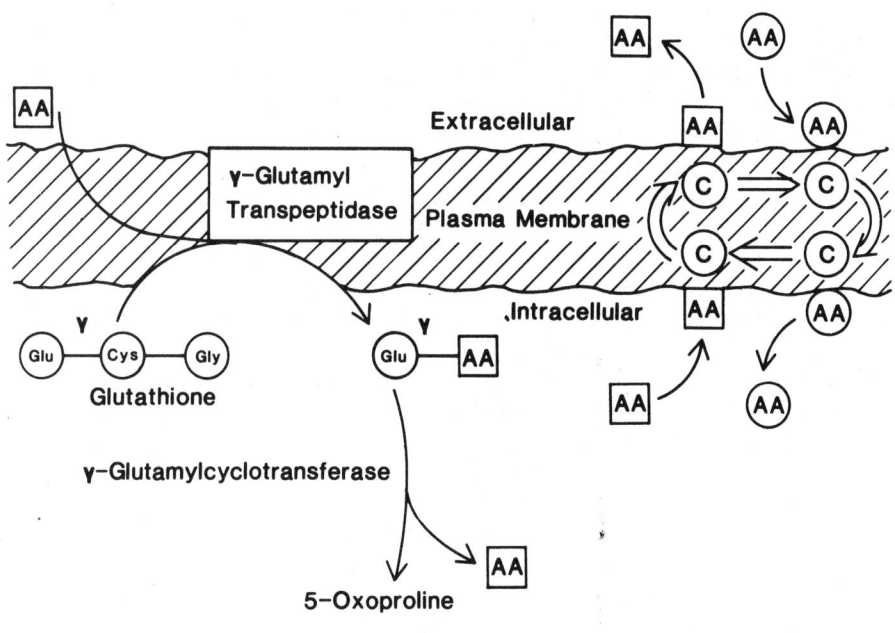

A   **B**

Figure 2. Examples of Mechanisms for Amino Acid Transport Across Endothelial Cell Membranes. A) Illustration of the role of the Gamma-Glutamyl cycle involvement in transport of amino acid [AA] across cell membranes. Cell membrane-bound gamma-glutamyl transpeptidase mediates the transfer of the gamma-glutamyl moiety from glutathione to an amino acid. The gamma-glutamyl residue acts as a carrier to facilitate the transcellular passage of the amino acid. The amino acid is released from the gamma-glutamyl-amino acid carrier intracellularly in a reaction mediated by gamma-glutamyl transcyclotransferase. 5-Oxoproline is used in a series of synthetic reactions to regenerate glutathione and continue the cycle. B) Illustration of a simple exchange of an extracellular amino acid (AA) with an intracellular amino acid [AA] by a transmembrane carrier protein (C).

addition, receptors for transferrin, a macromolecule known to be endocytosed by many cell types via a receptor-mediated mechanism (26), have also been identified on brain endothelium (27). The role of these macromolecules with respect to brain function, is for the most part, unclear. Thus, the physiological role of these transport systems that would offer additional evidence in support of their existence at the blood-brain barrie, is not known. It is known that insulin can alter appetite (28), and transferrin receptor distribution in the brain microvasculature has been correlated with the distribution of other neuromodulator receptors rather than with localization of iron in the brain (29). Transport of macromolecules by a receptor-mediated transcytosis process at the blood-brain barrier presents the possibility of using macromolecule-drug conjugates for drug delivery to the brain. Poznansky et al. (1984) have provided evidence that insulin-drug conjugates could become a practical drug delivery system (29).

Insulin and transferrin are among a number of proteins that when administered peripherally, may gain access to the brain environment and exert effects on the central nervous system. A drawback to their use as drug carriers to the brain is that they would also have interactions with peripheral receptors as well. An important aspect of drug delivery to the brain might involve selecting a peptide that has recognition sites or receptors confined to the brain microvasculature. Table II lists several peptides that are known to produce central nervous system effects after peripheral administration. It would be interesting to know which, if any, receptor populations for the individual peptides are confined to the brain microvasculature. If such a receptor population existed, selective delivery of drugs to the brain then might be possible with drug-macromolecule conjugates. Due to the lack of hard evidence for blood-brain barrier transcytosis, it has been suggested that the low blood-brain barrier extraction of some of these peptides is indicative of a reduced probability of actual trancytosis across the blood-brain barrier (31). This infers that the central effects of these peptides might be better explained by transendothelial signal transmission to the brain through other mechanisms (i.e. a second-messenger) without traversing the brain endothelium. Obviously, firm establishment of transendothelial vesicular transport of macromolecules as a recognized transport process at the blood-brain barrier must precede development of schemes for potential drug-macromolecule conjugate delivery to the brain.

The work of Simionescu et al. (1975), Palade et al. (1979), and Williams (1983) supports the hypothesis that a significant amount of macromolecule transport could be due to the formation of vesicles that shuttle bidirectionally between luminal and extravascular tissue sides of the endothelium (32-34). Figure 3 illustrates this process. According to this hypothesis, the initial process of endocytosis is a highly selective event involving interaction of the macromolecule with a recognition site on the surface of the endothelial cell. Subsequent

Table II. Peptides with Central Nervous System Effects after Peripheral Administration (30).
```
---------------------------------------------------------------
```
    Enkephalins
    Endorphins
    Melanocyte-Stimulating Hormone (MSH)
    MSH-Release Inhibiting Factor Number 1 (MIF-1)
    Thyrotropin Releasing Hormone (TRH)
    Luteinizing Hormone-Releasing Hormone (LHRH)
    Somatostatin
    Substance P
    Vasopressin
    Delta Sleep Inducing Peptide (DSIP)
```
---------------------------------------------------------------
```

sequestration and then transcytoplasmic vesicular transport of macromolecules is partially dependent upon the shape of the molecule, its charge, and the presence of carbohydrate moities (34-37). Since insulin endocytosis at the blood-brain barrier is receptor-mediated (25), this mechanism would appear relevant. There is, however, multiple mechanisms for macromolecules to traverse the endothelium. Possible mechanisms include, the formation of different sized multiple vesicles that link to form an effective transcellular pore, or the intercellular diffusion of macromolecules. Due to the lack of pinocytotic vesicles and the tight intercellular junctions in brain endothelium under normal conditions, the latter mechanisms would appear less important but can not be excluded as possiblities. A recent study by Solenski and Williams (1985) shows that insulin is specifically bound to capillary endothelium, sequestered in micropinocytotic vesicles, and internalized within free cytoplasmic vesicles (38). This evidence along with others (25, 39, 40) provides good evidence that receptor-mediated endocytotic mechanisms, for insulin at least, in peripheral endothelium as well as brain endothelium, do exist.

In Vitro Models

The study of carrier mediated and receptor mediated transendothelial transport as cellular events has been made feasible by recently developed <u>in vitro</u> model systems. The contribution of <u>in vitro</u> models as a complementary tool for studying blood-brain barrier functions (9) has been recently reviewed by Joo (1985). Here discussion will focus on the use of cultured endothelial cell monolayers as

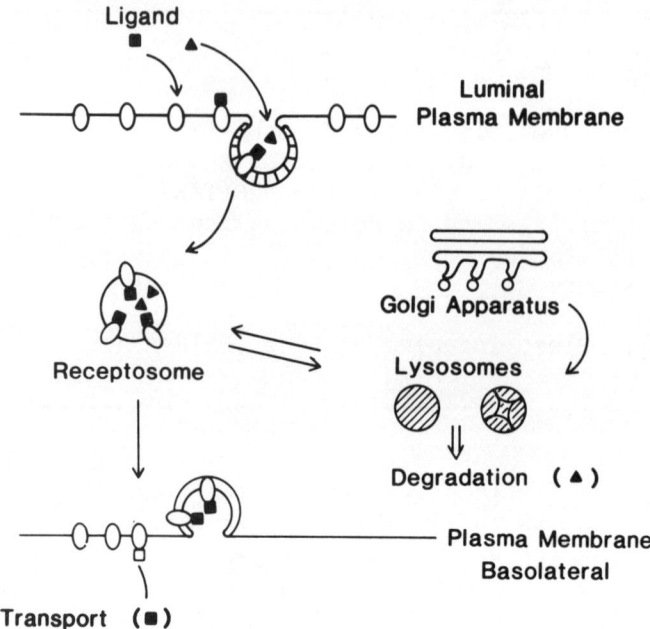

Figure 3. Receptor-Mediated Transcytosis. Macromolecules, or ligands, bind to a recognition site on the cell surface and are subsequently internalized. The internalized vesicle, receptosome, may be shuttled across the cytoplasm where interaction with lysosomes can occur. As a result of fusion with a lysosome, the contents of the receptosome can be processed by lysosomal enzymes. The receptosome, still bearing macromolecules, can then fuse with the plasma membrane on the opposite side of the cell where the contents are released.

in vitro model systems for characterization of transendothelial transport mechanisms.

In this laboratory, microvessel endothelial cells are isolated from the gray matter of bovine brains by enzymatic dispersion and centrifugation. Relatively large quantities of isolated brain microvessels are collected and then stored in DMSO and culture media at -70°C until needed. Thawed and seeded onto an appropriate growth surface consisting of fibronectin treated rat-tail collagen, the endothelial cells attach and grow to complete monolayers in approximately ten days (41). These monolayers have been characterized morphologically by electron microscopy. Similar to brain endothelium in vivo, isolated brain microvessel endothelial cells attach and grow on to form a single thin layer of closely apposed, overlapping cells with few pinocytotic vesicles (41). Alkaline phosphatase and gamma-glutamyl transpeptidase, specific markers for brain endothelium have been demonstrated in these monolayers both histochemically and biochemically (41,42). Compared to homogenates of gray matter, the cells of these monolayers are enriched in both marker enzymes. The catecholamine metabolizing enzymes (monoamine oxidase, catechol-O methyltransferase, and phenol sulfotransferase) associated with the blood-brain barrier in vivo and in vitro have also been demonstrated biochemically in these monolayers (42). Additionally, the endothelial origin of the cells in these monolayers has been further confirmed by the demonstration of specific markers of endothelium, Factor VIII antigen and angiotensin converting enzyme (41,42).

For transendothelial transport studies, complete monolayers grown on regenerated cellulose discs (approximate molecular weight cutoff of 160,000 Daltons) are placed between the chambers of a side-bi-side diffusion cell. The diffusion cells are so constructed as to provide for equal volumes in each of the sample chambers. A thermal jacket surrounds both sample chambers and can be thermostated by an external circulating water bath. Both chambers are also stirred with teflon stirring bars driven at a constant speed by an external drive console. One sample chamber of the diffusion cell is designated as the donor chamber and is pulsed with selected radiolabeled compounds. Subsequently, at various times, aliquots are removed from the other chamber, the receptor chamber, and analyzed by liquid scintillation spectrometry (43).

The neutral amino acid carrier of the blood-brain barrier, as indicated above, is of particular interest as a potential mechanism for selectively delivering neutral amino acid drugs to the brain. Primary (41-43) and serial (44-47) cultures of brain endothelium have been shown to possess a neutral amino acid carrier with characteristics similar to those of the in vivo blood-brain barrier transport system. The neutral amino acid carrier of primary cultures is bidirectional, concentration-dependent, and saturable. The apparent K_m for the carrier is 0.18 mM (43) which is in good agreement with the K_m (0.15 mM) for the amino acid carrier in vivo (15). Similarly, the amino acid carrier of these monolayers is not sensitive to inhibitors of active transport such as ouabain or sodium azide (43).

The transport of leucine, a marker for the neutral amino acid transport in primary cultures of brain endothelium, is inhibited by other amino acids as shown in Table III. The carrier is also stereospecific, and tends to be specific for large neutral amino acids as also shown in Table III. Methylation of aromatic amino acids in the alpha position is known to decrease the affinity of the amino acid for the carrier (48). Results summarized in Table III show that alpha-methylation of L-DOPA and tyrosine significantly reduces the ability of the respective compounds to inhibit leucine transport. It should be noted that selected amino acid drugs, L-DOPA, alpha-methyldopa, alpha-methyltyrosine, and baclofen, inhibit to some degree, leucine transport in this model system. The characteristics of alpha-methyldopa and baclofen transport across the monolayers of the in vitro system is the subject of future research in this laboratory.

Table III. Inhibition of ^{3}H-leucine (0.11 mM) transport across bovine brain microvessel endothelial cell monolayers. Monolayers grown on regenerated cellulose membranes were placed in a side-bi-side diffusion cell and the donor chamber of the diffusion cell pulsed with a mixture labeled leucine with or without the indicated unlabled amino acid. Experiments were carried out at 37°C with an incubation time of 2 minutes (43).

Amino acid	% Inhibition *
Large Neutral Amino Acids	
L-leucine	56
D-leucine	52
L-phenylalanine	64
D-phenylalanine	4
L-dihydroxy phenylalanine	66
D-dihydroxy phenylalanine	4
L-tyrosine	25
alpha-methyldopa	15
alpha-methyltyrosine	14
baclofen	23
Small Neutral Amino Acids	
L-alanine	10
glycine	0
methylamino isobutyric acid	1

* The concentration of indicated amino acids was 2.75 mM.

In a related project in this laboratory, preliminary results support the existence of a choline carrier in the monolayers of this model system. The transport properties of the in vitro choline carrier compare favorably with the in vivo blood-brain barrier choline carrier (49). Results from other experiments demonstrate a correlation between partition coefficient of several different molecules and flux of the molecules across the monolayer. These results also compare very well with related in vivo studies (50). The final results of current research projects will be the subject of future publications.

The transport macromolecules has not been studied in cultured brain endothelium. However, in vitro models of peripheral endothelium have been developed for study of macromolecule transport. Peripheral endothelial cell monolayers grown on human amnion (51) is restrictive to the passive transendothelial movemement of macromolecules and electric current. Relatively tight monolayers have also been grown up on semipermeable regenerated cellulose membranes (52). With the latter system model system, King and Johnson (1985) have shown that insulin undergoes transcellular transport by a receptor-mediated process (52). Application of brain endothelial cell monolayers for defining properties of receptor-mediated transport of insulin and other peptides is currently being investigated in this laboratory.

Conclusions

In this discussion we have briefly reviewed specific examples of carrier mediated and receptor-mediated processes that might be exploited in drug delivery schemes, and the potentially important in vitro model systems for characterizing these cellular events. The recent development of simple and relevant in vitro models of the microvascular endothelium represents a potentially useful tool for studying the cellular events related to transport. By studying the basic molecular interactions occuring during endothelial carrier mediated and receptor-mediated processes, novel mechanisms for physiologically selective delivery of drugs may evolve.

Acknowledgements

The authors gratefully acknowledge the support of INTERx, a subsidiary of Merck & Co., Lawrence, Kansas, The UpJohn Co., Kalamazoo, Michigan, and a Postdoctoral Fellowship (K.L.A.) from the American Heart Association, Kansas Affiliate, Inc., Topeka, Kansas.

References

1. Simionescu, N. and Simionescu, M., The cardiovascular system. In: "Histology" (Weiss, L. and Greep, R.O., eds.), McGraw-Hill Book Co., New York, 1977, pp. 373-431.

2. Smith, J.J. and Kampine, The microcirculation and the lymphatic system. In: "Circulatory Physiology," Williams and Wilkins, Baltimore, 1984, pp. 127-137.

3. Palade, G.E., Simionescu, M., and Simionescu, N., Structural aspects of the permeability of the microvascular endothelium, Acta Physiol. Scand., Suppl. 463, 11, 1979.

4. Reese, T.S. and Karnovsky, M.J., The structural localization of a blood-brain barrier to exogenous peroxidase, J. Cell Biol. 34, 207, 1967.

5. Brightman, M.W., Reese, T.S., Junctions between intimately apposed cell membranes in the vertebrate brain, J. Cell Biol. 40, 648, 1969.

6. Brightman, M.W., Morphology of blood-brain surfaces, Exp. Eye Res. 25, 1, 1977.

7. Bradbury, M.W.B., The blood-brain barrier, Circ. Res. 57, 213, 1985.

8. Meister, A., On the enzymology of amino acid transport, Science 180, 33, 1973.

9. Joo, F., The blood-brain barrier In Vitro: Ten years of research on microvessels isolated from the brain, Neurochem. Int. 7, 1, 1985.

10. Lai, F.M., Udenfriend, S., Spector, S., Presence of norepinephrine and related enzymes in isolated brain microvessels, Proc. Natl. Acad. Sci. USA 72, 4622, 1975.

11. Oldendorf, W.H. and Brown, W.J., Greater number of capillary endothelial mitochondria in brain than in muscle, Proc. Soc. Exp. Biol. Med. 149, 736, 1975.

12. Pardridge, W.M. and Oldendorf, W.H., Transport of metabolic substrates through the blood-brain barrier, J. Neurochem. 28, 5, 1977.

13. Pardridge, W.M., Strategies for drug delivery through the blood-brain barrier. In: "Directed Drug Delivery" (Borchardt, R.T., Repta, A.J., and Stella, V.J., eds.), Humana Press, Clifton, N.J., 1985, pp. 83-96.

14. Wade, L.A. and Katzman, R., Synthetic amino acids and the nature of L-DOPA transport at the blood-brain barrier, J. Neurochem. 25, 837, 1975.

15. Pardridge, W.M., Kinetics of competitive inhibition of neutral amino acid transport across the blood-brain barrier, J. Neurochem. 28, 103, 1977.

16. Markovitz, D.C. and Fernstrom, J.D., Diet and uptake of Aldomet by the brain: Competition with natural large neutral amino acids, Science 197, 1014, 1977.

17. Sved, A.F., Goldberg, I.M., and Fernstrom, J.D., Dietary protein intake influences the antihypertensive potency of methyldopa in spontaneously hypertensive rats, J. Pharmacol. Exp. Ther. 214, 147, 1980.

18. Nutt, J.G., Woodward, W.R., Hammerstad, J.P., Carter, J.H., and Anderson, The "on-off" phenomenon in Parkinson's disease, J. New Engl. J. Med. 310, 483, 1984.

19. De Montis, M.G., Olianas, M.C., Haber, B., and Tagliamonte, A., Increase in large neutral amino acid transport into brain by insulin, J. Neurochem. 30, 121, 1978.

20. Daniel, P.M., Love, E.R., Moorhouse, S.R., and Pratt, O.E., The effect of insulin upon the influx of tryptophan into the brain of the rabbit, J. Physiol. 312, 551, 1981.

21. Orlowski, M., Sessa, G., and Green, J.P., Gamma-Glutamyl transpeptidase in brain capillaries: Possible site of a blood-brain barrier for amino acids, Science 184, 66, 1974.

22. Samuels, S., Fish, I., and Freedman, L.S., Effect of gamma-glutamyl cycle inhibitors on brain amino acid transport and utilization, Neurochem. Res. 3, 619, 1978.

23. Cangiano, C., Cardelli-Cangiano, P., James, J.H., Rossi-Fanelli, F., Patrizi, M.A., Brackett, K.A., Strom, R., and Fischer, J.E., Brain microvessels take up large neutral amino acids in exchange for glutamine, J. Biol. Chem. 258, 8949, 1983.

24. Jonung, T., Rigotti, P., James, J.H., Brackett, K., Fischer, J.E., Effect of hyperammonemia and methionine sulfoximine on the kinetic parameters of blood-brain transport of leucine and phenylalanine, J. Neurochem. 45, 308, 1985.

25. Pardridge, W.M., Eisenberg, J., Yang, J., Human blood-brain barrier insulin receptor, J. Neurochem. 44, 1771, 1985.

26. Steinman, R.M., Mellman, I.S., Muller, W.A., and Cohn, Z.A., Endocytosis and the recycling of plasma membrane, J. Cell Biol. 96, 1, 1983.

27. Jefferies, W.A., Brandon, M.R., Hunt, S.V., Williams, A.F., Gatter, K.C., and Mason, D.Y., Transferrin receptor on endothelium of brain capillaries, Nature 312, 1984.

28. Hill, J.M., Ruff, M.R., Weber, R.J., and Pert, C.B., Transferrin receptors in rat brain: Neuropeptide-like pattern and relationship to iron distribution, Proc. Natl. Acad. Sci. USA 82, 4553, 1985.

29. Poznansky, M.J., Singh, R., Singh, B., and Fantus, G., Insulin: Carrier potential for enzyme and drug therapy, Science 223, 1304, 1984.

30. Kastin, A.J., Olson, R.D., Schally, A.V., and Coy, D.H., CNS effects of peripherally administered brain peptides, Life Sci. 25, 401, 1979.

31. Ermisch, A., Ruhle, H.-J., Landgraf, R., and Hess, J., Blood-brain barrier and peptides, J. Cerebr. Blood Flow Metab. 5, 350-357, 1985.

32. Simionescu, N., Simionescu, M., and Palade, G.E., Permeability of muscle capillaries to small heme-peptides, J. Cell Biol. 64, 586, 1975.

33. Palade, G.E., Simionescu, M., and Simionescu, N., Structural aspects of the permeability of the microvascular endothelium, Acta Physiol. Scand. Suppl. 463, 11, 1979.

34. Williams, S.K., Vesicular transport of proteins by capillary endothelium, N.Y. Acad. Sci. 416, 457, 1983.

35. Bower, D.B. and Williams, S.K., Exclusion of fibrinogen by capillary endothelium, Fed. Proc. 42, 580, 1983.

36. Simionescu, N., Simionescu, M., and Palade, G.E., Differentiated microdomains on the luminal surface of the capillary endothelium I. Preferential distribution of anionic sites, J. Cell Biol. 90, 605, 1981.

37. Simionescu, N., Simionescu, M., Silbert, J.E., and Palade, G.E., Differentiated microdomains on the luminal surface of the capillary endothelium II. Partial characterization of their anionic sites, J. Cell Biol. 90, 614, 1981.

38. Solenski, N.J. and Williams, S.K., Insulin binding and vesicular ingestion in capillary endothelium, J. Cell. Physiol. 124, 87, 1985.

39. Dernovsek, K.D., Bar, R.S., Ginsberg, B.H., and Lioubin, M.N., Rapid transport of biologically intact insulin through cultured endothelial cells, J. Clin. Endocrinol. Metab. 58, 761, 1984.

40. Jialal, I., King, G.L., Buchwald, S., Kahn, C.R., and Crettaz, M., Processing of insulin by bovine endothelial cells in culture, Diabetes 33, 794, 1984.

41. Audus, K.L. and Borchardt, R.T., Characterization of an in vitro blood-brain barrier model system for studying drug transport and metabolism, Pharm. Res., in press, 1986.

42. Baranczyk-Kuzma, A., Audus, K.L., and Borchardt, R.T., catecholamine-metabolizing enzymes of bovine brain microvessel endothelial cell monolayers, J. Neurochem., submitted.

43. Audus, K.L. and Borchardt, R.T., Characteristics of the large neutral amino acid transport system of bovine brain microvessel endothelial cell monolayers, J. Neurochem., submitted.

44. DeBault, L.E., Kahn, L.E., Frommes, S.P., Cancilla, P.A., Cerebral microvessels and derived cells in tissue culture: Isolation and preliminary characterization. In Vitro 15, 473, 1979.

45. DeBault, L.E., Henriquez, E., Hart, M.N., and Cancilla, P.A., Cerebral microvessels and derived cells in tissue culture. II. Establishment, identification, and preliminary characterization of an endothelial cell line, In Vitro 17, 480, 1981.

46. Cancilla, P.A. and DeBault, L.E., Neutral amino acid transport properties of cerebral endothelial cells in vitro, J. Neuropathol. Exp. Neurol. 42, 191, 1983.

47. Beck, D.W., Vinters, H.V., Hart, M.N., and Cancilla, P.A., J. Neuropathol. Exp. Neurol. 43, 219, 1984.

48. Pardridge, W.M. and Oldendorf, W.H., Kinetic analysis of blood-brain barrier transport of amino acids, Biochim. Biophys. Acta 401, 128, 1975.

49. Cornford, E.M., Braun, L.D., and Oldendorf, W.H., Carrier mediated blood-brain barrier transport of choline and certain choline analogs, J. Neurochem. 30, 299, 1978.

50. Oldendorf, W.H., Lipid solubility and drug penetration of the blood-brain barrier, Proc. Soc. Exp. Biol. Med. 147, 813, 1974.

51. Furie, M.B., Cramer, E.B., Naprstek, B.L., and Silverstein, S.C., Cultured endothelial cell monolayers that restrict the transendothelial passage of macromolecules and electrical current, J. Cell Biol. 98, 1033, 1984.

52. King, G.L. and Johnson, S.M., Receptor-mediated transport of insulin across endothelial cells, Science 227, 1583, 1985.

Chapter 9
Intestinal Aminopeptidase Distribution and Specificity: Bases for a Prodrug Strategy

Gordon L. Amidon and Kevin C. Johnson

College of Pharmacy
The Universty of Michigan
Ann Arbor, MI 48109-1065

Several aminopeptidases exist in the brush border region of the small intestine that assist in the terminal digestion of oligopeptides which arise from the partial digestion of protein by the action of pancreatic enzymes. Knowledge of these brush border enzymes could lead to novel ways to improve drug delivery through the use of amino acid prodrugs. Design and structural requirements of these prodrugs have already been discussed (1). The focus of the present review will be to give a general summary of the present knowledge of brush border aminopeptidases and some prodrug considerations.

Brush Border Enzymes and Their Specificities

An oligoaminopeptidase (EC 3.4.11.2) referred to as microvillus aminopeptidase, neutral aminopeptidase, aminopeptidase M and aminopeptidase N has been found in the brush border of the rabbit (2-3), rat (3-4) and man (3-10). This aminopeptidase is able to hydrolyze neutral N-terminal amino acids from peptides as well as synthetic derivatives of ß-naphthylamines and p-nitro-anilines such as L-leucyl-ß-naphthylamide and L-alanine-p-nitroanilide.

Aminopeptidase A (EC 3.4.11.7) or aspartate aminopeptidase (2-4,6-10) is able to hydrolyze acidic N-terminal amino acids (aspartic acid, glutamic acid) from peptides. A suitable substrate for this enzyme would be α-L-glutamyl-ß-naphthylamide or α-L-glutamyl-p-nitroanilide. This enzyme offers greater specificity due to the fact that pancreatic peptidases are usually not able to cleave peptide bonds formed by glutamic and aspartic acid (2).

Carboxypeptidase (EC 3.4.12.-) (2-4,6,8) is able to cleave C-terminal residues from peptides usually having a penultimate proline. N-CBZ-L-prolyl-L-alanine and Z-L-prolyl-L-leucine have been used as substrates.

Dipeptidyl-peptidase IV (EC 3.4.14.X) (2-9) is able to hydrolyze N-terminal dipeptides from peptides having penultimate proline, alanine or leucine residues. Substrates used to measure its activity include glycyl-L-prolyl-ß-naphthylamide and glycyl-L-proline-p-nitroanilide.

γ-glutamyltranspeptidase (EC 2.3.2.2) (3-5,7,9) is believed to play a role in the transport of amino acids and dipeptides across the brush border (3). L-γ-glutamic acid p-nitroanilide has been used as a substrate.

Two brush border peptidases, membrane Gly-Leu peptidase and zinc stable Asp-Lys peptidase, which have not been previously identified, hydrolyze glycylleucine and aspartyl-lysine in 5 mM Zn^{2+}, respectively (10).

Cytosol peptidases will not be discussed other than to say that they are more specific for the digestion of di- and tri-peptides. A more detailed review is available (3).

Structure and Biosynthesis

Brush border aminopeptidases are an integral part of the lipid bilayer of the microvilli which constitute the apical membrane of the enterocyte. These aminopeptidases are glycoproteins with the carbohydrate portion extending into the lumen to form the glycocalyx. The aminopeptidase can be liberated from the lipid bilayer with retained activity by either limited proteolysis with papain or extraction with a nonionic detergent such as triton X-100 (11,12) (Fig. 1). The corresponding proteinase and detergent molecular forms have hydrophilic and amphipathic characteristics, respectively. Limited proteolysis on the detergent form yields the proteinase form with the simultaneous release of a hydrophobic peptide. This hydrophobic peptide gives the detergent form its hydrophobic properties and is referred to as the anchor peptide (11).

A preparation of purified brush border can be obtained from homogenization of mucosal scrappings in the presence of EDTA (13,14). Under these conditions, the brush border spontaneously separates from the rest of the enterocyte. The resulting brush border fragments then form closed right side out vesicles. Negative staining gives a

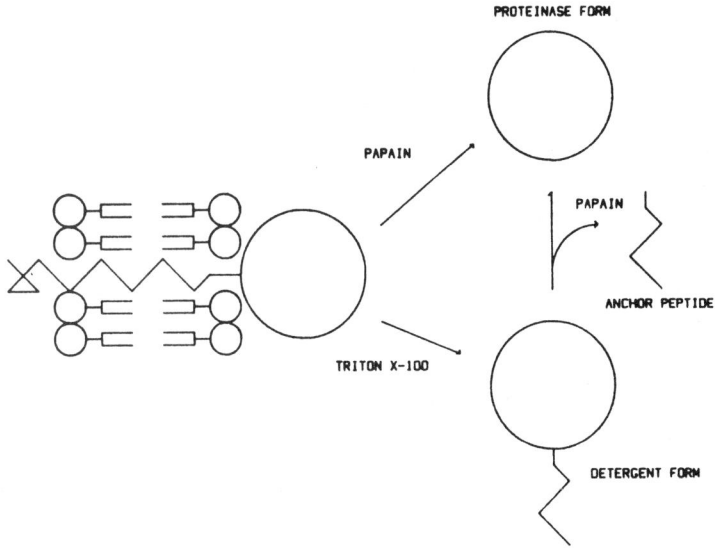

Fig 1 Scheme showing polar head (proteinase form), hydrophobic domain spanning the membrane (anchor peptide), and a cytoplasmic segment. Modified with permission from S. Maroux and D. Louvard, Gastroenterol. Clin. Biol., 1, 377 (1977).

granular appearance of the fuzzy coat or glycocalyx on the outer surface indicating that the vesicles are right side out (15). These vesicles provide an ideal preparation for the study of brush border aminopeptidases. With more vigorous homogenization, the microvilli can be sheared off from the apical membrane (13). The hydrophilic portion of the aminopeptidase can be released from the closed vesicle without affecting the lipid bilayer. At the same time, several enzymatic activities appear in solution. This provides evidence for the location of the active portion of the enzyme on the external face of the membrane (11,15).

Louvard et al. (16) have demonstrated that amino-peptidase is a transmembrane protein by taking advantage of the brush border membrane's ability to form closed vesicles. The experiment used the labeling reagent

4-fluoro-3-nitrophenyl azide to which was attached the macromolecule human Fab to prevent the label from diffusing into the membrane. This covalently coupled labeling reagent was trapped inside the closed vesicles as they formed. The reagent was then photolyzed <u>in situ</u> to generate a nitrene capable of reacting with any accessible group on the inner surface of the membrane (Fig. 2). The detergent form of the aminopeptidase was found to be significantly more labeled than the papain form, demonstrating that the enzyme spans the membrane and is exposed at the inner face of the vesicles.

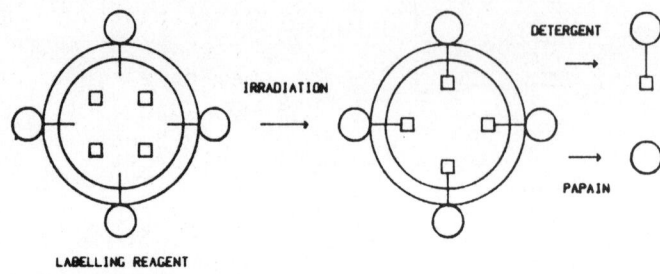

Fig 2 Scheme showing experimental design used to demonstrate that enzyme spans the membrane. Modified with permission from Louvard, Semeriva and Maroux (16).

Determinations of the N-terminal residues of aminopeptidases have shown the detergent and hydrophobic forms to be the same but different from the proteinase form (11). This suggests that the enzyme is anchored to the membrane by the N-terminus. The N-terminal sequence of the detergent form of rabbit aminopeptidase has been determined and shown to contain mostly hydrophobic amino acids (17). It was also shown to be different from the protease form which was rich in hydrophilic residues. There were many nonidentifiable residues, probably due to attached glycan chains which are abundant in the whole enzyme.

The N-terminal sequence of the detergent form is composed of two distinct parts. The first part contains two positive charges, one by the N-terminal tyrosine and one by lysine in position 4, and an uncharged hydrophilic serine in position 3. The other part starting after lysine is entirely hydrophobic up until the last identifiable residue glycine in position 14. The evidence for aminopeptidase N suggests that its structure is composed of approximately 20 hydrophobic residues spanning the membrane and sandwiched in between a positively charged N-terminal segment and a C-terminal hydrophilic segment (17).

The biosynthesis of aminopeptidases is carried out by polyribosomes attached to the endoplasmic reticulum (11). Several models have been proposed for the asymetric insertion of the enzyme into the membrane of the endoplasmic reticulum. A hypothesis that aminopeptidases may be processed similarly to secretory proteins arose from the discovery that a transmembrane glycoprotein of stomatitis virus also contained a hydrophobic N-terminal extension. In this case, a signal sequence initiates ribosome attachment, tunnel formation and the extrusion of the growing peptide chain into the cisternal space across the membrane. In the case of a bound aminopeptidase, the passage must be stopped before the protein is completely discharged into the cisternae (12).

A plausible model for the insertion of brush border aminopeptidase involves the recognition of the positive charge of the nascent protein chain by the negatively charged phospholipid polar heads of the endoplasmic reticulum membrane. The N-terminus charge may act as an electrostatic bolt which holds the initial residues of the growing chain on the cytoplasmic face of the membrane. The hydrophobic segment may then penetrate the membrane with the rest of the chain growing according to the "hair pin loop mechanism" (17) (Fig. 3). The synthesis is terminated with the bulk of the molecule on the extracytoplasmic face which will eventually become the external side of the brush border. The first steps of glycosylation occur to trap the molecule in the extracytoplasmic space. Glycosylation is completed in the Golgi apparatus before the final transfer to the plasma membrane (11).

Pulse-chase labeling studies on the biosynthesis of intestinal microvillar proteins maltase-glucoamylase, aminopeptidase A and dipeptidyl peptidase IV in pig have shown that intracellular transport proceeds in a membrane-bound state (18). Small intestinal explants were pulse-labeled for 10 min with [^{35}S] methionine and chased with nonradioactive medium. Initially, lower molecular weight

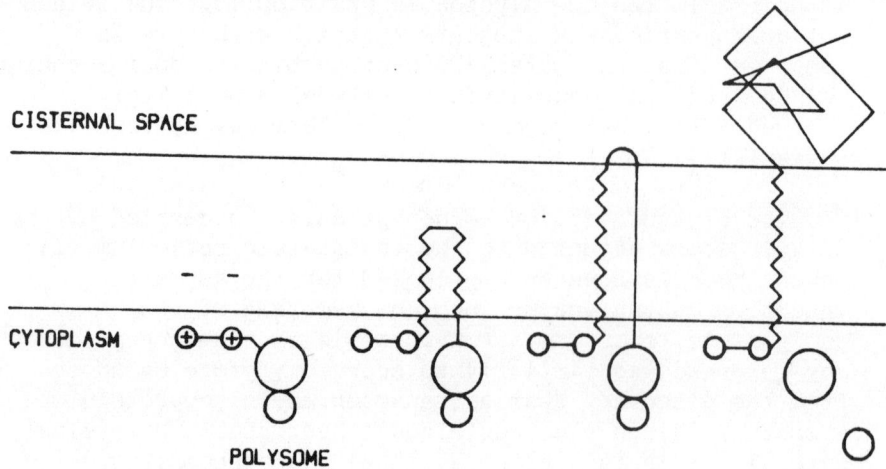

Fig. 3 Scheme for insertion of brush border aminopeptidase in membrane. Modified with permission from Feracci, Maroux, Bonicel and Desnuelle (17).

peptides were observed followed by higher molecular weight peptides. Only the higher molecular weight peptides persisted after 90-120 min of chase. These observations were made in Ca^{2+} precipitated membrane fractions representing intracellular and basolateral membranes. Only the higher molecular weight peptides were observed in the microvillar membrane, suggesting that the lower molecular weight peptides are transient precursor forms of the final enzymes. These lower weight forms were susceptible to endo-ß-N-acetyl-glycosaminidase H which is characteristic of intermediate glycosylation for proteins destined for cellular externalization. This evidence indicates the site of synthesis to be the rough endoplasmic reticulum with reglycosylation taking place in the Golgi complex to yield the mature enzyme. These observations are consistent with the "membrane flow" hypothesis (19).

There is general agreement that brush border aminopeptidases are synthesized in the rough endoplasmic reticulum and pass through the Golgi apparatus before being inserted into the plasma membrane. However, there are conflicting results as to whether they are transferred directly to the apical brush border membrane or arrive first in the lateral membrane before being rearranged to the brush border (11).

After a short pulse with [^{3}H] fucose, ultrastructural autoradiography showed vesicles labeled after the Golgi apparatus and before the plasma membrane. These vesicles have sometimes been observed to fuse with the brush border membrane. Using immunofluorescence, aminopeptidase N has been observed only in the brush border membrane and the Golgi apparatus. Histochemistry on the same sample showed active molecules in the brush border membrane, in the apical region of the lateral membrane and in a structure located under the terminal web (11).

Subcellular fractionation techniques can separate various membrane fractions by centrifugation through sucrose gradients. The membrane fractions are characterized by specific markers such as glycosyltransferases for the Golgi, Na+, K+ -ATPase for basolateral membrane and aminopeptidase for the brush border membrane. Aminopeptidase N of the rabbit enterocyte was found to be present in the basolateral membrane preparation in about 10% of the brush border amount. It cannot be ruled out that this amount came from the brush border by diffusion during cell homogenization. It has been shown that redistribution of brush border hydrolases over the entire cell surface occurs after disruption of the tight junctions. After intraperitoneal injection, [^{3}H] fucose labeling of glycoproteins demonstrated that at least 60% of the glycoproteins are incorporated first into the basolateral membrane fraction before reaching the brush border. Basolateral and brush border membranes prepared after injecting [^{35}S] methionine in a rabbit jejunum loop revealed that newly synthesized aminopeptidase N is first integrated in the basolateral membrane fraction, then migrates to the brush border membrane fraction. It has not, however, been definitely shown that the membrane containing the newly synthesized hydrolases is the lateral membrane. Microscopy and absence of different markers are low sensitivity criteria of purity, and do not rule out the presence of transporting vesicle contamination. The basolateral membrane needs to be more specifically purified to confirm the results (11).

Enzyme Distribution

The longitudinal distribution of aminopeptidases in the small intestine has been studied in man and rabbit.

Qualitatively, all studies are in good agreement. Skovbjerg (6) studied the distribution of carboxypeptidase (EC 3.4.12.X), microvillus aminopeptidase (EC 3.4.11.2), dipeptidyl peptidase IV (EC 3.4.14.X) and aspartate aminopeptidase (EC 3.4.11.7) in man. These enzymes were found to be present from the ligament of Treitz to the distal ileum. Microvillus aminopeptidase, dipeptidyl peptidase IV and aspartate aminopeptidase increased over the length studied, while carboxypeptidase showed no significant difference.

Triadou et al. (8) studied the distribution of neutral aminopeptidase (EC 3.4.11.2), acid aminopeptidase (EC 3.4.11.7) and dipeptidyl peptidase IV (EC 3.3.14.X) in man. Peptidase activity generally increased from the duodenum to the terminal ileum. The jejunal to ileal ratios for neutral aminopeptidase, acid aminopeptidase and dipeptidyl peptidase IV were 0.8, 0.4 and 0.5, respectively.

Sterchi et al. (9) studied the distribution of aminopeptidase M (EC 3.4.11.2), aminopeptidase A (EC 3.4.11.7) and dipeptidyl peptidase IV (EC 3.4.14.-) in man. Aminopeptidase A (Fig. 4a) and dipeptidyl peptidase IV (Fig. 4b) increase approximately 6- and 3-fold, respectively, from near the pylorus to the ileo-caecal junction, whereas aminopeptidase M (Fig. 4c) has no apparent increase in the distal gut.

Auricchio et al. (2) studied the distribution of oligoaminopeptidase, aminopeptidase A and carboxypeptidase in the rabbit small intestine. Oligoaminopeptidase, aminopeptidase A and carboxypeptidase increase approximately 6-, 7- and 3-fold, respectively, along the small intestine. The above studies indicate that the distal ileum plays an important role in the digestion of more complex substrates.

Auricchio et al. (4) studied the development of human and rat small intestinal brush border peptidases during fetal and neonatal life. Oligoaminopeptidase, aminopeptidase A, γ-glutamyltranspeptidase, dipeptidylaminopeptidase IV and carboxypeptidase were all found to be present in rat fetuses. The activities of human fetal intestinal peptidases were higher in the distal portion of the intestine than in the proximal portion although the differences were not statistically significant. With the exception of aminopeptidase A, peptidase activities were at or higher than adult activities. In a later study,

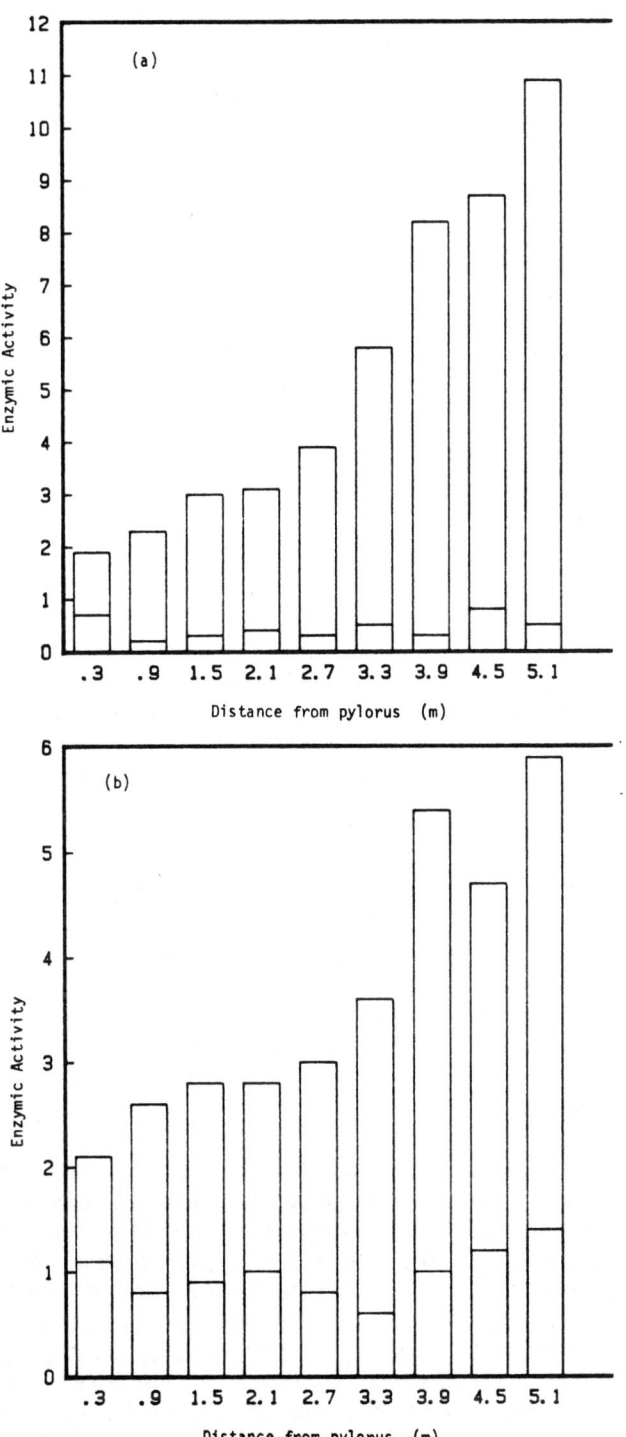

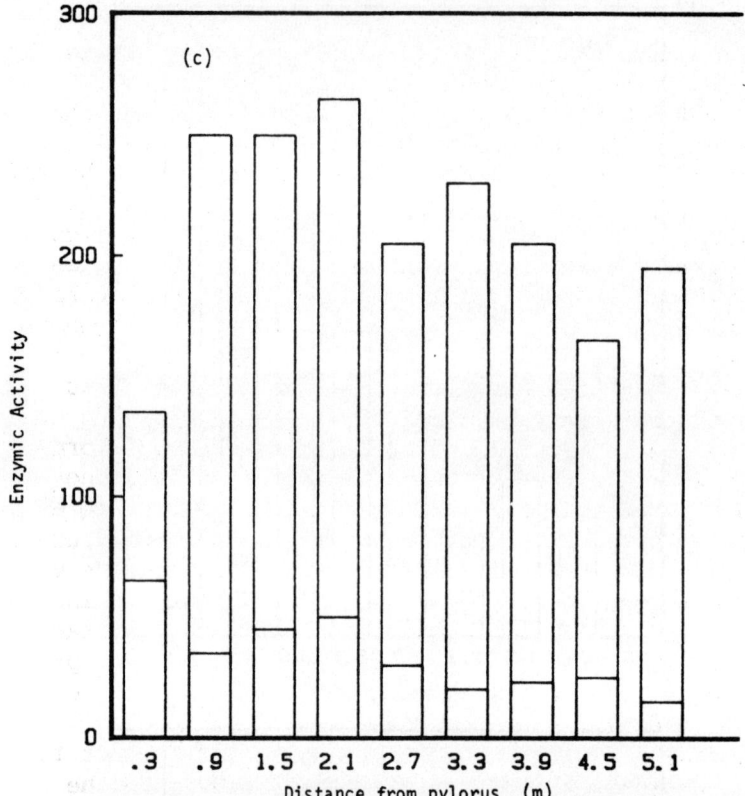

Fig. 4 Distribution of (a) aminopeptidase A, (b) dipeptidylpeptidase IV, and (c) aminopeptidase M along the human small intestine. Enzymic activity is expressed as μmol of substrate hydrolyzed/min per g of protein. Upper bar represents specific activity in particulate fraction; lower bar represents specific activity in soluble fraction. Reprinted by permission of Sterchi, Green and Lentze (9); and copyright (c) 19 The Biochemical Society, London.

oligoaminopeptidase and dipeptidylaminopeptidase solubilized by papain from 4th month human fetal brush borders had a faster anodal electrophoretic mobility in polyacrylamide and agar gel than adult peptidases. However, the specific activities were the same. The difference between adult and fetal forms of brush border peptidases could be due to differences in intracellular processsing of the carbohydrate moiety of these glycoproteins or post-translational modifications due to age-dependent variations of luminal agents that could modify the glycoproteins such as bacterial glycosidases or pancreatic enzymes.

Muira et al. (20) studied the distribution of aminopeptidase N and dipeptidyl aminopeptidase IV in the rat small intestine. Both enzymes are associated primarily with the brush border. Aminopeptidase N had a peak activity in the proximal to midregion whereas dipeptidyl aminopeptidase was more uniform with a broad peak of activity in the distal region. The distribution of aminopeptidase N was also studied along the villus-crypt cell axis and found to be highest in the villus. Mitotic figures are found in the crypts indicating rapid cell proliferation. The enterocytes have been shown to originate in the crypts and migrate up the villi to the tip where they are shed into the lumen (21). It has been suggested that the increased activity in the villus cells could be due to activation of inactive precursor forms synthesized in the crypt cells. However, with aminopeptidase N, a constant ratio of enzyme activity to enzyme protein measured by radioimmunoassay along the villus-crypt axis suggests that increased synthesis in the villus cells is responsible for the higher activity of aminopeptidase N. Skovbjerg (22) has also found a constant ratio of aminopeptidase activity to immunoreactive protein along the villus-crypt cell axis in human small intestine. Dipeptidyl aminopeptidase was found to have substantial activity in the crypt cells although it too had a constant ratio of activity to protein. In the distal regions of the intestine, there was an increase in the activity of cytoplasmic aminopeptidase N which was shown to be due to a distinct enzyme form. A soluble activity of dipeptidyl aminopeptidase IV was also observed but was shown to be immunologically identical with the same electrophoretic mobility of the brush border form.

The specific activity of both enzymes was different in isolated subcellular fractions. The value in the brush border was consistently 1.5 times higher than the total cell homogenates, the Golgi membrane activity was 75% of the homogenate, and there was a two-fold difference between the Golgi and brush border membrane activities. There may be inactive forms which are activated in the transfer from the Golgi to the microvillus membrane due to glycosylation. In summary, there was a constant ratio of enzyme activity to enzyme protein along the villus-crypt cell axis as well as the brush border membranes isolated from various regions of the intestine. However, there was also an apparent two-fold activation of enzymatic activity during the final transfer step from the Golgi to the brush border membrane (20).

Prodrug Strategy

The aminopeptidases provide a potential site for bioreconversion of amino acid prodrugs. The utilization of these enzymes was first proposed by Amidon et al. (23) in which an amino acid prodrug strategy was used to improve the absorption of poorly soluble compounds. By forming an amino acid prodrug, the solubility of an otherwise insoluble compound can be enhanced. At the same time, the membrane permeability is usually decreased as a result of introducing a charge into the molecule. This compromise can be overcome, however, if the prodrug is a substrate for a brush border aminopeptidase and is rapidly hydrolyzed near the brush border membrane to yield the highly permeable parent compound (Fig. 5). An added advantage of this approach is the formation of a nontoxic degradation product.

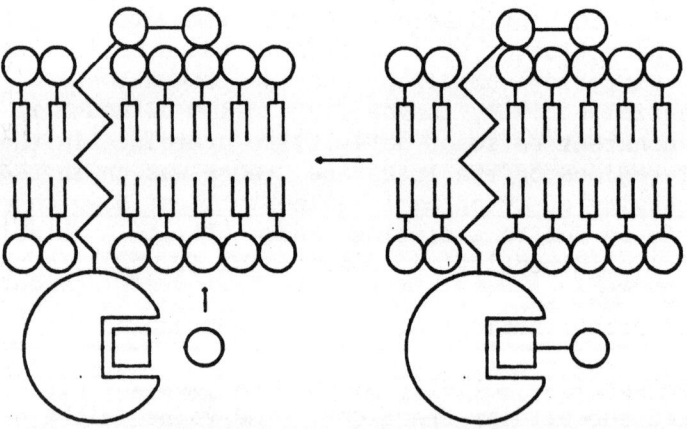

Fig. 5 Scheme demonstrating prodrug strategy. Circle-square combination represents amino acid prodrug, circle represents drug molecule, square represents amino acid.

Structural requirements of amino acid prodrugs have already been discussed in detail (1). In particular, drug molecules having free alcohol or amine functionalities to form esters and amides are potential candidates.

Competitive inhibitor studies have also demonstrated the importance of the free α-amino group and the L-configuration in the amino acid moiety as necessary substrate requirements for aminopeptidase activity. Amidon et al. (24-25) have studied the intestinal absorption of L-lysine-p-nitroanilide, L-alanine-p-nitroanilide and glycine-p-nitroanilide in the presence of competitive inhibitors in perfused rat intestine. L-lysine methyl ester, L-arginine-β-naphthylamide and L-arginine methyl ester decreased the permeability of L-lysine-p-nitroanilide, indicating that the hydrolysis site for lysine-p-nitroanilide prefers positively charged side chains. L-phenylalanine methyl ester, glycine methyl ester and L-alanine methyl ester containing nonpolar side chains did not inhibit the absorption of L-lysine-p-nitroanilide. When the free L-amino group was blocked in the case of N-acetyl-L-lysine methyl ester, inhibition was not observed as with L-lysine methyl ester. This demonstrates the requirement of a free L-amino group for inhibition. L-lysine itself does not show significant product inhibition at the concentrations employed, indicating that product inhibition is low (Fig. 6a).

Only L-alanine methyl ester was a good competitive inhibitor of L-alanine-p-nitroanilide. L-lysine methyl ester, L-phenylalanine methyl ester, L-arginine methyl ester and glycine methyl ester did not show significant inhibition, indicating that the hydrolysis site for L-alanine-p-nitroanilide is specific for small nonpolar amino acid side chains. β-alanine methyl ester and D-alanine methyl ester were not inhibitors demonstrating the requirement that the free amino group must be in the α-position and that proper sterochemistry is necessary. L-alanine amide and L-phenylalanine amide were not competitive inhibitors (Fig. 6b).

Glycine methyl ester was not an inhibitor of glycine-p-nitroanilide uptake suggesting a weak affinity of glycine for the hydrolysis site. L-lysine methyl ester was also not an inhibitor of glycine-p-nitroanilide (Fig. 6c).

The dipeptide L-prolylglycine inhibited the absorption of all three amino acid anilides whereas glycyl-L-proline did not (Fig. 6a,b,c). Glycyl-L-proline has been shown to have a high affinity for the intestinal peptide transport process and not to be a substrate or inhibitor of brush border aminopeptidase. The present results suggest that the amino acid anilides studied do not take part in direct uptake by the peptide transport process.

N-α-benzoyl-arginine-p-nitroanilide and N-α-succinyl-phenylalanine-p-nitroanilide were also shown to be poorly absorbed which is consistent with the brush border peptidase activity requirement of a free α-amino group (Fig. 6d).

The prodrug must also be sufficiently stable in solution to withstand the variations in pH in transversing the stomach to the site of reconversion in the small intestine. Hydrocortisone lysinate was synthesized as a potential amino acid prodrug of hydrocortisone (26). However, the pH rate profile indicates that the ester linkage is rapidly hydrolyzed at intestinal pH. Comparison of hydrocortisone free alcohol plasma levels in Beagle dogs from molar equivalent oral doses of hydrocortisone, hydrocortisone phosphate, hydrocortisone succinate and hydrocortisone lysinate were made (27). Hydrocortisone lysinate gave the most similar profile to hydrocortisone. This is probably due to rapid hydrolysis in the lumen to give free hydrocortisone or rapid bioconversion due to pancreatic and/or brush border enzymes. Hydrocortisone succinate shows lower levels which is consistent with its solution stability, its negative charge, and the lack of enzymatic activity specific for succinates necessary to reconvert the prodrug to the more membrane permeable parent compound. Hydrocortisone phosphate shows high initial blood levels which drop off quickly. This may be due to the predominantly upper small intestinal alkaline phosphatase distribution in dogs (27).

These results indicate that a successful amino acid prodrug must have adequate solution stability to avoid reconversion prior to proper orientation of the parent compound near the membrane, and substrate specificity for brush border aminopeptidases to insure that reconversion takes place. Knowledge of brush border aminopeptidases and their distribution is necessary for proper design of amino acid prodrugs as well as the species differences to draw correct inferences from animal experiments to human applications.

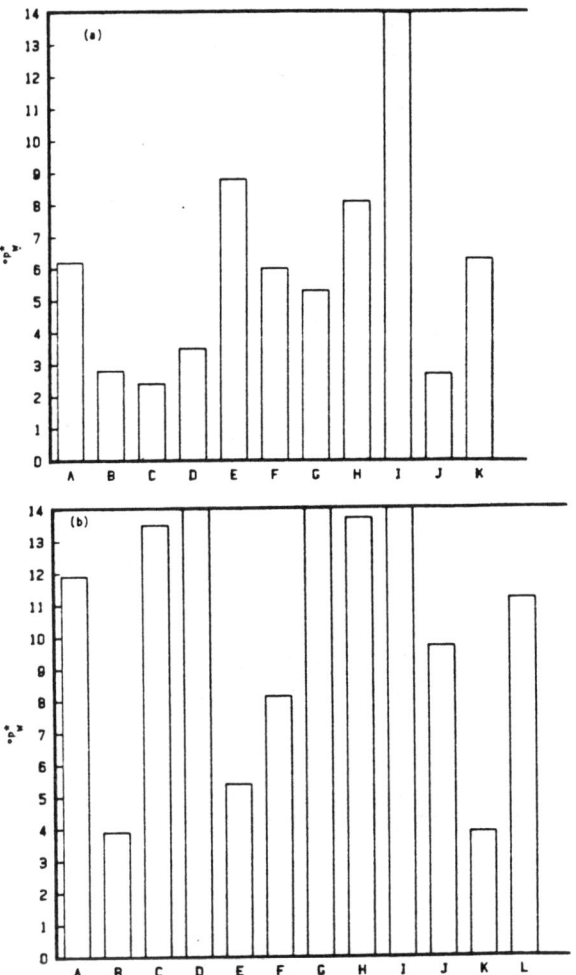

Fig 6 (a) Intestinal wall permeability ($°P_w^*$) of L-lysine-p-nitroanilide alone (A) and with L-lysine methyl ester (B), L-arginine-β-naphthylamide (C), L-arginine methyl ester (D), α-N-acetyl-L-lysine methyl ester (E), L-lysine (F), L-phenylalanine methyl ester (G), L-alanine methyl ester (H), glycine methyl ester (I), L-prolylglycine (J), or glycyl-L-proline (K). Reproduced with permission, copyright owner, the American Pharmaceutical Association (24).

(b) Intestinal wall permeability ($°P_w^*$) of L-alanine-p-nitroanilide alone (A) and with L-alanine methyl ester (B), β-alanine methyl ester (C), D-alanine methyl ester (D), L-lysine methyl ester (E), L-phenylalanine methyl ester (F), L-arginine methyl ester (G), glycine methyl ester (H), L-alanine amide (I), L-phenylalanine amide (J), L-propylglycine (K), or glycine-L-proline (L). Reproduced with permission, copyright owner, the American Pharmaceutical Association (25).

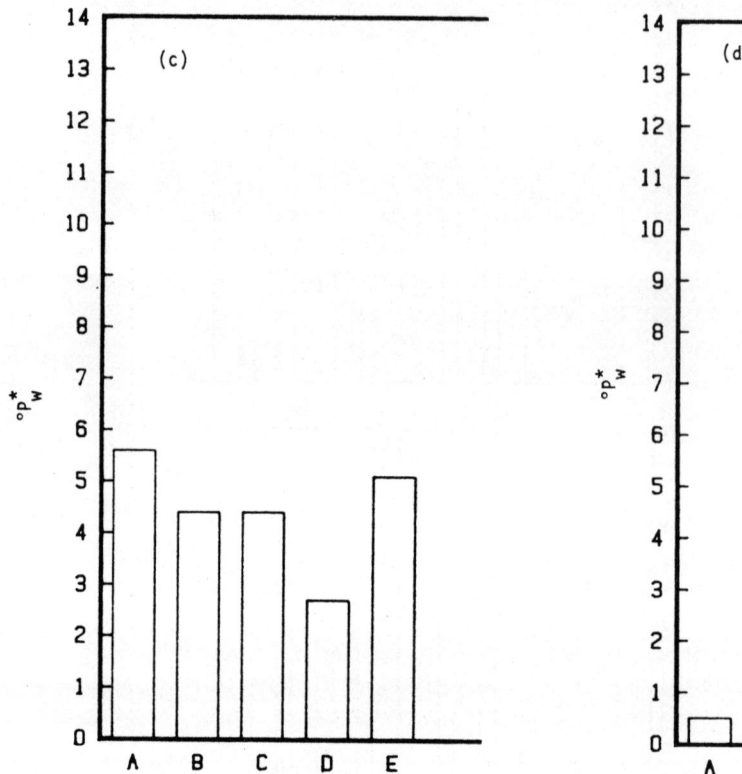

(c) Intestinal wall permeability ($°P_W^*$) of glycine-p-nitroanilide alone (A) and with glycine methyl ester (B), L-lysine methyl ester (C), L-propylglycine (D), or glycyl-L-proline (E). Reproduced with permission, copyright owner, the American Pharmaceutical Association (25).

(d) Intestinal wall permeability ($°P_W^*$) of N-α-benzoyl-arginine-p-nitroanilide (A) and N-α-succinyl-phenylalanine-p-nitroanilide (B). Reproduced with permission, copyright owner, the American Pharmaceutical Association (24).

References

1. G.L. Amidon, R.S. Pearlman and G.D. Leesman, Design of prodrugs through consideration of enzyme-substrate specificities. In: "Design of Biopharmaceutical Properties Through Prodrugs and Analogs," American Pharmaceutical Association, 1977, pp. 281-315.
2. S. Auricchio, L. Greco, B. De Vizia and V. Buonocore, Dipeptidylaminopeptidase and carboxypeptidase activities of the brush border of rabbit small intestine, Gastroenterology, 75, 1073 (1978).
3. S. Auricchio, "Developmental aspects of brush border hydrolysis and absorption of peptides. In: "Textbook of Gastroenterology and Nutrition in Infancy, Raven Press, New York, 1981, pp. 375-384.
4. S. Auricchio, A. Stellato and B. De Vizia, Development of brush border peptidases in human and rat small intestine during fetal and neonatal life, Pedatr. Res., 15, 991 (1981).
5. S. Auricchio, C. Caporale, F. Santamaria and H. Skovbjerg, Fetal forms of oligoaminopeptidase, dipeptidylaminopeptidase IV, and sucrase in human intestine and meconium, J. Pediatr. Gastroent. Nutr., 3, 28 (1984).
6. H. Skovbjerg, Immunoelectrophoretic studies on human small intestinal brush border proteins--the longitudinal distribution of peptidases and disaccharidases, Clin. Chim. Acta, 112, 205 (1981).
7. H. Skovbjerg, O. Noren and H. Sjostrom, Immunoelectrophoretic studies on human small intestinal brush border proteins, Scand. J. Clin. Lab. Invest., 38, 723 (1978).
8. N. Triadou, J. Bataille and J. Schmitz, Longitudinal study of the human intestinal brush border membrane proteins, Gastroenterology, 85, 1326 (1983).
9. E.E. Sterchi, J.R. Green and M.J. Lentze, The distribution of four peptide hydrolases along the small intestine of the adult human, Biochem. Soc. Trans., 9, 130 (1981).
10. N. Tobey, W. Heizer, R. Yeh, T. Huang and C. Hoffner, Human intestinal brush border peptidases, Gastroenterology, 88, 913 (1985).
11. S. Maroux and H. Feracci, Structure and biosynthesis of aminopeptidases, Methods Enzymol., 96, 406 (1983).
12. P. Desnuelle, Intestinal and renal aminopeptidase: a model of a transmembrane protein, Eur. J. Biochem., 101, 1 (1979).

13. A.J. Kenny and A.G. Booth, Microvilli: their ultrastructure, enzymology and molecular organization, Essays Biochem., 14, 1 (1978).
14. G.G. Forstner, S.M. Sabesin and K.J. Isselbacher, Rat intestinal microvillus membranes, Biochem. J., 106, 381 (1968).
15. D. Louvard, S. Maroux, Ch Vannier and P. Desnuelle, Topological studies on the hydrolases bound to the intestinal brush border membrane I. Solubilization by papain and Triton X-100, Biochim. Biophys. Acta, 375, 236 (1975).
16. D. Louvard, M. Semeriva and S. Maroux, The brush-border intestinal aminopeptidase, a transmembrane protein as probed by macromolecular photolabeling, J. Mol. Biol., 106, 1023 (1976).
17. H. Feracci, S. Maroux, J. Bonicel and P. Desnuelle, The amino acid sequence of the hydrophobic anchor of rabbit intestinal brush border aminopeptidase N, Biochim. Biophys. Acta, 684, 133 (1982).
18. E.M. Danielsen, H. Sjostrom and O. Noren, Biosynthesis of intestinal microvillar proteins--pulse-chase labeling studies on maltase-glucoamylase, aminopeptidase A and dipeptidyl peptidase IV, Biochem. J., 210, 389 (1983).
19. G. Palade, Intracellular aspects of the process of protein synthesis, Science, 189, 347 (1975).
20. S. Miura, I. Song, A. Morita, R.H. Erickson and Y.S. Kim, Distribution and biosynthesis of aminopeptidase N and dipeptidyl aminopeptidase IV in rat small intestine, Biochim. Biophys. Acta, 761, 66 (1983).
21. F. Moog, The lining of the small intestine, Sci. Am., 245, 154 (1981).
22. H. Skovbjerg, Immunoelectrophoretic studies on human small-intestinal brush-border proteins--relation between enzyme activity and immunoreactive enzyme along the villus-crypt axis, Biochem. J., 193, 887 (1981).
23. G.L. Amidon, G.D. Leesman and R.L. Elliott, Improving intestinal absorption of water-insoluble compounds: a membrane metabolism strategy, J. Pharm. Sci., 69, 1363 (1980).
24. G.L. Amidon, M. Chang, D. Fleisher and R. Allen, Intestinal absorption of amino acid derivatives: importance of the free α-amino group, J. Pharm. Sci., 71, 1138 (1982).
25. G.L. Amidon, M. Lee and H. Lee, Intestinal absorption of amino acid derivatives: structural requirements for membrane hydrolysis, J. Pharm. Sci., 72, 943 (1983).

26. K. Johnson, G.L. Amidon and S. Pogany, Solution kinetics of a water-soluble hydrocortisone prodrug: hydrocortisone-21-lysinate, J. Pharm. Sci., 74, 87 (1985).
27. D. Fleisher, B.H. Stewart and G.L. Amidon, Design of prodrugs for improved gastrointestinal absorption by intestinal enzyme targeting. In: Methods in Enzymology, Drug and Enzyme Targeting, Vol. 112, Academic Press, New York, 1985, pp. 360-381.

Chapter 10
Drug Delivery Systems Research from an Industrial Perspective

A. A. Sinkula

Pharmacy Research
The Upjohn Company
Kalamazoo, MI 49001

Introduction

Cost of R&D

The incentives to undertake pharmaceutical research and development continue to come under heavy pressure. Prominent among the "disincentives" are the ever increasing costs of health care, fewer research opportunities to generate new products, increased regulation, and the costs, in time and dollars, to conduct research. If research productivity and efficiency are measured as the introduction of new chemical entities (NCE's) to the U.S. marketplace in a timely manner, then the record of the past two decades causes concern. The early 1960's saw a decline of approximately 50% in the introduction of NCE's from the previous decade. This continued decline was less dramatic, though significant, during the mid-1960's to the mid-1970's. Trends to the present time continue to reflect this decline (1). Several factors are implicated in this lowered productivity, including rising R&D costs, alternative investment opportunities, decrease in the number of firms conducting pharmaceutical R&D, and erosion in effective patent life (2). Hansen estimated that, for the years 1963 to 1976, the average expense and opportunity costs to bring an NCE to market was $54 million[1] (3). Updated estimates revise this figure to $70 million (2). Further, the average effective lifetime of a patent for all NCE's introduced during 1977-1979 was slightly less than 10 years (4).

The inverse relationship between the number of NCE's (total/domestically discovered) introduced in the U.S. versus the

---

[1]This figure includes $30 million for research and $24 million for development.

associated R&D expenses for the years 1954 to 1979 is shown graphically in Figure 1. Clearly other means must be sought to exploit the development of drugs while containing the prohibitively high costs of such drug development.

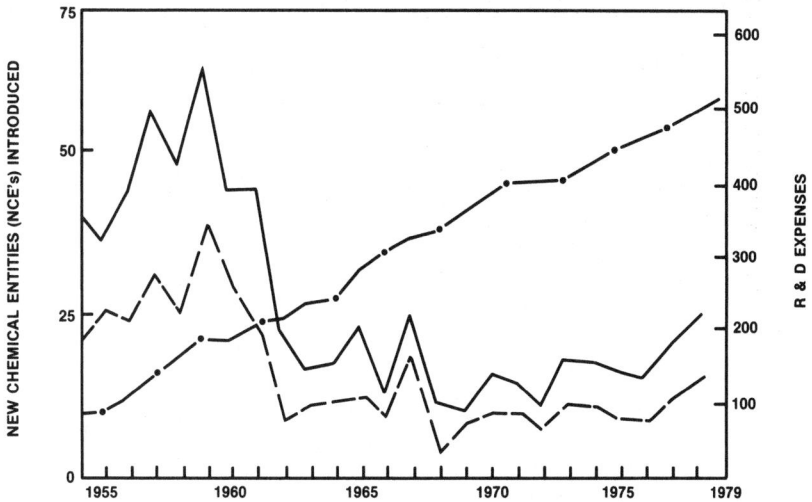

Figure 1. Relationship of U.S. New Chemical Entity Introductions (——) and Discoveries (----) to R&D Expenses (·-·-·). Adapted from ref. 5.

Alternatives

Several options are available to produce alternatives that serve to extend the utility of important NCE's currently on the market as well as provide important research advances for the next generation of drug delivery systems. Product improvements in existing NCE's can result in a) development of new claims b) improvement in therapeutic ratio and enhanced safety by directing drug to cellular and subcellular sites of therapeutic activity c) improvement of pharmaceutical shortcomings e.g. taste, pain on injection, gastric upset, diarrhea, stability, etc. d) improvement of biopharmaceutical properties, e.g. absorption, transport, metabolism, toxicity, etc.

The theme of this symposium centered on the bioreversible carrier and this approach has been utilized to provide novel and effective drug delivery systems that do not involve the de novo synthesis of new chemical entities. All of the aforementioned improvements in existing NCE's can be accomplished by the use of a bioreversible carrier - basically a generic term for a prodrug, soft drug, or similar biolabile chemical species. Bioreversible carriers are classified by the Food and Drug Administration as Chemical Type 2, i.e., the active moiety is marketed in the United States by the same or another manufacturer but the particular salt, ester, or derivative is not yet marketed in the United States by any drug manufacturer either as a single entity or as a part of a combination product (6). Bioreversible carriers are also referred to as pharmaceutical alternates. They are further subclassified according to therapeutic potential e.g., important, modest, or little or no therapeutic gain. Thus, depending on the choice of NCE and its designated use, a bioreversible carrier R&D program can entail the involvement of extensive technical resources and expertise. The elements involved in the development of bioreversible carriers to successful products are outlined in Scheme I. While the area of bioreversible carriers is now being recognized as a major facet of drug research, many problems still exist. These problems can be broadly classified accordingly.

(1) Lack of theoretical foundation
(2) Toxicity/safety criteria are difficult to establish
(3) Marketable delivery systems depend on the bioreversible carrier as well as the dosage formulation
(4) Clinical efficacy may involve intuitive interpretation
(5) Minimization of costs is critical

Theoretical

As distinct from the physical approach to drug delivery which is well grounded in theory (7), research activity with bioreversible carriers remains largely intuitive. Only recently have studies been directed toward developing physical models for the design, transport, and bioactivation of such entities in living systems (8-10). Also, elucidation of the pharmacokinetic parameters of bioreversible carriers has been recently studied and reviewed by Notari (11).

Toxicity/Safety

All drug entities, whether they are NCE's or bioreversible carriers, ideally possess a high therapeutic ratio prior to approval for use as therapeutic agents. Extensive toxicology, carcinogenicity and mutagenicity studies are conducted on every NCE in early stages of development (Scheme I). Eventually metabolic and efficacy trials are undertaken to further evaluate the safety and utility of each agent. Much of the same testing and evaluation must be performed on the bioreversible carrier and in this regard it can be considered a new drug entity. The carrier portion of the molecule is subjected to thorough metabolism studies to assure that it is non-toxic. This involves extensive assessment of the modified drug substance since its pharmacokinetic behavior may differ substantially from the parent drug molecule. All study protocols involving bioreversible carriers must be carefully designed to properly assess differences between the chemical species under investigation.

Formulation

The type of formulation that is used as the delivery system for a bioreversible carrier plays an important role in the therapeutic effectiveness of the drug. The nature of the carrier (salt, ester, soft drug) along with its physical state also affect fundamental drug properties such as duration of activity and distribution to various sites within the organism. One can expect delays in onset of action, for example, if the bioreversible carrier consists of one or more covalently bound - amide spacer groups and/or ester linkages that must undergo enzymatic hydrolysis prior to eliciting bioactivity. In addition, the release characteristics (disintegration, dissolution, partitioning of the carrier form of the drug from the physical dosage form) further complicate the behavior of such complex delivery systems in a predictable manner.

Clinical Efficacy

When an NCE is converted to a chemically bioreversible form, problems are increased because efficacy depends on regeneration of the NCE in vivo. The assurance that such reversibility occurs in a predictable manner presents the greatest challenge in this type of research. Even when the parent drug molecule is regenerated by enzymatic or non-enzymatic means in vivo, the predictability of the rate of hydrolysis must be consistent to provide adequate therapeutic drug levels over a large population of individuals. To add to the complexity of the problem, other agents containing potentially bioreversible linkages are reputed to be active per se, e.g., as the so-called bioreversible carrier. Certain topically applied anti-inflammatory steroid acetonide derivatives, for example, fall into this category and some question exists as to the bioactive form. Methodology must be developed to seek resolution to such ambiguous situations. Despite the somewhat empirical approach that has traditionally been taken to produce drugs via the bioreversible carrier, a remarkable number of such drugs are currently being marketed worldwide. Several major drug classes are represented and include steroids, antibiotics, neuroleptics, and antimalarials (12).

Cost

As discussed in the Introduction, the costs incurred in the development of an NCE currently surpass $70 million. One

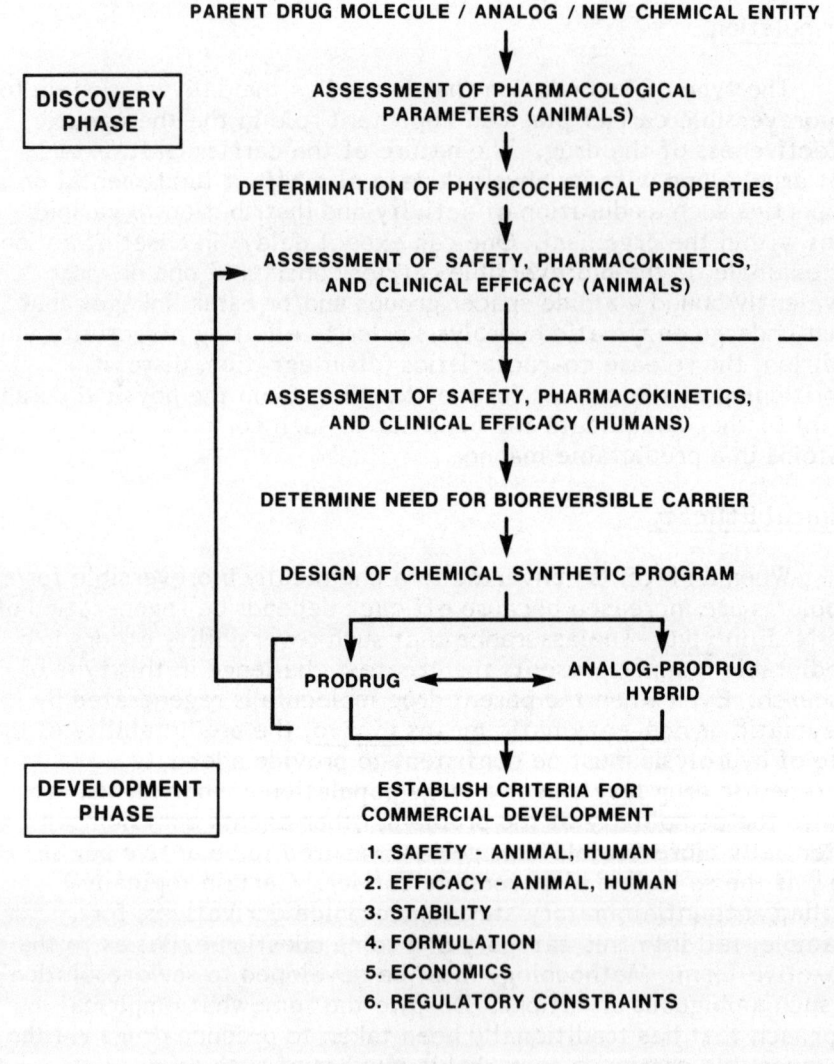

SCHEME I

Adapted from ref. 12.

alternative, already proposed, to extend and even enhance the utility of existing marketed drug products is by the application of the bioreversible carrier approach. This approach has been estimated to entail increased development times of 3-6 years and $1-3 million in additional costs (12). This is a small investment, however, if substantial benefits are derived in extending the useful life of many important drugs and potentially broadening their therapeutic efficacy and claims.

Other Industrial Perspectives/Concerns

The industrial approach to drug delivery systems research calls for a re-examination of the process that balances the high risks and costs involved in the development of new chemical entities versus the development of new and unique delivery systems as sources of new product generation. An increased awareness of the importance of drug delivery system research in the total process of drug research and development has been emphasized by Freund (13). Recent advances in cell biology and recombinant DNA technology enhance understanding of many underlying biological processes involved in the transport and site activation as such processes impact on drug delivery (14). While the emphasis of this symposium centered primarily on the research and development aspects of bioreversible carriers, the scope of an industrial drug delivery research program encompasses a broader range of concerns. Such programs must address issues that involve focus, balance, flexibility and integration as these issues relate to the conceptualization and implementation of modern drug delivery research. None of these issues are mutually exclusive but in fact are highly interdependent. Each will be discussed as they apply to industrial drug delivery research programs.

Focus - organization

Focus is concerned with the integration of disciplinary contributions to an interdisciplinary research program. All drug delivery research is assumed to be interdisciplinary in focus, i.e., drug delivery research projects are carried out within a single organizational unit that includes scientists with the necessary technical backgrounds to complete the research. Further, the unit organization promotes collaborative transactions between members of the group described as consultative (15). Within these research units are the disciplines necessary to undertake all tasks required to complete the research projects that contribute to the overall program objectives. These tasks are defined as cross-disciplinary and refer to task content rather than organizational form (16). Several factors are important in the design of such an interdisciplinary organization and include group size, evidence of team building activities, geographical integration of laboratory facilities, procedures that enhance/detract from the consulting mode of collaboration, etc. Importance is placed on intention rather than specific process (17).

Focus - disciplinary

Present and future drug delivery systems research must focus on and involve a blend of current theory and practice in molecular and cell biology as well as physical and organic chemistry. Recent advances in these disciplines as well as immunology, biochemistry, biophysics, and cell physiology have demonstrated an awareness of their importance to this area of interdisciplinary research. These fields of research now allow us to begin studies that will lead to an understanding of the underlying physiological, biochemical, and physicochemical processes governing the delivery of drugs. Developing an understanding of drug delivery from a biological perspective poses more questions than answers. For example, it is known that bioreversible carriers require the intervention of enzymes to regenerate the parent drug molecule in vivo and preparation of most candidates include this consideration in their initial design. Preliminary experiments validate this premise by in vitro enzyme hydrolysis studies. The extrapolation of such laboratory results to ultimate biochemical/enzymatic behavior in the host organism, however, remains a fertile area for investigation. The assumption is usually made that bioactivation will occur immediately prior to or at the site where active drug is needed to exert its therapeutic response and does not consider biochemical intervention during the entire transport process of the carrier. Thus metabolism and deactivation of the bioreversible carrier prior to interaction with appropriate receptors is disregarded or assumed to be of minor consequence. Doses are usually administered that will hopefully "swamp" the receptor with sufficient drug to ensure a response. Such drug design does not consider the biochemical implications of target selectivity or site specificity for drug delivery. An understanding of the physiological and morphological differences in cells associated with drug transport and delivery will enable investigators to tailor drug molecules that participate in the cellular transport process in ways that enhance efficacy. In certain cases, it may be necessary to transport the drug inter- or intracellularly, without metabolism occurring, to the receptor area of a target cell surface. For example, an orally administered cancer chemotherapeutic agent might pass the intestinal epithelial cell barrier intact with subsequent receptor mediated engulfment at a tumor surface with activation occurring within the tumor cell. The appreciation of the subtleties in cell physiology and morphology will add one more facet to the design of rational drug delivery systems. Further, the great strides made in understanding the molecular basis of immunoreactivity as it applies to immunotherapy suggests approaches to other challenges encountered in targeted drug delivery. The knowledge gained in understanding antigen/antibody interactions provides a means for site specific drug delivery through the use of monoclonal antibodies either directly attached to drug molecules or used as surface recognition agents on carriers such as liposomes. Finally, application of organic and physical chemistry to the synthesis of tailor made drug molecules and their incorporation into physical delivery systems completes the range of expertise needed to approach the complex problems of drug delivery from an interdisciplinary perspective. Very few programs of this scope exist within industrial laboratories at present.

Most challenges pertaining to the delivery of drugs in the host organism ultimately involve transport processes and phenomena. From the time that the drug is administered until a biological effect is achieved, forces are at work within the organism to maintain homeostasis against any foreign substance. Figure 2 outlines in schematic form the main phases of drug transport and action. The traditional approach taken in the development of drug delivery systems involves mainly the pharmaceutical phase. Assurance that disintegration and dissolution of the dosage formulation meet certain criteria in vitro can lead one to a false sense of security as to what occurs in vivo. It is only relatively recently that modeling of the pharmacokinetic processes involved in drug transport has achieved respectability. Such modeling however does not require a fundamental understanding of the biological processes occurring in vivo during drug absorption, distribution metabolism, and excretion. Presently very little is known about the biochemical, physiological, and immunological implications of the pharmacokinetic phase of drug transport and research in this area is required. Another area increasingly under study are those phenomena that occur during the pharmacodynamic phase of drug action. The sequence of events (19) that lead to the interaction of the ligand and receptor on the cell surface, with subsequent endocytosis, is shown in Figure 3. The series of interactions and processes that determine the ultimate fate of the drug, resulting in a biological response, occurs intracellularly. Many if not all of these important pathways that are so critical to a better understanding of drug design and the delivery of drugs are poorly understood. It is at this level of cellular activity that the important advances will be made in understanding the transport and mechanism of action of drugs. The mechanisms of how naturally occurring substances, e.g. proteins and nutrients, enter the cell are only partially understood. For example, after binding to the receptor occurs, the ligand-receptor complex collects in coated pits and is internalized to form vesicles. These vesicles fuse to form larger vesicles called endosomes. The endosomes undergo differentiation and uncoupling of receptor from ligand (CURL, compartment of uncoupling of receptor and ligand) by mechanisms that are only vaguely understood but probably mediated by a drop in pH from 7 to $\sim$5. The resulting tubular portion of the vesicle containing receptor material separates from the remainder of the vesicle and returns to the plasma membrane of the cell surface. Vesicles containing ligand fuse with lysosomes which degrade the ligand to metabolic products. Most of the studies carried out to the present time have emphasized understanding the ligand-receptor process with naturally occurring biochemicals, e.g. lipids. Investigation of drug-receptor interactions and the subsequent biochemical events remain a fertile area of research in drug delivery. Thus, processes affecting the transport, cell targeting and bioactivation of drugs must undergo intense study to provide a clearer understanding of how the delivery of drugs is governed.

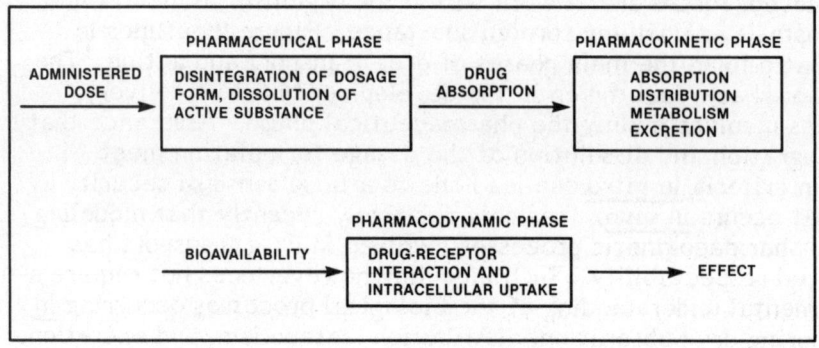

Figure 2. Main Phases of Drug Transport and Action. Adapted from ref. 18.

Attempts have been made to design drug molecules that will meet the needs for effective delivery to specific sites within the host organism. A composite molecule of this type is illustrated schematically in Figure 4. Chemically programmed into the molecular backbone are solubilizing groups that enhance the availability of the molecule for transport and a transport function that contains submolecular receptor recognition groups to direct the molecule to the cell surface. Also present on the backbone are functional groups that, with the use of spacer groups, can be utilized to attach all types of drug molecules.

These chemical drug delivery systems, with proper design, can be actively or passively transported and targeted to specific organs, tissues, or cells. This rational approach to the design of bioreversible carriers, grounded in a fundamental understanding of biochemistry, cell biology, immunology, and physical chemistry, represents the new frontier in industrial based drug delivery systems research.

Focus, as previously discussed, consists of both disciplinary and organizational elements. The successful blending of these elements into an industrial environment requires careful consideration as to what disciplines constitute a proper and effective research organization. While the importance of introducing "biology" into modern drug delivery systems research has been emphasized, closer examination is necessary to determine what disciplines within the realm of biology are central to this endeavor. The astounding progress made in cell biology, for example, involving the understanding of intracellular events affecting drug delivery and drug action are invaluable to future research efforts.

The concept of an industrial interdisciplinary drug delivery systems research group is so unique, however, that no precedent exists for its raison d'etre. Despite the lack of precedence for such a research group, one could infer that contributions from the chemical, biological, and clinical sciences would be necessary. Under each of these three broad disciplinary areas, specialty disciplines could be added based on specific research programs within any given industrial research laboratory. To effectively undertake drug delivery research using an interdisciplinary approach, a core group of disciplines must be represented.

In the area of biology, the following are considered important disciplines: immunology - to research the immunological basis for the delivery of drugs, e.g. targeting of drugs to specific sites via antibody-antigen interactions and other forms of site-directed drug carriers; cell biology - study mechanisms governing events at the cell surface and in the cell interior as they affect the delivery and therapeutic action of drug molecules; biochemistry - study membrane structure and morphology, receptors, and function and their influence on drug delivery; physiology - study the underlying mechanisms of transport and absorption of drugs through (across) biological barriers and membranes; pharmacology - study the organ and cellular response to drugs and drug delivery systems; toxicology - study implications of drug delivery systems and their effect on the therapeutic ratio; biophysics - examine mechanisms influencing and controlling plasma membrane fluidity, cell physics, cell adhesion, and cell conformation and their quantifiable changes in a drug environment.

Chemically based disciplines include: organic medicinal chemistry - responsible for synthesis of unique model compounds, including prodrugs, that will be studied as/or part of a delivery system; physical organic chemistry - study mechanisms of stability/degradation of drugs in unique delivery systems (liposomes, emulsions, devices, etc.); biopolymer science - conduct research in the use of new and unusual polymers as drug delivery systems including evaluation of biomaterials for purity and biocompatibility.

Finally, the availability of a clinical scientist to test concepts, formulations, and devices early in the implementation of a cross-disciplinary drug delivery research program in a clinical setting serves to focus the program on the most important end product - safe and effective drug delivery to the patient.

This group of disciplines blended into a programmatically focused effort can be viewed as a "complementary discipline" approach to drug delivery systems research. Each scientist contributes and shares his expertise in a collaborative manner to reach the research objective. Very little, if any redundancy or overlap should occur within the disciplinary responsibilities of the scientists. Because of the keen competition for scientific resources within the organization, each scientist's expertise may purposely not be overlapped but "gapped" in order to promote dialog and appreciation of related disciplinary expertise within the unit organization. The interdisciplinary gaps are thus filled by scientists constituting the complementary discipline core.

Flexibility

Flexibility denotes the ability to serve both present and future drug delivery needs within the existing organization. The idea of flexibility is closely interrelated with organizational balance and integration. Present drug delivery system needs involve emphasis on conventional and novel delivery systems and formulations. These present needs can be concisely stated in terms of mission statements that support the goals of the drug delivery system research organization:

1) Support the research and development of new drug entities through the design of drug delivery systems and formulations for toxicology and clinical testing.

2) Manufacture toxicology and clinical trial supplies to support the development of new drug entities.

3) Transfer new drug entity formulation, stability, and manufacturing technology to the appropriate individuals for final product development.

An organization must stand ready to be proactively involved in drug delivery system and formulation support for those new drug entities emanating from the discovery laboratories. This involvement should include early input in the candidate selection process. The influence of the pharmaceutical scientist in terms of supporting selection of a candidate possessing adequate stability in the formulated state as well as proper solubility characteristics can have a profound effect on the ultimate success of the drug candidate as a marketed

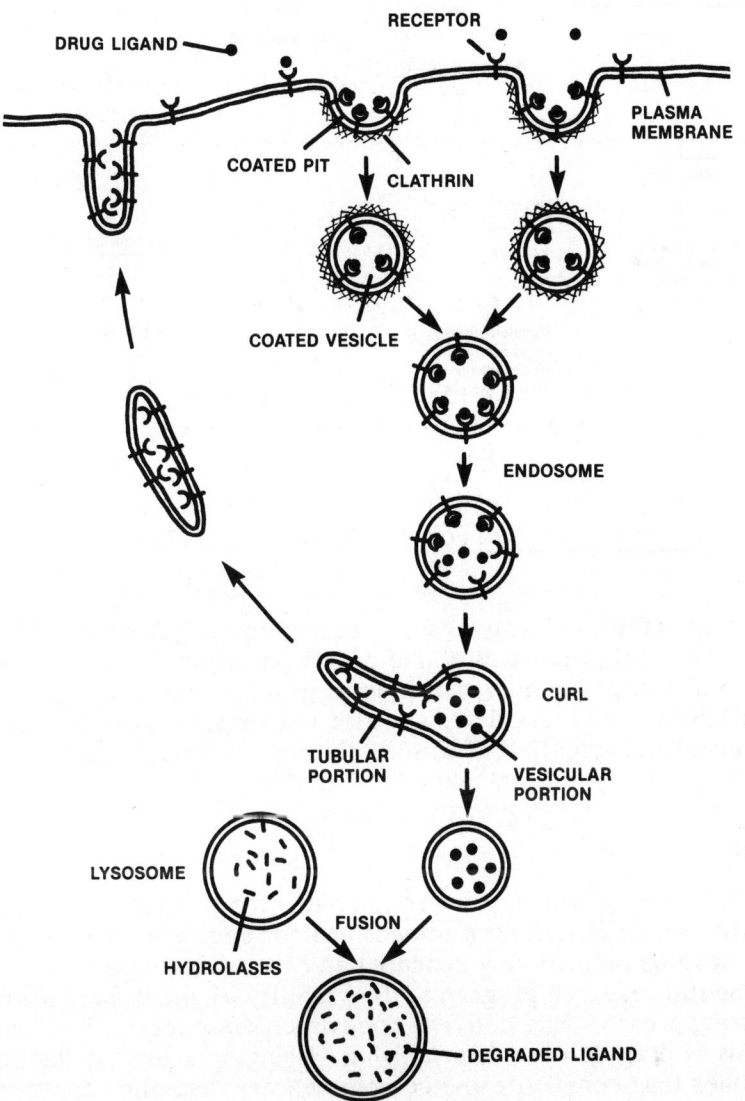

Figure 3. Ligand-Receptor Interaction and the Process of Endocytosis. Adapted from ref. 19.

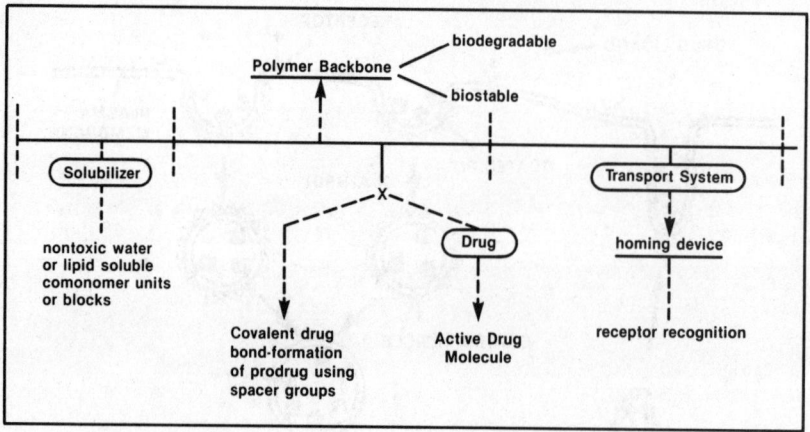

Figure 4. Schematic Representation of A Chemically Derived Drug Delivery System. Adapted from H. Ringsdorf, J. Polymer Sci: Symposium No. 51, 135 (1975).

product. Further, an early and continuing investigation into the physicochemical properties of the drug that influence release from the formulation, drug pharmacokinetic profiles, and ultimate bioavailability and bioactivity are also the responsibility of the pharmaceutical scientist. The scientist, as a member of an interdisciplinary research team, is obligated to share this critical information with colleagues in a timely manner in order to assure project success.

Future drug delivery needs complete the second part of the flexibility equation. If future needs are not addressed and nurtured by the development of new concepts and strategies based on fundamental research programs, the viability of the organization addressing present drug delivery needs soon disappears. The future in terms of drug delivery is promising. Using a variety of scientific disciplines that constitute the complementary discipline approach is necessary for addressing future needs. Combining biology, chemistry and clinical science into one strategic approach to study the problems confronting drug delivery and drug targeting is essentially the approach that industrial scientists must use to address the future of this area of drug research. The mission that guides future efforts in drug delivery systems research can be summarized in the following statement:

4) "Conduct basic research that will lead to an understanding of the underlying physiological, biochemical and physicochemical processes governing the delivery of drugs to support the future development of human and veterinary drug products."

Balance

Whereas flexibility is defined in terms of an extended temporal relationship to services provided in the organization, balance refers to the types of services rendered within a defined span of time. The immediate goal of the organization is to provide scientific support for the development and approval of new products for the market. A longer term goal is to undertake basic research in drug delivery that contributes to the discovery of drug candidates that eventually become new products. Balance is an important consideration in industrial drug delivery systems research because it modulates the amount of research, development, and technology that is undertaken at any point in time in the drug discovery and development process. The lines of demarcation between research, development, and technology are poorly understood and appreciated but are certainly not mutually exclusive. Perhaps research can best be understood by examining statement 4 on page 13. This statement reflects the fundamental approach taken to study processes influencing drug delivery and is concept and not product oriented. The result of this research is the generation of knowledge that can be applied to the design of systems and formulations for specific new drug entities. The systems and applications phase of the drug delivery research program can be designated as applied research, field-oriented research, or as development and is reflected in statement 1 on page 10. While the same degree of creative input is required here as in the concept or fundamental research phase of the drug delivery program, the focus is directed toward the physicochemical properties of the drug and their influence on drug performance. Therefore, the close attention to the formulation or device and its influence on the presentation of drug to the bioenvironment at the site of administration becomes of prime importance. The contribution of technology is one of systems refinement. Fine tuning the manufacturing process to develop the formulations and devices for testing are the primary goal of the technology phase and is summarized in statement 2 on page 10. In recent times, however, the initiation of a drug delivery project requires early input from the concept and applied research groups including the technology group. Since the integration and collaboration of all groups is crucial at early stages of the project, it becomes less a matter of definition than of understanding each contribution as it applies to the quality of the final product. Flexibility and balance within a drug delivery systems research program are schematically depicted in Figure 5.

Integration

Much research and development undertaken within the pharmaceutical industry is done in the context of the matrix organization. Management in such organizations is known as matrix management. The rationale for the use of a matrix organization (20) is satisfied if three conditions exist: 1) Need for dual focus - in the process of developing a drug for commercial use, there is a need for simultaneous decision making on both the technical aspects of the project as well as serving the resource needs of the project. There is thus a need to focus effort on two organizational tasks simultaneously and this can be accomplished through a matrix organization. Scientists working in this environment must be comfortable working with two bosses, e.g. line management and the project team leadership. The drug delivery scientist can be most effective in this setting if he understands the drug development process and the organization culture under which this process operates. 2) Need for efficient communications network - the vast amount of information generated during the research and development process requires high information processing capabilities among members of a drug development project team. The cross-disciplinary tasks involved in drug development are interrelated and a high degree of interdependence among project team participants is necessary to share information on a timely basis. Each scientist representative must possess the ability to effectively communicate the contribution and impact of their research to the goals of project. The drug delivery scientist plays a unique role in this regard because delivery system and formulation information and expertise is a "front-loaded" activity in the project, that is to say, the formulation is largely responsible for many early performance characteristics of the drug molecule, e.g. stability, bioavailability, low toxicity, enhanced bioactivity, etc. The importance of the formulation and drug delivery scientists contributions are important almost from the beginning of the project and are manifested in the preparation of suitable formulations for animal toxicology studies, Phase 1, 2, and 3 human clinical studies and the final marketed formulation. In many cases, the success, or lack thereof, of the delivery systems or formulation effort determines the success of the entire drug development program. As mentioned previously, the scientists knowledge of the drug development process and the impact of the organizations value system on the process are important factors in dealing with external forces that are unpredictable, e.g. regulatory requirements. Will the scientist recommend a more conservative approach to formulation research and development than the FDA guidelines suggest? Does one do more stability studies, for example, than are required? Does the project team adopt a strategy to assume risk and target for a skeleton NDA or assume little risk and seek a fully documented NDA? These questions and subsequent strategies taken

are a reflection of the organization culture and value system and
must be appreciated and accepted by the drug delivery scientist
working within its context. As important, the scientist must be able
to effectively communicate within such an organization. 3) Need to
effectively deploy and utilize scarce resources - two challenges
continually manifest themselves during the drug development
process, namely long-term resource commitment and rapid changes

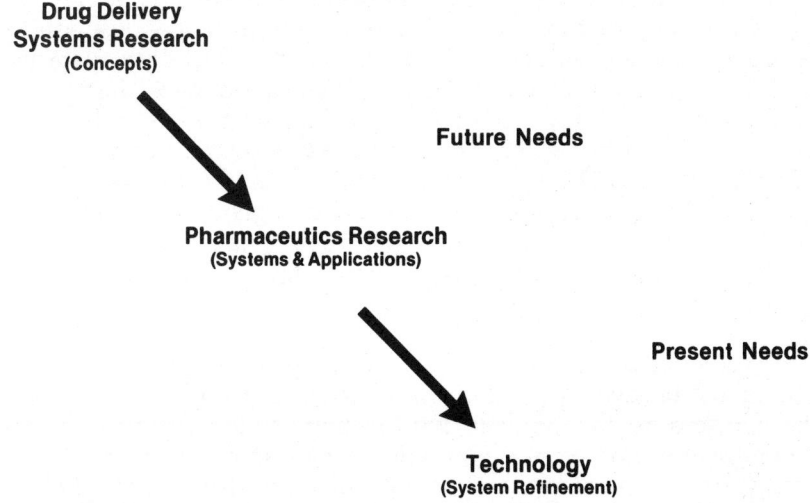

Figure 5. Balance Between Present and Future Needs for an
Industrial Based Drug Delivery Systems Organization.

in the external environment. Both have profound implications for
resource usage. Although every project cannot be supported for
peak loads, an adequate resource base must be provided to all
projects to ensure timely movement throughout the development
process. Prioritization of projects affords a method of allocating
resources equitably while the use of a matrix organization
modulates resource levels and needs during varying degrees of
resource intensity ("peaks and valleys") during the life of the
project. Most commonly, resources in greatest demand that lend
themselves to matrix management include Bulk Drug Preparation,
Pathology/Toxicology, Drug Metabolism/Pharmacokinetics,
Pharmacy/Formulation, and Biostatistics. Use of these resources as
support groups, with their own organizational structure, provides
critical services to the drug development team in a timely fashion.
The drug delivery scientist, being an integral part of this effort,
understands his role in the total effort.

Conclusions

The subject of drug delivery is receiving more attention in view of the challenges encountered in providing efficacious quantities of complex drug molecules to specific sites of action in a timely manner within the host organism.

Industrial drug delivery research programs are responding to these challenges with talent whose training involves a broad foundation of scientific expertise. Increased emphasis is being placed on training of scientists in the biological sciences, especially biochemistry and cell biology. The fact that drug delivery systems research is inter-disciplinary by its very nature mandate that programs now encompass the "complementary discipline" concept in which a wide variety of scientific talent reside in the same organizational unit. The intermix of programs and projects involving cell biologists, biophysicists, toxicologists, pharmaceutical scientists, chemists, engineers, etc. will require all involved scientists to broaden their technical knowledge in order to effectively participate in such programs.

Perhaps our perspective on the "drug delivery system" needs rethinking and broadening and our limited success in the past may in fact be due to a narrow perspective. In lieu of viewing the physical device or formulation or bioreversible carrier as the delivery system, we might consider the host organism, with its vast array of complex processes and facilitating mechanisms as the true delivery system. The physical form of the drug acts merely as the presentation of the drug for delivery by those biological processes so poorly understood at present. Ultimately what determines how, where, and to what degree a drug is delivered depends not so much on the device or formulation exclusively but rather on a combination of the physical chemical, the biochemical and immunological processes affecting the behavior of the drug or device within the organism. These are the most important fundamental challenges that beckon the industrial drug delivery research establishment.

Finally, industrial laboratories seek individuals who understand the role of drug delivery systems contributions to the total drug development process. The team approach to successful drug development is essential and the scientists must understand and appreciate the value systems of the project team as well as the total organization. The need for human relations and communication skills are critical to such interdisciplinary project success.

References

1. M.S. May, W.M. Wardell, and L. Lasagna, New drug development during and after a period of regulatory change: Clinical research activity of major United States pharmaceutical firms, 1958 to 1979, Clin. Pharmacol. Ther., 33, 691 (1982).
2. L. Lasagna, Will all new drugs become orphans?, Clin. Pharmacol. Ther., 31, 285 (1982).
3. R.W. Hansen, The pharmaceutical development process: Estimates of development costs and times and the effects of proposed regulatory changes. In: "Issues In Pharmaceutical Economics," Lexington Books, Lexington, Mass., 1979, pp. 151-187.
4. M. Eisman and W. Wardell, The decline in effective patent life of new drugs, Res. Management, 24, 18 (1981).
5. H.G. Grabowski, Public policy and pharmaceutical innovation, Health Care Financing Review, 4, 75 (1982).
6. Staff Manual Guide BD 4820.3, Food and Drug Administration, Bureau of Drugs, August, 1976.
7. M.J. Robinson, Sustained action dosage forms. In: "The Theory and Practice of Industrial Pharmacy," Lea and Febiger, Philadelphia, 1976, pp. 439-465.
8. W. Morozowich, M.J. Cho, and F.J. Kezdy, Application of physical organic principles to prodrug design. In: "Design of Biopharmaceutical Properties Through Prodrugs and Analogs," American Pharmaceutical Association, Washington, D.C., 1977, pp. 344-391.
9. C.D. Yu, J.L. Fox, N.F.H. Ho, and W.I. Higuchi, Physical model evaluation of topical prodrug delivery - simultaneous transport and bioconversion of vidarabine-5'-valerate I: physical model development, J. Pharm. Sci., 68, 1341 (1979).
10. C.D. Yu, J.L. Fox, N.F.H. Ho, and W.I. Higuchi, Physical model evaluation of topical prodrug delivery - simultaneous transport and bioconversion of vidarabine-5'-valerate II: parameter determinations, J. Pharm. Sci., 68, 1347 (1979).
11. R.E. Notari, Prodrug design, Pharmacol. Ther., 14, 25 (1981).
12. A.A. Sinkula, The chemical approach to achieve sustained drug delivery. In: "Optimization of Drug Delivery," Munksgaard, Copenhagen, 1982, pp. 199-210.
13. J. Freund, New drug delivery systems: scientific and corporate implications, Clin. Res. Practices and Drug Reg. Affairs, 1, 291 (1983).
14. C. Bezold, The Future of Pharmaceuticals: The Changing Environment of New Drugs, John Wiley and Sons, New York, 1981, p. 52.

15. S.E. Gold and H.J. Gold, Some elements of a model to improve productivity of interdisciplinary groups. In: "Managing Interdisciplinary Research," John Wiley and Sons, Chichester, 1983, pp. 86-101.
16. F. Rossini, A.L. Porter, D.E. Chubin, and T. Connolly, Cross-disciplinarity in the biomedical sciences: A preliminary analysis of anatomy. In: "Managing Interdisciplinary Research," John Wiley and Sons, Chichester, 1983, pp. 176-184.
17. S.R. Epton, R.L. Payne, and A.W. Pearson, Multidisciplinary, interdisciplinary - what is the difference? In: "Managing Interdisciplinary Research," John Wiley and Sons, Chichester, 1983, pp. 3-9.
18. E.J. Ariens, Drug Design, Vol. IV, Academic Press, New York, 1973, p. xi.
19. A. Dautry-Varsat and H.F. Lodish, How receptors bring proteins and particles into cells, Sci. American, 250, No. 5, 52 (1984).
20. S.M. Davis and P.R. Lawrence, The matrix organization - who needs it? In: "Matrix", Addison-Wesley Publishing Co., Reading, 1977, pp. 11-24.

INDEX

Acetals, 62
Acetaminophen esters, 5
Acetazolamide, 30
6'-Acetylpapaverine, 70
Acetylsalicylic acid, 67
Acid catalysis, 124
Acidic N-terminal amino acids, 243
Acyclovir, 67, 68
Acyloxyalkyl ethers, 16
Acyloxymethyl esters, 15, 79
Adrenaline, tissue concentration, 102
Adrenalone diesters, 101,101
Adrenalone diisovalerate, 100, 101
Adrenalone, tissue concentration, 102, 103
Alkaline phosphatase, 227
Allopurinol, 30, 41, 43, 53
Amides, 53
Amine carrier system, 229, 237
Amino acid esters, 18, 19
Amino acid prodrug
   membrane permeability, 254
   solubility, 254
   structural requirements, 254
Amino acid transport, 237
Aminoalcohols, 62
4-Aminobutyric acid, 67
Aminopeptidase A (EC 3.4.11.7), 243, 250
Aminopeptidase M, 243, 250
Aminopeptidase N, 243, 250, 251
Aminopeptidases, 252
   adult, 252
   development (fetal), 250, 253
   distribution, 249, 253
Ampicillin, 15
Antibodies as drug-carrier systems, 205
Aromatic amino acid decarboxylase, 227
Aspartate aminopeptidase, 243, 250

B-Glucocerebrosidase, derivatized, 221
Bacampicillin, 15

Barbital, 30
Barbituric acids, 67
Base catalysis, 124
Basic amino acid carrier system, 229
Benzocaine, 53
Benzodiazepines, 67
Berberine, 98
Bidirectional carrier systems, 228, 229
Biocompatibility, 207
Biological targeting, 97
Bioreconversion of amino acid prodrugs, 254
Bioreversible carrier, 263, 264
Bioreversible polymer-drug linkages, 198
   synthesis, 198
Blood-brain barrier, 98, 106 228, 229
Brain-specific delivery, 106, 108, 110
   tryptamine, 113
   tryptophan, 113
Brush border aminopeptidases
   biosynthesis, 247
   isolation, 244
   location, 244
   properties, 244
   structure, 244, 246
Brush border enzymes, 243
Brush border fragments, preparation, 244
Brush border membrane vesicles, 244, 245
Butyrylcholinestrerase, 227

CSF/plasma ratio, 106
Carbamates, 17
Carbamazepine, 27
Carbamoyl derivatives, 52
Carbohydrate-dependent recognition systems, 203
Carboxylesterase, 147, 150
Carboxypeptidase (EC 3.4.12.X) 244, 252
Carrier mediated transport, 228
   in vitro models, 233
Catalysis, intramolecular, 129
Catechols, 16, 67
Cathepsin B, degradation of copolymers, 199
Cell-specific targeting, 203

Cephalosporins, 79
Cerebrospinal fluid
  concentration, 106
Chemical delivery systems
  (CDS), 99, 100
Chemical modification, 97
Chloramphenicol succinate, 124
Chlorothiazide, 30
Chlorzoxazone, 30, 33, 37, 41
Choline carrier system
  in vitro, 237
  in vivo, 237
Coralyne, 70
Cromoglycidic acid, 15
Curl, 269
Cycloserine, 60
Cytosol peptidases, 244

Dexamethasone 21-sulphate, 20
Diethylstilbesterol, 80
Dihydroberberine, 98
Dihydro-2-PAM, 2
Dihydropralidoxime, 98
Dihydropyridine redox delivery
  system, 107, 109
Dihydrotrigonelline carrier
  system, 110
Diisovaleryl adrenaline, tissue
  concentration, 103
Diisovaleryl adrenalone, 100,
  101
  reduction-hydrolysis, 100,
    104
  tissue concentration, 103
5, 5-Dimethylhydantoin, 33
Dipeptidyl-peptidase IV
  (EC 3.4.14.X), 244, 250
Dipivalyl adrenaline, 101, 101
Disciplines, complementary,
  271, 272
Dopamine, 16, 53
  trigonelline carrier
    system, 110, 111
Double prodrugs, 66
Drug binding to macromolecules,
  effect of, 196
Drug delivery, 98
  receptor mediated, 217
  targeted, 270
Drug delivery systems,
  chemical, 270
Drug metabolism in the eye, 104
Drug selectivity, 96
Drug toxicity, 96

Electronic effects, 147
Enaminones, 60
Endocytosis, 269
  of polymeric drug-carriers,
    200
  receptor mediated, 230
Endosomes, 269
Endothelial cell monolayers,
  233
Endothelium
  brain, 227
  cerebral, 227
  continuous, 226
  discontinuous, 226
  fenestrated, 226
  microvascular, 226
  peripheral, 227, 228
Enol esters, 63
Enzyme catalysis, 146
  steric effects, 136
  substituent effects, 146
Enzyme kinetics, 152
Enzyme replacement therapy, 221
Enzyme specificity, 4
Enzymes, lysosomal in pinocytic
  vesicles, 197
Ephedrine, 24, 57
Epinephrine, 16, 100
Epinephrine dipivalate, 100,
  101
Epinephrine, dipivalyl ester,
  1, 2
Epithelial, active transport,
  227
Ester prodrugs, 14
Esterases, 148, 149
  specificity, 5
Estradiol, 16
  brain-specific delivery, 115
  redox chemical delivery
    system, 115
Exo-cytosis
  receptor mediated, 230

4-Fluoro-3-nitrophenyl azide
  reagent, 246
5-Fluorouracil, 30, 32, 40,
  41, 48, 81

GABA, redox chemical delivery
  systems, 114
Galactosamine, on fate of HPMA
  copolymers, 204

Gaucher's disease, 221
Glutamine-amino acid exchange, 230, 231
gamma-Glutamyl cycle, 230, 231
gamma-Glutamyl derivatives, 53
gamma-Glutamyl transpeptidase, 227
gamma-Glutamyltranspeptidase (EC 2.3.2.2), 244, 250
Glutarimides, 67
Glutethimide, 37
Glycine-p-nitroanilide, absorption, 255
Glycocalyx, 244, 245

Hammett relationship, 128
Hemisuccinates, 19
Hemolysis, methylpredinisolone esters, 158
Hexamethylmelamine, 31
Hexose carrier system, 229
HPMA copolymers, in vitro stability, 199
HPMA-oligopeptide copolymers, synthesis, 198, 199
Hydantoins, 21, 32, 58, 67
Hydrochlorothiazide, 30
Hydrocortisone, 17, 256
  lysinate, 256
  phosphate, 256
  succinate, 256
Hydrolysis, 129
Hydrophilicity-solubility relationships, 126
Hydroxide catalysis, 124
Hyperaminoacidemia, 230
  post-prandial, 230

4-Imidazolidinones, 67
IM irritation, methyl-prednisolone esters, 158
Insulin, receptor mediated transport, 230
Intercellular diffusion, macromolecules, 233
Intravenous injections, 122
Intrinsic toxicity, 96
Isoguvacine, 15
Isolated brain microvessel endothelial cells, 234

Ketals, 62

L-Alanine-p-nitroanilide, absorption, 255
L-Dopa, 53
L-Dopa transport, 229, 230
L-Lysine-p-nitroanilide, absorption, 255
LD-50, methylprednisolone esters, 158
LDL
  receptor, 218
  reconstituted, 218
LH, effect of estradiol CDS, 116
gamma-Lactones, 67
Ligand-receptor interaction, 269, 270
Ligands
  carbohydrate, 221
  hepatocytes, 219
  Kupfer cells, 221
  macrophage, 220
Liposomes with saccharide determinants, 219
Liposomes, in gene transfer, 220
Liver esterases, 150
Luteinizing hormone, effect of estrodiol CDS, 116
Lysosomotropic agents, 216

Machaelis-Menten kinetics, 152
Macromolecular drug carriers, 196
  biocompatibility, 197
  pinocytosis, 197
Macromolecular receptors, transcytosis, 232
Matrix management, 276
Melphalan transport, 229, 230
Membrane Gly-Leu peptidase, 244
6-Mercaptopurine, 41
Methyldopa, 15
alpha-Methyldopa transport, 229, 230
Methylprednisolone esters
  bioavailability, 153
  pharmacokinetics, 152
Methylprednisolone
  adipate, 130
  esters, 123, 127, 136, 142, 150, 152
  malonate, 130
  succinate, 130, 150
  sulfopropionate, 150
alpha-Methyltyrosine transport,

229
Metronidazole, 19, 20
Micellar prodrugs, 138
  stabilization, 141
Micellar solubilization, 139
Microvillus aminopeptidase, 243, 250
Mitrochondria, 227, 228
Monoamine oxidase, 227
Monocarboxylic acid carrier system, 229

N-(2-hydroxypropyl) methacrylamide (HPMA), 196
  copolymers, 196, 197
N-Acyloxyalkyl derivatives, 39, 58
N-Hydroxy-alkylation, 36
N-Hydroxymethyl derivatives, 32
N-Mannich bases, 21, 56, 81
Neutral amino acid carrier system, 229, 235, 236
  affinity of, 229
Neutral N-terminal amino acids, 243
Neutral amino acid transport, inhibition, 236
Neutral aminopeptidase, 243 250
New chemical entities (NCEs), 262, 263
Nicotinamide, 35
Nitrofurantoin, 33, 35
Nucleoside carrier system, 229

Oligoaminopeptidase (EC 3.4.11.2), 243, 250
Oligopeptides as drug-carrier linkages, 198
Ophthalmic drug distribution, 101
Organization
  balance, 272, 275
  flexibility, 272
  integration, 272, 276
  matrix, 276
Oxazolidines, 62
Oximes, 62

2-Pam, 1
  dihydro, 2
Pancreatic peptidases, 243
Paracetamol, 20
Parameter manipulation formulation, 184
  prodrug structure, 189
Parameters
  direct measurement, 177
  indirect measurement, 178
Parenterals, 122
Partition coefficient, 126
Penicillins, 14, 60
Peptide receptors, brain epithelium, 232, 233
pH-Hydrolysis rate profiles, 129
pH-Solubility dependence, 124, 125
Phagocytosis of polymeric drug carriers, 200
Phenylalanine nitrogen mustard, 229
Phenylbutazone, 63
Phenylephrine, 16
Phenylpropanolamine, 56, 60
Phenytoin, 20, 30, 33, 37, 41
Phosphate esters, 19, 79
Physical model approach, 164, 188
  cost effectiveness of, 189
  determination of parameters, 177
  efficacy studies, 186
  Laplace transforms in, 175
  linear kinetics, 176
  mathematics of, 172
  mechanics of, 165
  nonlinear kinetics, 176
  optimum parameter values, 189
  parameter manipulation, 183
  prediction of efficacy, 187
  sensitivity analysis, 91
Pilocarpine, 91
Pinocytic capture, non-specific, 202
Pinocytic vesicles, 197, 228, 230
Pinocytosis
  adsorptive, 197
  fluid phase, 197
  of polymeric drug-carriers, 200
  rates of, 200
Pivampicillin, 15
Polymer-drug conjugates, fate in vivo, 205
Potassium ATPase, 227
Pralidoxime, 98

Pro-prodrugs, 263
Prodrug, 97, 98
  chemistry, 2
  design, 121
  esterase-sensitive, 1
  patents, 12
  physical chemical parameters, 180
  regulatory requirements, 12
  solubility, 126
  strategy, 254
Protein mediated transport, 230, 231
Pulse-chase labeling studies, 247
Purine carrier system, 229

Quaternary carrier system, 107, 108

Receptor
  low density lipoprotein, 218
  saccharide, 218
Research
  cross-disciplinary, 267, 276
  disincentives, 262
  drug delivery systems, 267
  focus, 267, 268
  interdisciplinary, 267, 268
Rho, 147
Rolitetracycline, 27

Salicylamide, 25, 58
Serum esterases, 148, 149
  steric effects, 136
Shelf-life, 122, 138
Site specificity, 96, 98
Site-specific drug delivery, 100
Sodium ATPase, 227
Softdrug, 263
Solution stability, 124
  steric effects on, 135
Substituent effects, 128, 129, 133, 134, 147
Succinate esters, 123, 124
Succinimides, 67
Sulfamethoxazole, 53
Suldinac
  patient tolerance, 215
  pharmacotherapeutic patient tolerance, 214

Sulphate esters, 20
Sustained release in the brain, 106, 108

Taft relationship, 128
Taft-Ingold relationship, 134, 147
Taft sigma* constants, 128, 135
Taft steric parameters, 133, 147
Talampicillin, 15
Terbutaline, 41
Testosterone, 17
  brain-specific delivery, 115
  redox chemical delivery system, 115
Tetracycline, 27
Theophylline, 96
Therapeutic index, 96
Thiazolidines, 62
Thiols
  acylated, 4
  soft alkylated, 4
Thiophenol, 16
Toxicity
  intrinsic, 96
  methylprednisolone esters, 157
Transcytosis
  receptor mediated, 230
Transendothelial carrier systems, 226
Transendothelial signal transmission, 232
Transferrin receptors, transcytosis, 231
Transport
  cellular, 269, 270
  isolated skin graft studies, 280
  pharmacokinetic, 269
  receptor mediated, 230
    in vitro models, 243
Trigonelline carrier system, 110
Trimethadione, 67
Tyrosine, 15

Uracil, 37

Vidarabine, 20, 21
  choice of prodrug, 170
  2, 3-diacetate, efficacy
    studies, 186
  5'-esters of, 172
  factors limiting
    effectiveness, 168
  5'-monoesters, efficacy
    studies, 186
  5'-phosphate, 19
  prodrugs, 169
  inhibition of deaminase,
    170
  5'-valerate, 181
    efficacy studies, 186
    esterase lability, 182
  topical delivery, 167

Zinc stable Asp-Lys peptidase,
  244

BIOGRAPHICAL SKETCHES OF AUTHORS

Gordon L. Amidon

Dr. Gordon L. Amidon received his B.S. degree in pharmacy from the State University of New York, Buffalo (1967), M.A. degree in mathematics from The University of Michigan (1970), and his Ph.D. in pharmaceutical chemistry from The University of Michigan (1971). In 1971, Dr. Amidon joined the faculty at the University of Wisconsin where he also served as Assistant Dean for Educational Planning and Policy. In 1981 he took the position of Director of Pharmaceutical Research at Merck/INTERx. Dr. Amidon was appointed Professor of Pharmaceutics at The University of Michigan in 1983. He is Chairman of the Joint Program Board of the SmithKline Beckman/University of Michigan Program for Therapeutics Systems Research and also serves as Director of Research for SmithKline Consumer Products.

Dr. Amidon is nationally known for his research in the field of solubility, transport phenomena, prodrugs and drug absorption. He has published extensively in journals, co-authored one book, and contributed chapters to several books. His awards include being the recipient of the Ebert Prize of the American Pharmaceutical Association in 1974, 1980, and co-recipient in 1984. He was elected a Fellow of the APhA/Academy of Pharmaceutical Sciences in 1981. Dr. Amidon has served as Vice Chairman (1982), chairman elect (1983) and chairman (1984) of the Basic Pharmaceutics Section of the Academy of Pharmaceutical Sciences. He is a member of the American Pharmaceutical Association, Academy of Pharmaceutical Sciences and the American Association for the Advancement of Science.

Bradley D. Anderson

Bradley D. Anderson, Associate Professor of Pharmaceutics, College of Pharmacy, University of Utah, Salt Lake City, Utah, was born November 23, 1948. He attended the University of Kansas where he received his bachelor's degree in Chemistry in 1971. After graduation he was employed as a quality control chemist for a division of Cutter Laboratories, Inc. until 1974. In 1974 he returned to The University of Kansas and in 1973 received a Ph.D. degree in Pharmaceutical Chemistry. Dr. Anderson then joined the Pharmacy Research unit of the Upjohn Company, Kalamazoo, Michigan where he spent over 5 years as an industrial research scientist. In April 1983 he joined the faculty of the Pharmaceutics Department at The University of Utah.

As an industrial researcher and now as an academic scientist Dr. Anderson has engaged in research in a variety of areas. He has published numerous research articles in solution thermodynamics, kinetics and mechanisms of drug degradation, drug formulation optimization, and the design of physicochemical properties through prodrug formation and has several patents and patents pending in the prodrug area.

Dr. Anderson is a member of the APhA, The Basic Pharmaceutics Section of the Academy of Pharmaceutical Sciences, and is currently serving as Vice-Chairman of the Basic Pharmaceutics Section of the Academy. He also has served on the Ebert Prize selection committee. In addition to his Academy responsibilities, Dr. Anderson is a member of the American Association for the Advancement of Science, Phi Lambda Upsilon, and Rho Chi.

Kenneth L. Audus

Born November 11, 1954, Watertown, South Dakota. Education: B.S., Chemistry, 1980, the University of South Dakota; Ph.D., Pharmacology, 1984, The University of Kansas School of Medicine. Present Position: Research Fellow of the American Heart Association - Kansas Affiliate, in the laboratory of Dr. Ronald T. Borchardt, Department of Pharmaceutical Chemistry, The University of Kansas. Research Interests and Experience: Characterization of drug transport and metabolism in brain microvessel endothelial cell monolayers (an _in vitro_ blood-brain barrier model). Receptor identification and characterization. Steady-state, lifetime, and differential phase fluorometry to probe membrane structure and ligand-receptor interactions.

Nicholas Bodor

Dr. Nicholas Bodor is a Graduate Research Professor in the Department of Medicinal Chemistry at the University of Florida in Gainesville. He is also Vice President for Research of Pharmatec, Inc. Before coming to the University of Florida, Dr. Bodor was Director of Medicinal Chemistry Research at INTERx Research Corporation in Kansas and an Adjunct Professor at the University of Kansas in Lawrence. His main research interests include design of drugs with improved therapeutics index, design of new chemical-delivery systems, computer assisted drug design, drug transport and metabolism, and theoretical and mechanistic organic chemistry. He has published over 120 research articles and has over 95 patents. He is a Fellow of the Academy of Pharmaceutical Sciences and a member of numerous professional organizations. He is also a consultant for a number of major pharmaceutical companies.

Ronald T. Borchardt

Ronald T. Borchardt was born February 18, 1944, in Wausau, Wisconsin. Education: B.S. 1967, School of Pharmacy, University of Wisconsin; Ph.D. 1970, Department of Medicinal Chemistry, University of Kansas. Research and Professional Experience: 1969-1971, Senior Assistant Scientist, Laboratory of Chemistry, National Institute of Arthritis and Metabolic Diseases; 1971-1981, Assistant, Associate Professor of Biochemistry, University of Kansas; 1981-present, Summerfield Professor of Biochemistry and Director, The Center for Biomedical Research, University of Kansas, 1983-present, Summerfield Professor and Chairman, Department of Pharmaceutical Chemistry and Courtesy Professor, Department of Medicinal Chemistry, University of Kansas. Honors: Established Investigator of the American Heart Association, 1974-'79; University of Kansas Mortar Board Outstanding Educator, 1980; MASUA Honor Lecturer, 1980-81; Sato Memorial International Award - Pharmaceutical Society of Japan, 1980; Dolph C. Simons, Sr. Research Award in the Biomedical Sciences, University of Kansas, 1983. Research Interests: Biochemistry and chemistry of S-adenosylmethionine-dependent methyl-transferases; CNS epinephrine and hypertension, the mechanism of action of neurotoxins; metabolic and transport properties of isolated gastrointestinal mucosal cells and capillary endothelial cells (Blood Brain Barrier).

Hans Bundgaard

Hans Bundgaard is Professor of Pharmaceutical Chemistry at the Royal Danish School of Pharmacy, Copenhagen, Denmark. He received his M.S. in Pharmacy in 1968 and a Ph.D. was obtained in 1973. A Dr. Pharm. degree was obtained in

1978. His main research interests include design of prodrugs, stability and chemical reactivity of drugs and physicochemical aspects of drug delivery. He has written about 160 scientific papers and edited a number of monographs on these subjects. He is a member of the Editorial Board of Int. J. Pharm. and various other pharmaceutical journals.

Robert A. Conradi

Robert Conradi received his baccalaureate degree in biochemistry at the University of Illinois in 1974. He then worked one year at the university before taking a position in a small Illinois firm studying polymeric drug delivery systems. In 1978, Mr. Conradi joined the pharmacy research unit at the Upjohn Company, Kalamazoo, MI. At Upjohn his work has focused on using the prodrug approach to optimize physical and chemical properties of drugs. He has co-authored 10 research articles and is a member of the American Chemical Society and the American Scientific Affiliation.

Ruth Duncan

Dr. Duncan has been a Research Fellow at the University of Keele since 1979 (her work is funded by the British Cancer Research Campaign). She was awarded a B.Sc(Hons) in Zoology from the University of Liverpool (1975) and Ph.D. in Biochemistry from the University of Keele (1979). Principal areas of research interest and expertise include, endocytosis and lysosomal function, lysosomtropic drug delivery and the use of soluble synthetic polymers as targetable drug carriers. Publications cover all these areas. Memberships include the British : Biochemical Society, Society for Cell Biology, Society for Experimental Biology and the Controlled Release Society. Dr. Duncan is also a member of the Editorial Board of the Journal of Controlled Release.

Takeru Higuchi

Dr. Higuchi is University Regents Professor of Chemistry and of Pharmacy at The University of Kansas, President of INTERx Research Corporation and Vice President of Merck Sharp & Dohme Research Laboratories. A native of Los Altos, CA, he received the AB degree in chemistry from the

University of California at Berkeley in 1939 and a Ph.D. degree in physical and organic chemistry from the University of Wisconsin in 1943. He has received honorary D.Sc. degrees from the University of Michigan, Eidgenossische Technische Hochschule Zurich, the University of Illinois, and the Philadelphia College of Pharmacy and Science; an honorary citation from Wisconsin University and the Citation for Distinguished Service from KU. He has spent his professional life as a pharmaceutical scientist-educator closely identified with industrial research. Before joining the KU School of Pharmacy in 1967 where he served as Chairman of the Department of Pharmaceutical Chemistry, he was Edward Kremers Professor of Pharmaceutical Chemistry at the University of Wisconsin. His research interests include the physical chemistry of pharmaceutical systems, pharmaceutical analysis, molecular complexation, transport processes and mathematical analysis, novel drug delivery concepts, and thermodynamics of nonaqueous solutions. He has published over 300 papers relative to these interests and has served as major professor to over 130 Ph.D. graduates. Dr. Higuchi was founder of APhA's Academy of Pharmaceutical Sciences and served as its first president. In 1981, the Academy established a Takeru Higuchi Research Prize and Endowment Fund to recognize the highest accomplishments in the pharmaceutical sciences. Dr. Higuchi is a recipient of many awards administered by APS including the Remington Medal, the Kolthoff Gold Medal, and the Ebert Prize.

Kevin C. Johnson

Mr. Kevin C. Johnson received his B.A. degree in chemistry from Kalamazoo College in 1980. During the summer of 1980, Mr. Johnson was employed by The Upjohn Co., Kalamazoo, MI, as a research assistant under the direction of Dr. Bradley Anderson. He began his graduate studies in pharmaceutics at the University of Wisconsin, Madison, under the direction of Dr. Gordon L. Amidon. Mr. Johnson transferred to the University of Kansas in 1981 and is currently enrolled in the Pharmaceutics program at The University of Michigan, College of Pharmacy, where he expects to receive his Ph.D. degree in December, 1985.

Mr. Johnson has contributed several monographs to be published in: The Chemical Stability of Pharmaceuticals; participated in several annual graduate student research meetings; and presented a poster session at the APhA/APS meeting in Miami, FL (1983).

T. Y. Shen

Dr. T. Y. Shen is a native of China. He received his Ph.D. and D.Sc. in organic chemistry from the University of Manchester, England. After coming to the U.S. in 1950, he did postdoctoral research at Ohio State University and Massachusetts Institute of Technology. He joined Merck Sharp & Dohme Research Laboratories as a senior research chemist in 1956. He is currently Vice President, in charge of Membrane and Arthritis Research. His pioneer research in the area of non-steroidal antiinflammatory agents led to the discovery of indomethacin, sulindac and diflunisal. His earlier interests also included the synthetic study of antiviral nucleosides and immunopharmacological agents. More recently he has investigated cell membrane receptors for saccharides and lipid mediators as potential therapeutics targets. He has over 200 U.S. patents and over 150 scientific publications to his credit.

Dr. Shen has been serving on the Editorial Boards of the Journal of Medicinal Chemistry, Prostaglandins and Medicine, Medicinal Research Reviews and Clinica Europea Journal. Among his professional recognitions are the New Jersey Patent Award 1975, Scientific Medal of University of Pisa 1976, Rene Descartes Medal of University of Paris 1977 and the first Alfred Burger Award if Medicinal Chemistry of the American Chemical Society of 1980.

Anthony A. Sinkula

Anthony A. Sinkula, Director, Pharmacy Research and Drug Delivery Systems Research, The Upjohn Company, is a native of Wisconsin. He received a B.S. in Pharmacy (1959) from the University of Wisconsin and an M.S. (1961) and Ph.D. (1963) in Medicinal Chemistry from the Ohio State University. he was a National Institute of Mental Health Fellow from 1960-63. His major research interests involve the application of prodrug chemistry and biology to the optimization of therapeutic properties of drugs. He has been an invited participant at national and international meetings and symposia on prodrugs and novel drug delivery systems. He has authored over 80 papers, reviews, chapters and patents and is co-editor of the book, <u>Physical Chemical Properties of Drugs</u>. Memberships include the American Pharmaceutical Association and Academy of Pharmaceutical Sciences.

3 5282 00117 5127